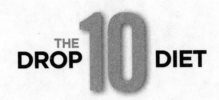

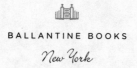

BALLANTINE BOOKS

New York

THE DROP **10** DIET

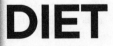

ADD TO YOUR PLATE
TO LOSE THE WEIGHT

LUCY DANZIGER

Beth Janes and the Editors of *SELF* Magazine

Author's Note: *The Drop 10 Diet* proposes a program of exercise recommendations for the reader to follow. However, you should consult a qualified medical professional (and, if you are pregnant, your ob/gyn) before starting this or any other fitness program. As with any diet or exercise program, if at any time you experience any discomfort, stop immediately and consult your physician.

As of press time, the URLs displayed in this book link or refer to existing websites on the Internet. Random House, Inc., is not responsible for, and should not be deemed to endorse or recommend, any website other than its own or any content available on the Internet (including without limitation at any website, blog page, information page) that is not created by Random House.

Published in the United States by Ballantine Books, an imprint of The Random House Publishing Group, a division of Random House, Inc., New York.

BALLANTINE and colophon are registered trademarks of Random House, Inc.

ISBN 978-0-345-53162–9
eBook ISBN 978-0-345-53163-6

Printed in the United States of America on acid-free paper

www.ballantinebooks.com

2 4 6 8 9 7 5 3 1

FIRST EDITION

Book design by Casey Hampton

Contents

Introduction

About five years ago, I decided to clean up my eating. I wanted to lose 10 pounds, get faster at running, biking, and swimming, and be heart-healthier, too. I didn't dislike my body, but I wanted to look better in jeans, especially after seeing a photo of myself from behind—it's not a view I usually see, and it wasn't pretty.

I have always hated dieting—it feels so contrary to the idea of being a self-empowered woman in a world where we should be able to do anything our brothers and fathers can do. Why not eat out of the same bag of chips as my husband or big bro? Why not share the earned muffin after a run, the dessert at the end of a long, tiring day? And yet I wasn't feeling great. I had low energy, and even with an exercise regimen that included forty-five minutes of cardio a day, I wasn't seeing results.

Then one day I decided to eat healthier. It was that simple. I cut down on sugary carbohydrates and chose foods that "paid me back" in terms of the amount of nutrients they delivered per calorie. It wasn't a diet in the traditional, restrictive sense—nothing was totally off-limits. I began to educate myself and learned that the fiber count in bread and cereal matters—and not just to the elderly, but to me and would-be healthy eaters of all ages. I looked at labels for the first time, checking for more than calories: I wanted to know where they came from and how much saturated fat was in there, and I focused on things like the ratio of protein to carbs in energy bars (something I'd never checked before). But mostly, I stopped eating foods that had labels. I bought more whole foods, like fresh vegetables and fruits, nuts, and low-fat yogurt and cheese. I followed the advice of *Self* magazine: If a packaged food stays fresh on the shelf for weeks or months, there's probably something in there that you don't want in your body.

I established a basic rule when it came to portions: If I could grow a food, I could eat unlimited amounts of it. Now I live in an apartment on a busy street in the middle of New York City. So of course I wasn't literally growing crops. But my aunt and uncle had a farm in Georgia, and although they harvested more hay than crops, I understood the concept. They also raised goats and cattle, and there were chickens in the barn whose eggs were always being poached by sneaky predators. I knew what a farm was all about, and I even had a garden of my own behind my weekend house when I was old enough to have my own babies. There, I grew oversize zucchini, tiny tomatoes, cucumbers, snap peas, and even broccoli and eggplant. My garden always has had more weeds than veggies, but working in it ingrained the idea that food you can grow is the best food for your body. You can enjoy foods from the earth to your heart's content with little risk of calorie overload. Plus, by the time you fill up on ratatouille, my favorite summer vegetable stew, you don't have a lot of room for greasy garbage.

Meal after meal, I filled my plate with what I later learned are superfoods (because they are so full of nutrients), and the weight started to fall off. People would ask me, "What diet are you on?" And when I answered that it wasn't a diet per se, it was a way of eating—they didn't like to hear it. Everyone wanted a quick fix, a magic detox, a cleanse that would solve their weight and health problems. They thought that was simpler than being told to choose the right foods. But in fact, eating healthfully for life is the simplest thing to do. I never counted a single calorie, I never measured a single portion, and I certainly didn't go on a restrictive diet. But by shifting my choices, I naturally curtailed my intake of cookies, brownies, cookie dough, and hot-fudge sauce out of the jar in the fridge.

The most amazing thing is how quickly I shed the extra weight. I lost 10 pounds in about five weeks, starting on July Fourth weekend in

2007. By August 15, I was at my race weight from college, when I rowed crew! I kept going, and by back-to-school season in September, I was down another 7 pounds—so I'd lost 17 pounds in one summer! For the next few months, my rate of loss slowed, but by Christmas I had peeled off 22 to 25 pounds (even with the extra sweets and holiday treats I was enjoying). I've gone up and down a little since then—once even getting a bit too thin in my face, so I bumped up my portions and added back more treats. But I've settled into a zone where I feel healthy and energetic, and I enjoy what I'm eating.

People often assume that my exercise level is the reason I can maintain my weight, but I know otherwise. Yes, I trained for two Ironman triathlons, but even with all the swimming, biking, and running, I didn't lose weight. And when I wasn't training (I was sidelined with a stress fracture for months), I didn't gain. I know that it has more to do with what I eat—my exercise fluctuates, but most of the time my diet is consistent. I eat the superfood way about 80 percent of the time and splurge on extras the rest of the time. When I go out to eat Mexican with friends, I help myself to chips (with plenty of salsa) and have a margarita, too. I eat chocolate nearly every day (the dark variety is actually a superfood!), so my diet is far from strict. I couldn't stay on a diet. I can stay heart-healthy, and in a healthy weight zone, eating this way for the rest of my life. Now, thanks to this book, so can you. Happy eating!

THE SUPERFOODS

1

1 Welcome to the Last Weight Loss Program You'll Ever Need

What if there were a whole new way of eating that could slim you down, enhance your health, increase your energy, and help you feel full, satisfied, and happy with the food on your plate? Now there is—and you're holding the key. By following the diet and advice in this book, you can change your body, your health, and your life—all without giving up foods you love or ever feeling deprived. Whether you want to lose 10, 20, 50 pounds, or more, these pages contain the easy tools to help you achieve your goal in a way that fits your lifestyle.

Are you in your twenties and establishing your own independent, adult eating habits? In your thirties and struggling to lose baby weight? In your forties and wondering when you'll ever find the time to eat well? Or are you fifty-plus and looking to achieve your optimal weight in order to stay healthy? Whatever your age, food preferences, or lifestyle, the simple solution is to add more superfoods to your plate and watch the pounds melt off. That's it. No fads, extreme calorie cutting, or banned foods—in fact, by continuing to eat your favorite treats, you are more likely to win at weight loss. All you'll give up is extra, unwanted pounds.

Here's the secret: We've identified thirty everyday foods that contain specific ingredients scientifically proven to help turn on your body's fat-burning powers, rev up your metabolism, tame your appetite, and curb overeating. Eat more of these superfoods, and your body is primed to drop extra weight. Best of all, *you* choose how you lose. Add some or all of the superfoods to your current diet (we'll give you tons of easy tips) or follow our step-by-step meal plan (with recipes or no-cook options—you pick) to shed 10 pounds in five weeks. Have more to lose? Keep going until you reach your personal target. When you're done, use our easy tips to tweak the plan so you can easily maintain your healthy new habits and weight loss for good.

Ready to get started? Say hello to the first day of your slimmer, superfoods way of life!

Redefining Diet

On the Drop 10 plan, you can forget everything you think of when you see or hear the word *diet*. Deprivation? It doesn't apply here. Hunger pangs? Not on the menu. Cravings? We help you indulge them and show you how doing so will improve your odds of meeting your weight loss goals. This plan is like no other: We actually encourage you to eat more in order to weigh less. So many diets fail because they ask you to change everything at once and put your favorite foods off-limits; some ask you to drastically reduce calories, cut out entire food groups, or even skip solid food all together. (A cleanse? That's for the shower!) The Drop 10 diet works because it helps you trim down with every bite you take, not by telling you to stop taking them. From here on, diet—and this one in particular—is not a four-letter word, and it's not something you are "on" or that you "break." It's the total of everything you feed your body, and it offers an incredible opportunity to live life at your healthy best. And that means slimmer and happier, too.

Why This Plan Will Work for You

Studies show that in a depressing 63 to 80 percent of cases, dieters end up gaining back the weight they lose and often more. They typically either cannot sustain restrictive programs or find that menu plans are not practical in the real world—in *your* world, where you need to grab a fast lunch at work, juggle feeding yourself and your family at night, and fit in fun get-togethers with friends. By not taking into account how you live, most diets set you up to fail at every turn. But the flexible Drop 10 diet creates opportunities for you to succeed with every bite, thanks to three key, groundbreaking elements:

1. *The superfoods that fight fat.* This program hinges on thirty delicious, fat-fighting foods that you'll *want* to add to your diet. They're ordinary items, some of which may be in your kitchen right now. But each possesses extraordinary properties that work against fat to help you lose weight. (You can skip ahead if you can't wait for the incredible details on how they do it!) But that's only part of the story. The foods are wholesome and packed with nutrients; by eating more of them, you will automatically begin crowding out the processed snacks and meals that are a staple of the American diet and play a huge role in our obesity crisis and related health struggles. Bottom line: These foods give you thirty chances to get ahead in weight loss simply by eating, not by saying no!

2. *A customizable program that puts you in charge.* This carefully designed plan fits into your life, not the other way around. You have distinct time demands and food, cooking, and exercise preferences. You've got family commitments and lifestyle priorities that only you understand. We get that—it's why you call the shots. You pick and choose from the tools on these pages to build a personal eating and exercise program that takes into account your likes and dislikes, strengths and weaknesses, and everything else that makes you unique—including the foods you crave. That's right: Nothing is off-limits! You can simply add superfoods to your existing menus and add favorite superfood recipes to your usual rotation, or go all the way with the full meal-by-meal Drop 10 plan, which is based on 1,600 stomach-filling, delicious calories per day. But even here, you choose from an extensive and tasty selection of easy breakfasts, lunches, snacks, and dinners. They create your base diet of 1,400 calories, which frees up 200 calories a day for anything you want—you'll still lose weight. You can also save up four days' worth of your

MEET THE THIRTY SUPERFOODS FOR WEIGHT LOSS

We analyzed hundreds of rigorous studies and consulted top scientists and nutrition experts to determine the best slimming superfoods. In addition, to make the plan as easy to follow as possible, we factored in . . .

- Accessibility. You'll find most, if not all, of the foods at your local grocery store.
- Affordability. What good is a diet if it's so pricey that after reaching your goal, you can't afford to celebrate by buying new (skinnier) skinny jeans? Sure, particular foods on the plan may not be the cheapest in the store, but taken as a whole, this diet will work with any budget, especially considering how you'll naturally begin to spend less on the processed foods that drive up supermarket bills.
- Flavor and variety. Bland gets boring fast, so we selected foods that are tasty enough to inspire stick-to-itiveness. The list spans all food groups, including carbs such as whole-grain pasta (yes, pasta!) and yummy treats like chocolate (yep, chocolate!). Eat one superfood or eat them all. With every bite, you improve your body and health!

Thirty Superfoods for Weight Loss

- Almond butter
- Apples
- Artichokes
- Avocado
- Blueberries
- Broccoli
- Cherries
- Coffee
- Dark chocolate
- Edamame

- Eggs
- Goji berries
- Kale
- Kiwifruit
- Lentils
- Mushrooms
- Oats
- Olive oil
- Parmesan
- Peanuts

- Pomegranates
- Popcorn
- Pumpkin seeds
- Quinoa
- Sardines
- Steak
- Sweet potatoes
- Whole-grain pasta
- Wild salmon
- Yogurt

treat calories and "spend" them all at once—you'll still slim down! (Drinks and nachos with friends? Dig in. Pizza night with the family? Enjoy an extra slice!) As you'll read in the pages to come, Drop 10 has already helped dieters just like you shed the weight they wanted to. Now it's your turn!

3. *Research to back it all up.* For more than thirty years, *SELF* magazine has been committed to bringing readers proven, effective ways to improve their health and well-being. Our editors and experts constantly scour journals and spend hours researching and testing strategies in order to separate hype and trends from what truly delivers results. But the ideas and methods in this book are backed by science. You can read it in these chapters, but you'll also see the proof as the inches begin to disappear.

The Science of Superfoods

The idea of eating to lose turns the traditional approach to dieting on its head. And that's exactly why this plan will help you: If most diets fail and more than two-thirds of Americans are overweight or obese, it's clear that something in our current approach to dieting is not working. Isn't it time to rethink the battle of the bulge? Researchers all over the world have been doing just that, exploring how food itself can help you become a diet success. Here's a rundown of what we know about the superfoods:

- *Specific nutrients trigger fat and calorie burning.* Over the past several years, research has begun to pour in showing that certain foods could aid in weight loss or are associated with being slim. For example, a 2005 study from the University of Tennessee in Knoxville finds that adults on a weight loss diet who ate yogurt lost 61 percent more fat overall and 81 percent more belly fat than those on a similar eating plan that didn't include yogurt. As it turns out, eating calcium-rich dairy foods suppresses two hormones that influence how your fat cells do their job; in other words, when they're low, your body favors fat burning and resists fat storing. Another exciting discovery: a special type of fiber found in sweet potatoes and lentils, called "resistant-starch carbo-hydrates," which increases the production of certain peptides and hormones that turn up your body's furnace, compelling it to burn more fat and calories. Who needs gimmicky shakes and supplements? Mother Nature, it seems, was the original weight loss guru.

- *Superfoods stymie fat production in your body.* It's often said that weight loss is all about taking in fewer calories than you burn. And while that is certainly true, there's more to the story. Gaining and losing weight is a complex process in the body, more complicated than just adding and subtracting calories. Some foods (nuts, avocados, whole grains) actually discourage your body from packing on fat, whereas others (refined carbohydrates such as white bread) encourage it.

  Here's why: When you eat, your body breaks down the food to get at the glucose (or sugar) molecules it needs to burn for energy. As glucose enters your bloodstream, your pancreas pumps out insulin to ferry the sugar out of blood and into cells that use it for fuel. In an ideal diet, this happens slowly and continuously over several hours; your body releases small amounts of glucose into your blood, and a low, steady stream of insulin takes it to cells. But when you eat highly processed, fast-digesting foods, loads of glucose flood your blood at once, causing insulin levels to rise sharply and spurring your body to store those calories as fat instead of burning them. To make matters worse, the faster you digest food, the hungrier you become for more energy within an hour or two of eating, triggering cravings for sugary treats. The result: You start snacking (and gaining). The way to stop this runaway fat production is with foods that slow digestion and release glucose a little at a time, keeping insulin levels steady and your body's cells humming along at a cruise-controlled, calorie-in, calorie-out pace that naturally curbs hunger.

  Most of the weight loss superfoods slow digestion with fiber (complex carbohydrates that take your body longer to pull apart into usable components), healthy fats, and protein. Some foods contain all three. Take nuts, for instance: Studies find that people who consume nuts lose more weight when dieting, are less likely to experience significant weight creep over time, or are leaner than those who don't, even though nuts are high in fat and calories. What gives? The crunchy combination of fats, protein, and fiber spends more time in your gut, keeping insulin levels steady.

• *Superfoods curb hunger and overeating.* Taking in a variety of slow-digesting foods that are high in protein, healthy fats, and fiber not only keeps insulin levels steady, but it also keeps you feeling fuller, longer—key for controlling hunger and stabilizing the number of calories you consume. Say you eat a protein-rich egg along with yogurt and fresh blueberries (all superfoods!) for breakfast. By midmorning, your stomach isn't rumbling and you feel just as energized as you did a few hours earlier. You're a lot less likely to raid that box of doughnuts at work or hit the vending machine, right? Likewise, if lunch consisted of wild salmon, broccoli, and quinoa, not only would you not succumb to a three p.m. slump, you'd more easily drive right past that fast-food joint on the way home and instead make healthier, lower-calorie dinner choices. Suddenly, by eating more nutrient-dense, delicious foods, you'll effortlessly eat fewer calories overall while gaining more vitamins and energy.

Superfoods and Your Health

Fruits and vegetables, whole grains, calcium-rich dairy, lean protein, fish—the range of foods on our list provides all the macronutrients (protein, fiber, healthy unsaturated fats) plus the vitamins, minerals, antioxidants, and other phytochemicals you need for your body to function and be healthy. But they also exert specific positive effects on cholesterol, blood pressure, digestion, your immune system, and more.

Take the unsaturated fat in fish, nuts, and avocados. It lowers levels of LDL, or "bad" cholesterol, while raising levels of HDL, the "good" type that sweeps up lipoproteins from the lining of blood vessels, where they might otherwise build up and contribute to blocked arteries. Or consider fiber: Researchers at the Karolinska Institute in Stockholm, Sweden, discovered that women who eat more than 4½ servings a day of whole grains had a 35 percent lower risk for colon cancer. The reason: Fiber speeds the passage of stool through the colon, limiting your body's exposure to potentially carcinogenic waste.

The health benefits of superfoods are undeniable. Yet fewer than 1 in 10 eat the recommended 1½ to 2 cups of fruit and 2½ cups of vegetables daily. We consume only about half the minimum 25 grams of fiber we need per day, and only about 10 percent of us get the amount of heart-healthy seafood a year that the American Heart Association recommends to lower your risk for cardiovascular disease. (Fish should be on your plate at least twice a week.) As a result, we're unhealthier than ever: Heart disease is now the number one cause of death. And diabetes rates are skyrocketing: As many as 1 in 3 Americans could develop the condition by 2050 if trends continue, according to the Centers for Disease Control and Prevention.

The Drop 10 diet helps you painlessly increase your intake of health-promoting foods. But that's not the only way it can cut your risk for disease and help you feel healthier. Shedding excess pounds alone makes drastic improvements to health. (Being overweight or obese is linked to a host of chronic conditions, including diabetes, heart disease, and depression.) The best part: You needn't whittle down to a size 2. Lightening your load by even a few pounds can turn things around for you significantly, in the short and the long term. What the research reports:

- *Diabetes.* Losing a scant 2 pounds may cut your chances of developing type 2 diabetes by 16 percent, according to a study from the Colorado School of Public Health.
- *High blood pressure.* Overweight people who lost 15 pounds or more reduced their risk for hypertension by as much as 28 percent, researchers at the Boston University School of Medicine find.
- *Inflammation.* A modest weight loss of about 13 pounds is enough to bring inflammation levels down to those found in lean people. Inflammation is central to the body's ability to heal and to fight bacteria; a poor diet and excess body fat can put this process into overdrive. Once inflammation becomes chronic, it attacks healthy

cells and causes damage that may contribute to heart disease and other conditions.

- *Back pain.* After trimming nearly 10 pounds, study participants reported significantly less upper-back, lower-back, and hip pain, research from the University of Cincinnati indicates.
- *Self-confidence:* Losing only 5 percent of one's body weight—about 8 pounds for a 165-pound woman—leads to a significant increase in self-esteem, reports a study in the journal *Health and Quality of Life Outcomes*.

Your Personalized Drop 10 Plan

Knowing which superfoods to eat is only part of the effective Drop 10 diet plan. Even more important is finding easy ways to incorporate them into your current eating habits. In this book, you'll find multiple strategies for harnessing the superfoods' superpowers and customizing the plan to fit into your life.

Want to Do the Bare Minimum?

If you're not ready to jump fully into a formal diet with meal-by-meal menus, you can test the superfood waters one bite at a time. In the first several chapters, as you learn more about each of the amazing superfoods, you'll sample ways to integrate each one into your existing diet immediately. Pick a few of your favorites and start munching!

Want to wade in a bit further? Look for the day-by-day tips in chapter 9 for how to start working more of the superfoods into each of your usual meals and snacks. Follow only the tips and enjoy only the foods you like, or try a tip each day, slowly adopting more and more eating habits that will help you drop pounds now and keep them off for life. Either way, you will effortlessly sneak slim-down goodies into your daily life and lose weight, because adding the nutrient-rich items to your plate helps you naturally cut calories, saturated fat, and fat-promoting refined carbs without feeling as if you're giving up a thing—or even following a diet at all.

SECRETS OF THE SUPERFOODS
How ordinary foods help you fight fat and win!

The Superfood	The Slimming Ingredient(s)
Almond butter	Unsaturated fat, protein, fiber
Apples	Fiber
Artichokes	Fiber, resistant-starch carbohydrates
Avocado	Monounsaturated fat, fiber

Weight Loss Superpowers Explained	Bonus Health Benefits
The combo of healthy fats, protein, and fiber squash hunger and cravings, while the fat prevents spikes in blood sugar and insulin—a key factor for stymieing hunger and abdominal fat. (Sharp rises in insulin levels drive excess calories to become fat.) Fiber also may prevent your body from absorbing some calories from meals, because some of the almond's fat passes through unabsorbed.	Healthy fats and other nutrients in this spread may help lower cholesterol, improving heart health, decreasing your risk for diabetes, and protecting your brain. Almonds are also packed with vitamin E, which helps keep skin hydrated and guards against sun damage.
An apple's 4 to 5 grams of fiber and its water content fill you up on relatively few calories (about 95). The dense fruit is also psychologically filling: The size and crunch contribute to feelings of satiety, so you end up eating less overall.	Thanks to antioxidants that neutralize damaging free radical molecules, noshing on apples is linked to a reduced risk for cardiovascular disease, some cancers, and even asthma, and it may help ward off Alzheimer's disease.
RSCs are a fiber-like starch that may trigger peptides that increase fat and calorie burning and help regulate your appetite. Artichokes' resistant starch also doesn't break down like other types of carbs. As a result, they're more filling.	Artichokes rank first among veggies in antioxidant content. Those and other healthy nutrients may help defend against cancer and heart disease.
Avocados put the brakes on overeating in two ways: The healthy fat is satiating, and its oleic acid (a type of fat) activates the body to produce more of the appetite-taming hormone cholecystokinin (CCK). Fiber and fat also work together to keep insulin levels steady, discouraging fat storage.	Heart-healthy fats in avocados lower LDL ("bad") cholesterol while raising your HDL ("good") levels, reducing your risk for heart disease. The veggie is also rich in a number of vitamins and minerals, including bloat-busting potassium.

The Superfood	The Slimming Ingredient(s)
Blueberries	Fiber, anthocyanins
Broccoli	Fiber, vitamin C
Cherries	Fiber, anthocyanins
Coffee	Caffeine

	Weight Loss Superpowers Explained	Bonus Health Benefits
	Like apples, blueberries are full of filling fiber (4 grams per cup), which helps pull fat through the digestive tract, possibly preventing some from being absorbed. Their antioxidant anthocyanins, the compounds that give the fruit their blue hue, may also trigger increased fat burning.	The berries, which tout potent antioxidant activity, may decrease the inflammation that contributes to heart disease and other conditions. Anthocyanins may also mop up free radicals, help brain cells fire faster, and ward off skin cancer and wrinkles.
	Broccoli delivers more nutrients in fewer calories than most other common veggies; it has just 31 calories per chopped cup. One of the most notable boons for weight loss is broccoli's filling fiber, which stabilizes blood sugar and insulin and slows down eating and improves digestion. The veggies' vitamin C may also enhance fat burning.	Cruciferous vegetables like broccoli have been linked to lower rates of cancer (experts think they contain chemicals that turn on the body's natural detoxifying enzymes), while its vitamin C and beta-carotene help keep skin healthy and smooth. You'll net heart and vision benefits, too.
	Cherries' color-providing anthocyanins may increase enzymes in fat cells that encourage fat burning and help keep belly fat at bay. Cherries may also enhance how the body metabolizes sugar. Meanwhile, all types of cherries are rich in hunger-taming fiber.	Antioxidant-rich cherries may help fight inflammation, ease muscle pain after exercise, improve sleep, and keep your brain and heart healthy.
	The buzz on coffee: The amount of caffeine per 1 cup temporarily revs your metabolism by 15 percent. Caffeine also helps block signals of muscle fatigue, making exercise feel easier so you can work out harder or longer (and burn more calories!) without feeling the extra exertion.	Coffee is healthy from head to toe. Research suggests it may lower the risk for Alzheimer's and Parkinson's diseases, depression, heart disease, breast cancer, skin cancer, and diabetes. Caffeine may also help your brain process information more quickly.

The Superfood	The Slimming Ingredient(s)
Dark chocolate	A rich, indulgent cacao
Edamame	Protein, choline, fiber
Eggs	Protein, choline, vitamin D
Goji berries	Protein, fiber, vitamin C

Weight Loss Superpowers Explained	Bonus Health Benefits
Eating dark chocolate (think about 70 percent or more cacao) may lower levels of cortisol, a stress hormone associated with increased appetite and weight gain, especially in the spare-tire area. And new research has found that indulging in the treat may reduce cravings for sweet, salty, and fatty foods.	Compounds in dark chocolate may help improve blood flow to the brain and cognitive performance. They also may lower blood pressure, reduce the risk for hypertension, and may improve skin hydration.
Edamame is a low-fat, cholesterol-free source of protein, which keeps you full and may rev up calorie burning. Meanwhile, it delivers the B-vitamin choline, which helps block fat absorption and breaks down fatty deposits. You also get nearly four times the filling fiber from the beans than from tofu.	Isoflavones in edamame protect your heart and bones, and there's some evidence that eating soy could lower your risk for breast cancer. Research suggests the beans may also quell PMS-related cramps, headaches, and breast tenderness.
Eggs' high-quality, satiating protein reduces hunger for hours and may even cause you to eat less the entire day. In addition, your body burns more calories digesting protein-rich foods than those higher in carbs and fat. You'll also take in vitamin D, which may enhance weight loss, and fat-blocking choline.	Eggs deliver numerous nutrients that keep your system and your skin healthy, including selenium and biotin, a B vitamin. Plus they're one of the few natural sources of vitamin D, adequate levels of which may help guard against osteoporosis, high blood pressure, depression, and cancer.
Eighteen different amino acids make these tart, chewy berries a surprising source of protein, giving them a hunger-curbing edge over other fruit. Fiber also helps suppress appetite, while vitamin C may encourage fat burning.	Like other berries, gojis are chock-full of protective antioxidants; research suggests the fruit's nutrients may keep the immune system functioning, help prevent sun-induced skin damage, fight cancer cells, and benefit eye health.

The Superfood	The Slimming Ingredient(s)
Kale	Fiber, vitamin C
Kiwifruit	Vitamin C
Lentils	Fiber, resistant-starch carbohydrates, protein
Mushrooms	Water, flavor
Oats	Fiber

Weight Loss Superpowers Explained	Bonus Health Benefits
Kale packs a serious nutritional punch. For just 34 calories per raw chopped cup, you'll get filling fiber along with vitamin C, which may increase fat burning.	Like its leafy-green cousin broccoli, kale may turn on your body's natural detoxifying enzymes to help ward off lung and stomach cancers; plus, it's a great source of skin-saving vitamins A and C and carotenoids that may protect your eyes.
One kiwi contains nearly a full day's quota of vitamin C, which may play a part in your body's ability to burn fat. Research shows that the more deficient a person is in the vitamin, the heavier she tends to be.	Kiwis may help lower triglycerides, a type of fat that circulates in blood, and improve bowel function. And unlike most other fruit, kiwi contains vitamin E, which along with C keeps skin glowing and smooth.
Keeping blood sugar and insulin from spiking is important in your fight against fat; lentils do it with plenty of soluble fiber and protein, both of which slow digestion and keep you satiated. Meanwhile, RSCs influence satiety signals and boost fat burning.	The fiber in lentils helps lower cholesterol, while their high levels of folate and magnesium promote healthy heart function. Lentils have also been linked to a lower risk for diabetes and some cancers.
Mushrooms contain a scant 20 or so calories per cup, but they're physically dense and meaty, plus they contain natural flavor compounds similar to MSG (the salt-based flavor enhancer), all of which may help you feel more satisfied. Swapping fungi for beef, for example, may lead you to consume hundreds of calories less without feeling any hungrier or less satisfied.	Out of all veggies, mushrooms have the highest amount of selenium, which may protect against some cancers. They also contain beta-glucan and chitin, two types of fiber that absorb fat and carry it out of the blood, cutting your risk for heart problems. Plus, beneficial bacteria or nutrients within 'shroom cell walls may strengthen your defenses against disease.
Oatmeal ranks as one of the most satiating foods, making it a top pick for fighting cravings (as long as you pick the plain stuff, not the packets with added sugar). Beta-glucan, the fiber in oats, keeps your body's blood sugar and insulin levels steady, helping to fight fat, specifically around your middle.	The powerful beta-glucan in oats not only lowers blood cholesterol and helps prevent heart problems, it also seems to boost your immunity. What's more, oats contain about half a day's worth of manganese, a key mineral for bone health.

The Superfood	The Slimming Ingredient(s)
Olive oil	Monounsaturated fat
Parmesan	Calcium, protein
Peanuts	Protein, fiber, monounsaturated fat
Pomegranates	Fiber
Popcorn	Fiber

Weight Loss Superpowers Explained	Bonus Health Benefits
Like avocados and almonds, olive oil (all types, not just extra-virgin) has satiating healthy fats. Research suggests that swapping them for saturated fat helps people lose weight and that following the Mediterranean diet helps maintain weight loss. Monounsaturated fat may also facilitate fat oxidation and prevent fat storage.	Olive oil's "good" fats bestow multiple health benefits like lower cholesterol and a lower risk of heart disease; plus, they help your body absorb fat-soluble vitamins. Extra-virgin olive oil is also rich in disease-fighting antioxidants and other nutrients.
Compared with other cheeses, the pasta topper contains one of the highest amounts of fat-fighting calcium. And thanks to its strong flavor, you're likely to feel more satisfied by a single serving.	Calcium is a boon for bones, teeth and nerve function. Hard cheeses like Parmesan also tend to have less lactose, so they're a great choice for people who are sensitive to dairy.
Technically a legume, peanuts are thought of as nuts and taste more like them. What sets them apart: They contain more satiating protein than any other nut. That, along with their fiber and fat, make these nibbles a perfectly balanced, appetite-taming food. No wonder multiple studies link eating peanuts with weight loss.	Peanuts contain off-the-chart amounts of resveratrol, an antioxidant compound also found in red wine, plus other nutrients that may lower your risk for cardiovascular disease, cancer, and age-related cognitive decline.
The juice gets all the glory, but fresh pom seeds, called arils, may be better for your waistline. Low in calories and high in fiber, they fill you up and satisfy your sweet tooth without packing on pounds like foods with added sugar can.	Pomegranate seeds and juice are loaded with antioxidant polyphenols and other compounds that may protect against cancer and inflammation, promote heart health, and lower the risk for Alzheimer's disease.
Believe it or not, this snack food counts as a belly-filling, insulin-steadying whole grain; 3 cups of the plain, air-popped variety delivers nearly 4 grams of fiber for just 93 calories. (Oil-popped, butter-drenched corn has much more fat and calories.)	Eating a diet rich in whole grains like popcorn is a healthy move that can reduce your risk for cardiovascular disease, stroke, and diabetes, as well as colon and breast cancers.

The Superfood	The Slimming Ingredient(s)
Pumpkin seeds	Protein, fiber, unsaturated fat
Quinoa	Protein, fiber, resistant-starch carbohydrates
Sardines	Protein, omega-3 fatty acids, calcium, vitamin D
Steak	Protein, iron

Weight Loss Superpowers Explained	Bonus Health Benefits
Whether toasted at home or bought hulled, these crunchy seeds pack the stomach-filling trifecta—protein, fiber, and healthy fat—making them an ideal snack or salad topper to help you avoid hunger and cravings. Protein also burns through more calories during digestion than do fat and carbs, while fiber cuts down on the amount of calories you absorb from food.	The seeds' magnesium may help prevent headaches by relaxing blood vessels in the brain. The seeds also contain phytosterols, compounds that could lower cholesterol and fend off certain cancers.
This whole grain packs the dynamic duo of fiber and protein to keep insulin levels steady and hunger at bay. Plus, the RSCs may ramp up fat burning. And unlike most other grains, quinoa is a complete protein, delivering all the essential amino acids (protein's building blocks) necessary for building the lean muscle that keeps your metabolism humming.	As with all heart-healthy whole grains, eating quinoa can help lower your cholesterol. The vitamin-rich superfood may also lower your risk for certain cancers and promote clear skin and healthy digestion.
Meet the unsung heroes of the sea. Sardines' omega-3 fatty acids may help you burn fat, build muscle, and improve your insulin sensitivity, which could work against belly fat. The seafood's protein fills you up, and you'll take in plenty of fat-fighting calcium and vitamin D. Recent research links higher levels of D when dieting to greater fat loss, especially in the belly.	Omega-3s are true health all-stars: They've been shown to lower cholesterol, disease-causing inflammation, and the risk for heart attack and stroke; plus, they can protect your eyes, alleviate depression; quell anxiety, improve brain function, rejuvenate your skin, and calm symptoms of arthritis.
Just 3½ ounces of lean beef provide 21 grams of protein, which is essential when dieting because it helps you build and retain the muscle mass that stokes calorie burn. You'll also get easy-to-absorb iron, a mineral that assists blood cells in carrying energizing oxygen to organs and tissue.	Iron's role in oxygen transport may help give skin a glow, too. Steak is also brimming with zinc, a crucial mineral for wound healing and immune function.

The Superfood	The Slimming Ingredient(s)
Sweet potato	Fiber, resistant-starch carbohydrates
Whole-grain pasta	Fiber, protein, resistant-starch carbohydrates
Wild salmon	Protein, omega-3 fatty acids, vitamin D
Yogurt	Vitamin C

Weight Loss Superpowers Explained	Bonus Health Benefits
With more fiber than white potatoes, these orange powerhouses help thwart insulin spikes and, thus, fat and hunger. Plus, they contain RSCs, which stimulate appetite-suppressing hormones and may increase fat burning and energy expenditure.	Sweet potatoes are bursting with nutrients that keep you healthy, including the antioxidant beta-carotene, which may protect your heart, ward off cancer, and keep your skin smooth.
Healthy whole-wheat and other 100% whole-grain pastas supply a hearty helping of protein and fiber, a one-two satiating punch that curbs overeating and halts snack attacks. Fiber also reduces the amount of calories you absorb, while RSCs may increase fat burning, shrink fat cells, and help regulate your appetite.	Fighting heart disease, diabetes, cancer—and even zits—whole-grain foods like pasta are all-around smart picks for your health. They may also boost concentrations of serotonin, low levels of which are linked to depression.
Salmon contains copious amounts of omega-3s, which may increase fat burning during exercise and help your body maintain calorie-burning muscle mass. The fish's fat content and protein also make it ideal for staving off between-meal munchies.	You'll gain the same head-to-toe, inside and out, health-promoting benefits from salmon's omega-3s as those listed above for sardines. Go for wild salmon, though, which may contain fewer pollutants than farmed varieties.
Often touted as a perfect weight-loss food, low-fat and nonfat yogurt (both Greek and regular) fill you up to fight hunger. Plus, yogurt is loaded with calcium, which may fire fat burning and discourage fat storage. Research has shown that people who eat yogurt while dieting lose more fat—and more belly fat—than those who don't.	Bones, teeth, and nerve function all get a boost from calcium. Many brands of yogurt also supply live, active cultures (aka probiotics or healthy bacteria) that aid digestion and are linked to a stronger immune system and a lower risk for gum disease, and even some cancers.

Ready to Dive in to a More Formal Diet and Lose 2 Pounds a Week?

The full Drop 10 diet, which begins on page 222, consists of a five-week meal plan of simple, delicious, and satisfying recipes and ideas for superfood-packed breakfasts, lunches, snacks, and dinners. (Plus, you get 1,400 calories a week to eat anything you want!) Far from rigid, this plan offers several options and multiple ways you can customize it. Here's what to expect:

1. *Easy meal prep.* Some meals cook quickly; others require no cooking whatsoever. The plan also includes meals and snacks perfect for eating on the go, prepping ahead of time, or throwing together in fewer than 60 seconds (seriously). Whatever you've got on your schedule, this plan will accommodate it, while providing the ideal balance of carbohydrates, protein, and healthy fats to keep you satiated and hunger-free.

2. *A flexible menu.* You can follow the plan as rigidly or as loosely as you like; try a new breakfast, lunch, snack, and dinner each day for five weeks, or make only the meals that excite you, repeating your favorites several times over the five weeks. Lunches and dinners also contain about the same calorie counts, making them interchangeable. It's all part of our commitment to creating opportunities for you to succeed. This diet isn't about how well you can stick to a plan; it's about helping you find your personal sweet spot for weight loss by eating more fat-shredding health powerhouses in place of nutrient-empty, fattening foods.

3. *Freedom to eat your sweet, salty, savory, and fatty favorites.* As promised, the Drop 10 diet encourages you to eat the foods you love. Not only will you be much happier, but you'll also be more successful in making long-term changes to your eating habits. Here's how the plan works. Your goal each day is to stay around 1,600 calories. To do it, you choose from our extensive list of delectable and filling meals and snacks to make up your base diet of 1,400 calories a day. That leaves roughly 200 bonus calories a day to use however your taste buds see fit. Eat one 200-calorie goody every day, or roll over your calories for up to four days, allowing

you to splurge on food and drinks with as many as 800 calories in one sitting. (Saving up an entire week's worth of bonus calories may trigger cravings, so try to keep it to four days.) Think of these calories as "happy calories"—the tastes that make you smile and enjoy eating. Love ice cream? Craving salty fries? How about a cupcake? There's room to have them all throughout the week. Or if you know you're going out for, say, margaritas on Saturday, save up a few days' worth and have two to really put a grin on your face. How you spend your happy calories is between you and your getting-flatter-by-the-week stomach! Indulge and the pounds will still disappear.

Need Even More Inspiration?

We know this plan is your ticket to diet success, and the proof is in the people! Throughout this book, you'll read motivational stories of people just like you who have dropped 10 or even 20 or more pounds following the Drop 10 diet. Go ahead, flip to page 65 or 102 now. We dare you to not feel inspired! Get started today and you're that much closer to attaining the trim, healthy body of your dreams.

Superworkouts that Supercharge Weight Loss

Fat falls off even more quickly and easily when you combine a diet program with exercise. But the workouts you'll find in chapter 13 are not your average sweat sessions. Think of each as the fitness equivalent of a superfood—they've been proven to torch serious calories, rev metabolism, target a muffin top, and more. And just like the eating plan, the superworkouts are flexible; regardless of your current fitness level, schedule, or gym membership status, you'll find multiple options to help you reap the better-body rewards. Out of shape? Short on time? Hate to exercise? It's no sweat! We've got two magic bullets for serious slimming:

- Fat-targeting cardio workouts. Select from multiple activities that sizzle extra calories and zero in on fat. You'll learn how to incorporate intervals—short, go-all-out spurts interspersed with minutes at a slower pace—into your workouts. They accelerate weight loss, especially in the belly area, more than slow-and-steady cardio does.

- Body-toning, metabolism-stoking strength exercises. Building lean muscle triggers your body to burn more calories, even when you're sitting still. Plus, it creates a swimsuit-worthy, sculpted frame. A win-win! You'll find plenty of moves from which to pick favorites, whether you want to work out at home, outside, or in the gym.

Prep for Success: Get Ready to Get Slim!

Before you launch into the plan, try one or all of these warm-up strategies to set the stage for winning at losing. By completing simple to-dos, you'll achieve an immediate sense of accomplishment—your first success that will motivate you to stay on track. Building on little triumphs, even the small ones here, creates momentum that can carry you to a leaner, healthier you.

- Clear kitchen clutter. You needn't toss out all your treats—remember, you're allowed to indulge! But do clean out and organize your fridge (especially those produce drawers), freezer, and pantry. Ditch anything that's old or stale or that you just won't eat or, on the flip side, can't stop eating. (You can't be tempted to overdo it on what's not there!) Do whatever you need to do to make room for the fat-busting fare to come.
- Stock up on staples. Supplying your pantry with vinegars, dried herbs, and other essentials will make preparing slimming meals and eating healthfully a snap.
- Build a get-slim toolbox. You'd be surprised how the right kitchen gadgets can make chopping, cutting, and cooking less of a chore and, yes, more fun. (Try it, you'll see!) Weight loss bonus: Research shows that the more you cook and eat meals at home—that is, where you control ingredients and calorie content—the more

successful you're likely to be at losing weight and keeping it off. So if you don't already have them, invest in good-quality knives, including chef's, paring, and bread knives (Chicago Cutlery and Victorinox Swiss Army are two affordable, reliable brands), a set of measuring cups and spoons, and a large cutting board. (It doesn't matter what type of board you choose, although silicone boards are usually dishwasher safe, whereas wood and eco-friendly bamboo typically need to be washed by hand.) Also stock durable glass or plastic storage containers so you can prep healthful meals and snacks ahead of time. With yummy, slimming fare ready just behind the refrigerator door, you're less likely to succumb to fast, fatty options.

- Recruit a buddy—or two or three. There's strength (and success!) in numbers. Dieters who have support from their friends are more likely to keep the weight off than those who fly solo, reports a study from the *Journal of Consulting and Clinical Psychology*. Why not make losing weight with the Drop 10 diet a challenge among a few pals and family members? Mutual encouragement and a little get-healthy competition can go a long way in motivating you to start and stay on the plan.

- Ask for help. If your nearest and dearest don't want to join in, enlist their support in your journey. Line up people you can call to discuss struggles and celebrate milestones, but also be specific about what you want or need from those closest to you. For example, suggest to your mom that she offer salad along with her usual big Sunday family dinners. Or float the idea to your husband that if he wants to spoil you, he might give you a foot massage versus a treat from the ice-cream parlor again.

- Pick a hero. Think about the people you know, and choose one or two you truly admire, not for their svelte physique, but for their ambition or perseverance or positive attitude. Keep thoughts of these people in your back pocket, so to speak, and whenever you feel yourself faltering, draw on them for inspiration and imagine them encouraging you to continue to strive.

- Carve out time to shop. Bare cupboards are a big, fat fat trap. Inevitably there will be times when you come home tired and hungry. Without a kitchen stocked with healthful alternatives and ready-to-go snacks, you're more likely to dial for an extra-large pizza dinner. Before embarking on week one, evaluate your schedule and establish a time when you'll hit the supermarket each week to load up on supplies.

- Make movement a must. Schedule exercise as diligently as you do work, family, and social engagements. (Seriously, put workouts in your calendar, and keep those appointments as you would any other!) Whether you go for a walk or follow the fun, fat-sizzling routines in chapter 13, you'll see better results on the scale in pounds and in the mirror in the form of a more toned, sculpted body.

LOG YOUR MEALS, LOSE MORE WEIGHT!

Tracking meals and snacks in a journal makes you more aware of what you put in your mouth, which goes a long way toward preventing mindless munching. One study in the *American Journal of Preventive Medicine* finds that dieters who kept daily records of what they ate lost twice as much weight as dieters who didn't. There's no right or wrong way to do it; the important thing is that you get the information down somewhere. Think about what will be most convenient for you. You can jot down meals in a small notebook you keep in your handbag, in an online calendar tool, or on your smartphone. Simply separate entries by days as you would a regular journal, then after eating anything, jot down what you ate, how much, the approximate number of calories, where you were, and how you felt. If a meal or snack isn't part of the eating plan or listed among the treats in chapter 12, check labels or look up calorie content online at NutritionData.Self.com. Periodically review your journal to see if you can spot any danger zones in your eating. You may detect a pattern of afternoon stress snacking on the job, for instance, and decide to pack a healthy pick to reach for instead.

Make a Pledge

You sign contracts for all sorts of things, why not make a positive pact with yourself? Write one up, or use the template below to state your weight loss intentions, then clip it out and hang it where you'll see it every day. Concentrate on the reasons you want to lose weight for yourself, not any external pressure you may feel. This type of internal, personal motivation, especially when nurtured over time, was associated with greater weight loss success, reports the *Journal of Nutrition Education and Behavior.* Yes, you can do it!

Promise to myself

On this date, _____, I commit to a happier, healthier, slimmer me. I want to take charge of my diet for myself—for the health I'll build, the energy I'll gain, and the self-confidence I'll develop. To do that, I vow to . . .

- Make smart choices. I will think about what I feed my body before every meal and snack, and how what I eat will benefit my health and my goals. That includes not feeling deprived but enjoying my favorite foods with awareness.
- Be kind to myself. I recognize that no one is perfect and that I may encounter setbacks. I will not beat myself up or feel guilty. Instead, I will learn from roadblocks. I will look at each meal and each day as an opportunity to start fresh and recommit to my goals.
- Believe in myself. I am responsible for my success. I am strong enough to make healthy changes in my life—and stick to them!—and I am tough enough to weather the ups and downs. *Bring it on!*

Signed,

_____

drop 10 inspiration

"Being healthy is a wonderful feeling."

NAME: Michelle Reichenbach

AGE: 37

OCCUPATION: Scheduling system data analyst at a hospital

FAMILY STATUS: Married, one stepdaughter

HEIGHT: 5 feet 3 inches

STARTING WEIGHT: 218

DROP 10 WEIGHT: 196

LOST: 22 pounds in seven weeks

My story: "I have asthma, and every pound makes it worse, so health and self-image were my motivators to get started."

Biggest challenge to losing weight: "Commitment and having a true plan to follow. I also lacked the ambition to exercise."

Why Drop 10 clicked: "The food tastes great! I tried a plan with prepackaged meals, but it was expensive, and the foods lacked flavor and sometimes left me hungry. And not being allowed a variety of real foods made me crave everything. With Drop 10, having the menus for the week was a huge help—knowing what each meal was going to be kept me from eating junk. I also realized that exercise holds a big key to any diet success. The workout was very challenging, but exercising made me feel energized."

How my body changed: "At my last checkup, my pulmonologist tested my asthma and it was a lot better. Next we will look at cutting down on medication."

Success tip: "Preparation is key! When I make one meal, I measure out the ingredients for another so the prep time is cut down. I'm going to continue with this plan because it gets results."

2 Super Fruits

. . . .

APPLES

. . . .

The Slimming Story

An apple a day helps excess pounds fall away! How the fruit does it is simple: Apples fill you up, so you're hungry for fewer calories overall. You can partly thank the slow-to-digest, stomach-satiating fiber you take in with every bite; it also helps stabilize blood sugar levels and curb sugar cravings. Even better, fiber helps ferry out some of the fat and calories you take in from other foods and which your body would otherwise absorb and pack onto belly and thighs! (Read more about fiber's magical fat-fighting abilities on page 38.)

> **ONE BAD APPLE CAN SPOIL THE BUNCH**
>
> Compared with a smooth-skinned, crisp apple, a bruised, punctured, or overly ripe piece emits more ethylene, a natural gas given off by fruit that hastens the ripening of others nearby. For that reason, toss or quickly eat overly ripe apples and those with battered skin.

But roughage alone doesn't explain apples' pound-peeling properties. Apples are what experts call a "low-energy-dense food," meaning they serve up a lot to chew on for not a lot of calories. Even though water makes up the majority of that volume (an apple is about 86 percent H_2O), you feel satisfied on relatively few calories (about 95 for a medium piece of fruit). In fact, most fresh fruits and veggies are low energy dense and may help you lose weight. But apples are particularly effective because they're also psychologically filling: Crunchy and weighty, they require more chewing and so seem more substantial. How 'bout *them* apples?!

The Amazing Proof

- People who ate an apple fifteen minutes before lunching on cheese tortellini consumed 187 fewer calories in total than those who snacked on nothing beforehand, according to a study from Pennsylvania State University in University Park.

→ **Trim-Down Tip:** Going out to eat? Munch an apple on your way to the restaurant and you're likely to leave lighter than you would have otherwise—and with leftovers.

- Women who ate about a cup of dried apples daily (the equivalent of about two pieces of fresh fruit) for a year lost an average of 3.3 pounds, even though they made no other changes to their diet or exercise routines, researchers from Florida State University in Tallahassee report.
- In a similar study published in the journal *Appetite,* researchers directed a group of women to eat three small apples, three pears, or three oatmeal cookies every day; each snack totals 200 calories and has 6 grams of fiber. After ten weeks, people in the apple group lost more than 2 pounds without tweaking their diet in any other way; the pear group lost less and the cookie eaters' scales didn't budge.

→ **Trim-Down Tip:** Keep your kitchen or office stocked with fresh apples for when a snack attack hits. Or place a bowl by the front door so you can grab one on your way out. Seeing the fruit reminds you to eat it!

Apples Defend Against an Apple Shape

In 2008, researchers working for the U.S. Apple Association ana-lyzed food consumption data and determined that people who regularly eat apples and applesauce have a smaller waistline than those who don't. They're also likely to have lower blood pressure and reduced levels of C-reactive protein, a sign of inflammation in the body. (Inflammation is necessary for healing cuts and other injuries, but when it rages unchecked, it may contribute to disease, including cancer.) When elevated blood pressure and excess fat around the abdomen occur along with higher levels of blood glu-cose and triglycerides, a type of fat in the blood, it may signal metabolic syndrome, a cluster of symptoms that increases the chance of stroke, diabetes, and heart problems. Experts aren't ex-actly sure what initially triggers the syndrome—it's a bit of a chicken-or-egg question—although obesity and inactivity are two key risk factors. The research does make one thing clear, however: Apple eaters were 27 percent less likely to be diagnosed with the syndrome, suggesting that adding apples to your diet can help keep both your body healthy and your stomach slim.

Four More Reasons to Eat Apples

1. *They fight cancer.* Apples' fiber and antioxidant compounds may help ward off certain cancers, including breast and colon cancer. Researchers from Jagiellonian University Medical College in Kraków, Poland, for example, determined that eating an apple a day slashes colon cancer risk by 35 percent. Have two or more and it seems to cut the risk in half.

→ **Trim-Down Tip:** Don't pitch the peel! Not only does an apple's skin contain antioxidant polyphenols, but it also delivers about double the fat-blocking fiber.

2. *Your ticker hearts apples.* Apples' stellar combo of antioxidants and fiber may lower cholesterol and improve heart health, too.

Studies show eating the fruit lowers LDL cholesterol (the "bad" type, which contributes to heart disease) and increases levels of HDL (or "good" cholesterol, which may reduce your risk). Apples may also help lower blood pressure and inflammation. It's no surprise, then, that women who ate apples and/or pears at least twice per week were 13 to 15 percent less likely to die of heart disease compared with those who ate them less often, according to a study in *The American Journal of Clinical Nutrition.*

3. *You might breathe easier.* The antioxidants in apples seem to impart anti-inflammatory, antiallergenic, and other benefits that could improve air flow in your lungs. In fact, people who eat two or more apples a week were 32 percent less likely to be asthmatic, researchers at King's College in England report.

4. *It's smart for your brain.* Apples' potent antioxidants boost levels of acetylcholine, a neurotransmitter that helps brain cells fire speedily, facilitating the processing of information. The chemical also fights the oxidative damage that hinders memory and learning and contributes to Alzheimer's disease. (Think of that damage like rust on a bicycle: The more there is, the more it affects functioning.)

WANT TO EAT MORE APPLES STARTING TODAY?

When you're snacking or setting out appetizers, ditch the crackers and instead use apple slices as a base for dips, hummus, cheese, and peanut butter. They pair just as well with everything and provide a similar hearty crunch.

DON'T LIKE APPLES?

Eat them with stronger, complementary flavors. Try stirring slices into a bowl of yogurt and sprinkling with cinnamon. Or mix shredded apples into spiced oatmeal, or hide thin slices in a hearty turkey-and-Cheddar sandwich.

→ **Trim-Down Tip:** An apple today—or in twenty-one days! Stock up on apples every time you're at the market; although you don't need to refrigerate the fruit, if you do, an apple can stay fresh for three weeks—or possibly longer.

Going Apple Picking?

If you're overwhelmed by your choices in the apple section of the market, follow these easy steps to help you choose the right variety for you.

- Listen to your taste buds. You've got to eat apples to reap their waistline rewards, so if there's a particular type you find more a-peeling than others—one that will encourage you to munch more often—buy that kind. Similarly, if you're budget-conscious and want to go with what's on sale, do it. All varieties contain healthy phytonutrients and antioxidants, although Fuji, Red Delicious, Gala, Liberty, and Northern Spy apples tend to contain more than other varieties commonly eaten in the United States.
- Look for local and in-season choices. The less time apples spend between the tree and your stomach, the more concentrated their nutrients.
- Opt for organic if you can. Conventionally grown apples have among the highest concentrations of pesticides of any fruit—an unfortunate fact that has earned apples the top spot on the Environmental Working Group's "dirty dozen" list of produce that you're better off buying organic. (Go to ewg.org for the full list.) If you can't afford organic or don't have access, know that only 3 to 4 percent of products had pesticide levels of concern, according to a report by the Food and Drug Administration (FDA), and that most experts agree that eating fruit and vegetables however they're grown is optimal for good health. Wash conventionally grown apples well: Scrubbing the skin (try a fruit or vegetable scrubber) removes dirt and may reduce pesticide residue.

FIBER: A PROVEN WEAPON IN THE FIGHT AGAINST FAT

What if every time you ate, you could protect your waistline from a percentage of the fat and calories you consume but still keep all the taste? It sounds too good to be true, but that's exactly what fiber does. Men who eat at least 34 grams of fiber a day absorb up to 6 percent fewer calories, according to studies, while women who eat up to 24 grams daily absorb 90 fewer calories, according to a study in the *Journal of Nutrition.* That's nearly 10 pounds a year—poof—gone! By eating! How does fiber manage to pull off this disappearing act? It packs up and speeds a portion of the food you eat through your digestive tract before you absorb all of its calories.

That's only one of a few ways this supernutrient—and the twenty-one superfoods that contain it—helps you trim the fat. Fiber is the part of plants—fruits, veggies, whole grains, and legumes—that your body can't digest. There are two main types, and both play a role in your weight-shedding endeavors.

Soluble fiber: Called soluble because it dissolves in water, this is the type of fiber that makes oatmeal filling and keeps lentils soft inside. It's also plentiful in many fruits and veggies. In your stomach, soluble fiber doesn't actually dissolve into nothing; rather, it forms a gel-like substance that slows the digestive process, forcing your body to spend more time breaking down food into usable sugar molecules. Low-fiber foods, such as white bread, break down quickly, sending sugar surging into your bloodstream, so you feel a quick energy boost followed by a crash. (Think about the time it takes to chew and swallow an apple versus taking a swig of a sugary soda—same idea.) By delaying digestion, you prevent those spikes in blood sugar and, thus, insulin, a hormone that tells your body to store calories as fat. Plus, the longer food takes to digest, the longer it stays in your system and the longer you feel full, which means fewer cravings and less overeating, both during and between meals.

Insoluble fiber: This is what your grandma was referring to when she said her fiber muffins will keep you, um, regular. It is plentiful in the coarser and chewier parts of plants and grains. It doesn't dissolve; it actually absorbs water and adds bulk to your stool, helping shuttle waste more easily through your intestines. Insoluble fiber works with soluble fiber to keep you full and lock up and ship out a portion of the calories you eat, saving you from absorbing the full load.

Ready to Roughage It? Read This First.

- Focus on total grams. Don't worry about getting a certain amount of each of the two different types of fiber; if you're eating a spectrum of fiber-rich foods (like the superfoods for weight loss), you'll get what you need. Instead, aim to increase your total fiber intake to at least 20, and preferably 35, grams per day.
- Take your time when adding fiber to your diet. Although you're probably eager to start filling up on the nutrient, taking in loads more than usual right away can cause gas, bloating, and cramps. A better strategy: Gradually increase your fiber totals by incorporating a few more grams into your diet every day or so, giving your body the time it needs to adjust.
- Stay hydrated. Fiber and water go hand in hand; H_2O helps roughage pass smoothly through the digestive system and keeps you from getting constipated or bloated. So as you begin eating more fiber-rich foods, be sure you're drinking enough, and perhaps even add a glass to your usual routine. A good marker is actually your urine. If it's pale, you're on the right track; but if it's dark and you don't need to go that often, start guzzling.

apple nutrition by the numbers

95
calories per 1 medium-size apple

14
percent of your daily value of vitamin C

4
grams of fiber

BLUEBERRIES

The Slimming Story

These sweet, juicy berries are true blue for anyone with pounds to lose. One cup packs about 4 grams of fiber—around the same as an apple—into a diet-friendly 84 calories. Because it takes your body longer to digest fiber, blueberries help you feel full, putting the kibosh on overeating. And as fiber packs and moves waste through your digestive tract and out of your body, it takes some fat and calories with it for extra trimming. Fiber works with blueberries' water content and lack of fat to make the fruit low energy dense, too, meaning you can eat a large, satisfying portion but take in relatively few calories.

Blueberries also contain other potential pound-shedding players called "anthocyanins," the powerful antioxidants that give the petite orbs their vivid hue. Preliminary research in animals suggests that the compounds turn on genes that activate proteins known to trigger fat burning and discourage fat storage. Blueberries also seem to improve how the body uses sugar, stabilizing its insulin response. This result helps regulate fat burning and storage as well—especially in the belly, where excess weight raises the risk of metabolic syndrome. So although more research is needed to confirm whether eating the fruit has the same effect on, say, a human muffin top, you've got nothing to lose by adding anthocyanin-packed blueberries to your diet—oh, except excess weight!

The Amazing Proof

- After researchers at the University of Michigan in Ann Arbor fed pudgy, prediabetic rats whole blueberry powder (the equivalent of about 1½ cups of blueberries a day for a human), the rats lost abdominal fat and improved their glucose and insulin sensitivity.

→ **Trim-Down Tip:** Fresh berries not available? Buy frozen. They won't go bad, and because the fruit is usually frozen shortly after picking, the blueberries may hang on to more of the potentially slimming antioxidants that otherwise can diminish over time. Add the iced morsels directly to hot dishes such as oatmeal, or, to thaw quickly, place in a colander and run under cool water.

- Reams of research over the past few decades reveal that eating more fruit (and veggies) can lead to greater success on the scale. One reason: the low energy density of produce. Studies routinely show that when people add more low-energy-dense foods such as blueberries to their diet, they eat fewer calories throughout the day yet don't report feeling deprived or starving. They're still eating a large weight or volume of food, which is likely emotionally and physically satisfying.

→ **Trim-Down Tip:** Instead of topping cereal, ice cream, or some other dish with blueberries, start with a bowl of berries and then add the other food; by switching the ratio, you'll take in more of the fruit and get a weight loss boost.

Four More Reasons to Eat Blueberries

1. *You'll score brain benefits.* Powerful antioxidants and other phytonutrients in blueberries can help brain cells fire faster and protect against cellular damage and inflammation that lead to age-related cognitive decline. Animal research also suggests the fruit restores cells' normal "housekeeping" duties, which slow as you get older, possibly interfering with brain function. Older adults who drank 2 cups of blueberry juice a day for twelve weeks improved their scores on verbal learning and memory tests by 41 percent and 33 percent, respectively, according to a study from the University of Cincinnati.

2. *Antioxidants in blueberries may fight cancer.* Out of all commonly consumed fruit, blueberries contain the highest level of antioxidants, according to the United States Department of Agriculture (USDA). The potent phytochemicals protect against cell damage that could potentially contribute to cancer.

3. *Your heart loves blueberries.* Anthocyanins and other nutrients in blueberries work in a few different ways to keep your cardiovas-

cular system ticking healthfully. They fight the inflammation and cell damage that can contribute to heart problems, and anthocyanins specifically seem to upregulate nitric oxide, which signals blood vessels to relax, increasing blood flow. The molecule also helps inhibit the buildup of platelets and cells in vessels.

4. *You could ward off tummy trouble and urinary tract infections.* The fiber and antioxidants in blueberries help fight inflammation in the intestines that may lead to stomach cramping and diarrhea, according to researchers from Lund University in Sweden. When it comes to UTIs, cranberries usually get all the applause, but blueberries may prevent the painful infections in the same way: Proanthocyanidins in the fruit stop bacteria from clinging to cells in the bladder—the first step in the development of a UTI. If you can stop the adhesion, the germs wash harmlessly out of your body.

→ **Trim-Down Tip:** Start your day with blueberries and yogurt. Doing so can help you avoid getting an upset stomach and a muffin top. The waist of a breakfast eater is nearly 2 inches slimmer than that of a person who skips, according to a study in *The American Journal of Clinical Nutrition.*

Dried Fruit Dos and Don'ts

Got a sweet tooth? Think of dried fruit as mind candy—literally. Most types of dried fruit are sweet enough that they can fool your sugar cravings, but they're loaded with fiber, fat-free, and just as portable and easy to eat as actual candy. Before digging in, keep these dos and don'ts in mind:

- Do watch for added sugar. Packaged dried fruit often has added sugar or other caloric sweeteners you don't need and probably won't miss. Check ingredients before buying, and skip over brands that list sugar.
- Do limit serving sizes. Dried fruit is concentrated with nutrients and fiber, but minus the water, it's denser in calories, too. Stick to portions no larger than ¼ cup.

- Don't forget about the fresh stuff. Part of what makes fruit so effective at squashing hunger is its water content, which adds weight and volume and works with fiber to keep you full and satiated. Snacking on dried fruit is better than not snacking on fruit at all, but pick fresh produce over dried more often than not.

....

→ **Trim-Down Tip:** Even if you won't follow the full Drop 10 meal plan, set a goal to eat more fruits and veggies in general. Then keep a bag of dried fruit in your desk drawer or at home. Having a healthier option on hand can remind you of your goal and encourage you to stick with it.

....

FIGHT WEIGHT CREEP BY EATING!

Adults who increased their intake of fruit and low-fat or skim milk gained less weight over time than those who skimped on the two, reports a study in *The American Journal of Clinical Nutrition*. A good way to get more of both: a quick blueberry smoothie. In a blender, combine $1/2$ cup blueberries, $1/2$ cup of any other fruit (we like banana), 1 cup skim milk, and $1/4$ cup ice.

Buy, Buy Blueberries

Headed to the market? Use these tips to find the best fruit:

- Say no to stains. Skip over containers of blueberries that look stained, which indicates the fruit inside may be bruised or moldy. What you want: firm, plump, smooth-skinned berries.
- Consider color. The bluer the hue, the riper the fruit. Although reddish berries aren't quite ripe for eating raw, you can use them for cooking or baking.
- Go organic if possible. Like apples, conventionally grown blueberries tend to have higher levels of pesticides than other fruit.

WANT TO EAT MORE BLUEBERRIES STARTING TODAY?

Frozen blueberries and almonds make a tasty grab-and-go snack. Prep a couple of individual portions to keep in the freezer so you're always prepared: Combine $1/2$ cup fresh blueberries and 1 tablespoon almonds in a zipper sandwich bag and freeze. Let thaw five minutes before munching.

DON'T LIKE BLUEBERRIES?

Sneak them into a filling smoothie; blend fresh or frozen blueberries with several other flavorful ingredients to mask the taste while still reaping blueberries' slimming superpowers. One recipe to try: Blend $1/4$ cup ice, $1/4$ cup strawberries, $1/4$ cup blueberries, 6 ounces nonfat vanilla yogurt, 1 tablespoon pomegranate juice, 2 tablespoons almond butter, and 1 teaspoon honey.

Trim-Down Tip: To keep blueberries fresh for up to ten days, keep them in the refrigerator in their original package or a sealed storage container and wait to wash them until just before you eat—excess moisture could cause them to spoil sooner.

blueberry nutrition by the numbers

84
calories per cup of blueberries

24
percent of your daily value of vitamin C

4
grams of fiber

CHERRIES

The Slimming Story

Start popping these bright bites, and life while dieting is just a bowl of, well, cherries. Both the tart and sweet varieties are bursting with antioxidants that may jump-start fat burning. The compounds, including anthocyanins, which impart the fruit's scarlet hue, boost enzymes that seem to help the body oxidize fat. Research also suggests they work to increase the uptake of sugar into muscles, which use it for energy. That's important, because the more efficient your body is at moving sugar out of the bloodstream and into cells, the lower your risk for metabolic syndrome, which is linked not only to diabetes and heart disease, but also to obesity and a wider waistline.

Cherries also help whittle your waist with fat-fighting fiber: A cup of the sweet variety serves up approximately 3 grams. (Tart cherries contain only 1.6 grams.) And thanks to the fruits' high water content, that cup feels weighty and substantial, so you're physically and emotionally satisfied with the snack. Sweet cherries offer an extra advantage: Their lip-smacking flavor may help quiet a craving without the calorie dump.

→ **Trim-Down Tip:** Whether you can't end dinner without dessert or you're trying to break an afternoon candy binge habit, try swapping your usual treat for cherries and let the natural sugars satisfy your sweet tooth for a slim 87 calories per cup.

Skip This Cherry Bomb

Plucking a maraschino cherry out of a Manhattan or whiskey sour (or Shirley Temple!) and popping it into your mouth is part of the fun of drinking the cocktails. Maraschinos, unfortunately, are highly processed and often contain high-fructose corn syrup and artificial coloring. Skip the added sugar and drop a few fresh or muddled (lightly smashed) sweet cherries into your drink instead.

> ### WAIT TO WASH!
>
> Rinse cherries only immediately before you eat them. Moisture left on them can promote rot, wasting the juicy, fat-fighting eats and the money you spent on them.

The Amazing Proof

- Obese rats fed the human equivalent of 1½ cups of tart cherries for twelve weeks metabolized sugar better, weighed less overall, and had 18 percent less fat mass than those who didn't consume the fruit, a study from the University of Michigan in Ann Arbor reports.

→ **Trim-Down Tip:** Tart cherries are typically sold as dried fruit; before buying, check ingredients to make sure there aren't any added sweeteners.

- In a study from Michigan State University, mice were fed a fatty diet along with purified anthocyanins and ursolic acid (a natural anti-inflammatory) derived from Cornelian cherries, a variety similar to the tart cherries found in the United States. After eight weeks, the animals gained 24 percent less weight than rats that chowed the same diet but without the cherry compounds.
- Women with diabetes who drank about 1½ ounces of a highly concentrated tart cherry juice every day for six weeks lost 6 pounds and lowered their blood pressure, according to a study published in *Nutrition & Food Science*.

→ **Trim-Down Tip:** You can buy tart cherry juice, sometimes called Montmorency (a type of cherry), at your local grocery store. Choose brands with no added sugar and 100 percent cherry juice. (Manufacturers often sell a blend.) A word of warning: Fruit juice is high in calories, so instead of drinking it straight, sip a slimming spritzer by combining an ounce or two with a full glass of sparkling water.

Four More Reasons to Eat Cherries

1. *They help ease muscle soreness and arthritis pain.* Cherries' potent concentration of antioxidants has anti-inflammatory powers that mimic the way ibuprofen works (although to a lesser degree). Studies of marathon runners and weight lifters find that those who drank tart cherry juice before and after exercise reported less postexercise pain and loss of strength compared with those drinking a placebo.

2. *Cherries are a treat for your ticker.* The phytochemicals in cherries may affect the production of lipids in the body and help lower your cholesterol. Plus, eating about 2 cups of cherries daily reduced a marker of inflammation, another cardiac risk factor, by up to 25 percent, according to research published in *The Journal of Nutrition.*

3. *You could help ward off cancer.* Cherries' powerful antioxidants, including anthocyanins, mop up free radicals and may jump-start your immune system, which could give the fruit the potential to protect against cancer. Preliminary animal and cell studies show that cherry compounds can inhibit tumors and the growth of colon cancer cells.

4. *They'll keep your brain sharp and help you snooze more soundly.* As with other antioxidant-rich fruit, cherries' compounds fight the oxidative damage that injures neurons and may increase risk for memory loss, dementia, and Alzheimer's disease. Tart cherries are also a natural source of melatonin, a hormone your body makes that helps regulate sleep.

RED ALERT!

Tart cherries are highly acidic, so if you take medication for acid reflux or are prone to heartburn, snack on the sweet varieties.

WANT TO EAT MORE CHERRIES
STARTING TODAY?

Swap in dried sweet or tart cherries in place of raisins. For example, eat cherries plain as a snack, add them to trail mix, or sprinkle them on a green salad or in chicken salad, in yogurt, or on cereal.

DON'T LIKE CHERRIES?

Puree or finely chop sweet cherries and mix into whole-grain muffin and bread recipes.

→ **Trim-Down Tip:** Don't let jet lag weigh you down. Snack on dried cherries in flight to fight its effects after you land. Sweet dreams—of a slimmer you!

Cherry-Pick the Best Fruit

Whether you're shopping at the grocery store, a farmers' market, or an orchard, remember the three R's:

Red: Choose varieties of cherries that are bright or dark red in color. They contain more fat-fighting anthocyanins than yellow-red Gold or Rainier cherries.

Robust: Opt for cherries that already look ripe—large and juicy—but are still slightly firm to the touch. Cherries won't continue to ripen once off the tree.

oRganic: Okay, so this is not technically an R, but close enough! Conventionally grown cherries are number sixteen on the Environmental Working Group's list of produce that tends to have higher levels of pesticides than other similarly raised fruits or vegetables. When you can, choose cherries farmed without chemical help.

cherry nutrition by the numbers

87
calories per cup of pitted sweet cherries

10
percent of your daily value of vitamin C

3
grams of fiber

GOJI BERRIES

The Slimming Story

More proof that good things come in small packages: these tiny, tart, and chewy berries. Bright red-orange gojis, aka lycium fruit or wolfberries, have been a staple of traditional Chinese medicine for centuries, but what primarily make them an Rx for weight loss are their eighteen amino acids, which deliver a hefty dose of hunger-taming, fat-fighting protein. Just how much protein are we talking? A 1-ounce serving of berries, which you buy dried, contains 4 grams—ounce for ounce, the same as a hard-boiled egg.

Protein does a lot more to help you reach your weight loss goals than stave off the munchies. Simply digesting protein burns double the calories your body expends breaking down fat and carbohydrates. Protein also provides the building blocks needed for lean muscle mass; the more muscle you maintain, the speedier your metabolism—that is, you burn more calories every day, even when you're doing nothing.

Protein aside, gojis also deliver many of the same skinny-making nutrients as their superfruit peers. A 1-ounce serving packs 3 grams of fiber, which teams with protein to keep you satiated, slows digestion, and steadies your blood sugar and insulin levels, discouraging the production and storage of excess fat. You'll net about 20 percent of your daily recommended intake of vitamin C, too, helping your body burn fat for fuel.

The Amazing Proof

- Upping your daily intake of protein with gojis is a smart way to get more of this filling nutrient without loading up on unwanted dietary fat. In a study from Purdue University in West Lafayette, Indiana, women on a low-cal diet ate either 30 percent or 18 percent of their calories from protein. All lost weight, but the high-protein group felt generally fuller than the other group, plus happier than even before they started dieting. The lower-protein group's mood took a downturn. (No wonder—who doesn't get cranky when she's hungry!?)

- In a similar twelve-week trial published in the journal *Obesity Research,* subjects who ate meals consisting of 25 percent protein felt fuller throughout the day, had weaker late-night cravings, and thought less about food than those who got meals with only 14 percent protein.

→ **Trim-Down Tip:** Snack on gojis postworkout. Try this mix, which you can stash in your gym bag: 2 tablespoons goji berries, ¼ cup whole-grain cereal, 2 tablespoons almonds. A combo of carbs and protein is the best muscle-building fuel.

- Gojis also supply you with fat-sizzling vitamin C. Studies show that the lower one's blood levels of the vitamin, the more body fat one is likely to have, and the more one is likely to weigh. Researchers aren't exactly sure why but think it's because vitamin C is necessary for the body to produce carnitine, a compound that shuttles fat into cells that burn it for fuel.

→ **Trim-Down Tip:** Goji berries are a food chameleon; they go well with just about anything. Add them to salads, wraps, or other dishes to pack more vitamin C and protein into every meal.

Four More Reasons to Eat Goji Berries

1. *You'll reap all the health and beauty benefits of carotenoids.* Goji berries are bursting with this group of vitamins, including beta-carotene, and with that comes a plethora of healthy advan-

> WANT TO EAT MORE GOJI BERRIES
> STARTING TODAY?
>
> Keep this filling trail mix on hand for anytime snacking. Mix ¼ cup of dried goji berries with ¼ cup raisins and ¼ cup walnuts.

tages. The vitamins are important for healthy immune function, they're potent antioxidants that may help protect against cardiovascular disease, and they encourage smooth, clear skin.

→ **Trim-Down Tip:** Eating gojis with the good-for-you fats in nuts and salad dressings helps your body better absorb the berries' carotenoids.

2. *Goji berries may bolster skin's natural SPF.* In an animal study from the University of Sydney in New South Wales, Australia, mice were given the human equivalent of 4 ounces or more of goji berry juice or various control drinks daily, then exposed to ultraviolet light. After a week, the goji-gulping mice showed significantly less inflammation and greater protection against the sun's ability to suppress the immune system.
3. *Compounds in goji berries show anticancer activity.* Preliminary research suggests that the polysaccharides in gojis may ramp up the body's immune response to cancer cells. In lab studies, for example, fractions of the compounds inhibited the growth of cells from certain cancers, including that of the breast.
4. *You could see benefits for your eyes.* Goji berries are rich in the carotenoid zeaxanthin, which eyes use as protection against UV damage that could otherwise lead to macular degeneration.

Where to Buy Goji Berries

Look for gojis with other dried fruit in the produce or snack food aisle of the supermarket. If yours doesn't carry the berries, check either a larger chain or smaller neighborhood health food store, or buy them online.

→ DON'T LIKE GOJIS?

Hide them in your dessert. Blend 2 tablespoons goji berries, 1/2 cup low-fat ice cream, and 1/4 cup skim milk for a shake that will help you stop body jiggle.

goji berry nutrition by the numbers

100
calories per ounce of goji berries

20
percent of your daily value of vitamin C

3
grams of fiber

4
grams of protein

KIWIFRUIT

The Slimming Story

More than a quick way to brighten your fruit salad, kiwis are lean, green, fat-fighting machines. With more vitamin C per ounce than even an orange, a single large kiwi serves up 84 milligrams, 107 percent of your day's quota. Vitamin C may increase your body's fat-burning potential by stimulating the production of two enzymes you need to make carnitine, a compound that transports fat molecules from fat tissue into cell mitochondria, where it's burned for energy when you exercise—even if you're only out for a stroll. Researchers speculate that too little carnitine, possibly due to too little vitamin C, may inhibit your body from using fat as fuel. As it turns out, studies have found that the concentration of C in blood is inversely related to body fat: The heaviest people tend to have the lowest levels. Eating plenty of C-rich foods such as kiwi is one way to deposit more of the vitamin into your blood, ensuring your fat-burning potential stays high.

As if its vitamin C content weren't impressive enough, kiwi wraps additional pound-peeling nutrients into its petite package. You'll take in 2 grams of stomach-filling fiber, which works to transport some of the calories you eat through your system before they end up on your frame. And, like other fruit, kiwi is a low-energy-dense food, meaning it is high in water and low in fat, filling you up for a mere 42 calories each. Plus, ounce for ounce, the fuzzy fruit contains nearly as much potassium as a banana. Potassium is belly-bloating sodium's nemesis: It latches on to salt and helps flush the excess out of your body so you look (and feel) less puffy. Bikini shopping, anyone?

The Amazing Proof

- People with marginal levels of vitamin C burned 10 percent less fat per pound of body weight while walking than those with normal levels of the nutrient, a study at Arizona State University in Mesa reveals. They also felt more tired. But—get this—when researchers gave the subjects vitamin C supplements (500 milligrams), their fat burning increased fourfold!

→ **Trim-Down Tip:** You needn't pop pills to raise your levels of C; taking in about 200 milligrams a day from food (the amount in two or three kiwis) may give you the same fat-burning fire, the study's lead author says.

• Kiwis pack more nutrition into fewer calories than most other fruit. Kiwis are tied for first (with guava) among thirty-three popular fruits in a nutrient-density test by researchers at Rutgers University in New Brunswick, New Jersey, who averaged the percentages of recommended daily values of nine critical vitamins, minerals, and fiber (including potassium and vitamin C) in 100 grams of fruit. And kiwis came in fourth in terms of how many calories it "costs" to get 1 percent of your daily quota of the vitamins.

Four More Reasons to Eat Kiwifruit

1. *They're a green light for your heart.* After eating a kiwi twice a day for twenty-eight days, study subjects lowered their levels of triglycerides (a heart-harming fat in the blood) by 15 percent and reduced the buildup of platelets in arteries by 18 percent, cutting the chances of developing blood clots, reports a study from the University of Oslo in Norway.
2. *Kiwis keep skin young and smooth.* Think of the fruit as edible skin care. Antioxidants in kiwi mop up skin-damaging sun-induced free radicals; plus, its vitamin C helps your skin

→ KOOL KIWI FACT

Once known as a Chinese gooseberry, the kiwi was renamed by a California produce importer who thought the furry brown orbs from New Zealand resembled that country's national bird, the kiwi.

WHEN IS ORGANIC WORTH IT?

Eating organic produce is certainly appealing—who wouldn't want to lower her exposure to pesticides, even levels that are deemed safe? Plus, organic eats may be more nutritious than conventionally grown fruits and vegetables because they are fresher and you can eat the peels. But relax—you don't need to break the bank to eat well. Follow these easy rules:

- Eat fruits and veggies, period. Studies link a higher intake of produce to a lower risk for many diseases, regardless of how it is grown.
- Not buying organic? Go local and seasonal. Some nonorganic produce shipped from afar may contain additives to help the food survive the trip. Eating in-season fruit ensures you're getting the freshest food, too.
- If you're going to eat the peel, go organic. Some pesticides coat the outer layer (the peel), so removing it reduces residue. But many peels are nutritious, so for thin-skinned veggies and fruits, choose organic and eat them whole. Apples, blueberries, and cherries, for example, are the three superfoods for weight loss that are high on the Environmental Working Group's list of produce that tends to hang on to pesticides. On the flip side, don't bother shelling out extra for organic when it comes to fruit with thick skin, such as pomegranates and kiwis.

make more supportive collagen, which, when strong, firm, and healthy, creates a smoother complexion. Indeed, people who eat plenty of C-rich foods have fewer lines than those who take in less, a study in *The American Journal of Clinical Nutrition* reveals.

3. *You'll boost your immunity and help fight off cancer.* The abundant vitamin C in kiwi bolsters your defenses against common bugs and possibly even cancer. A potent antioxidant, the vitamin works to thwart the effects of cancer-causing free radicals, and

WANT TO EAT MORE KIWI STARTING TODAY?

Sweet and juicy, kiwi makes a natural (and naturally deli-cious) substitute for jelly or jam, which tends to have added sugar and excess calories. Try it: Place sliced kiwi in a peanut-butter sandwich or enjoy on toast.

DON'T LIKE KIWI?

Slip the fruit into a tropical salsa with other bold flavors and you'll never know it's there. Combine 1 diced kiwi, 1 diced mango, 1 diced red bell pepper, 2 tablespoons lime juice, and 1 tablespoon chopped fresh cilantro. Eat with tortilla chips or spoon over grilled steak, chicken, pork, or fish.

population studies suggest that those who eat foods high in the vitamin may have a lower risk for certain forms of the disease. (Trials show that supplements do not reduce risk as well as C-loaded food can, so eat up!)

4. *The fruit may calm tummy trouble.* Munching two kiwis per day alleviated constipation and improved bowel function in people with irritable bowel syndrome, according to a study in the *Asia Pacific Journal of Clinical Nutrition.* Researchers credit kiwi's fiber content and an enzyme in the fruit that may stimulate re-ceptors in the colon, triggering a natural laxative effect.

It's Easy Going Green

Follow these tips for buying, storing, and eating kiwis:

- Use the press test. A ripe piece of fruit will feel slightly soft when you press it gently with your finger. If it's firm, let it sit out for a day or two to ripen.
- Skip organic. Kiwis are on the Environmental Working Group's "clean 15" list of produce—meaning they tend to contain among the lowest amount of pesticides—so buy conventional to save money.

- Ripen at room temperature. Once they are ripe, transfer kiwis to the fridge, where they can last four to seven days.
- Eat immediately after slicing. Kiwis contain the enzyme actinidin, which acts as a food tenderizer when exposed to the air. If you wait too long after cutting, your fruit will turn mushy. For the same reason, add kiwis to fruit salad or other dishes right before serving.
- It's okay to eat the skin. Yep, it's edible—and good for your diet. Munching a kiwi with the skin on triples your intake of waist-whittling fiber. Simply wash, slice, and *mmm*. How's that for fuzzy logic?
- Or skip it. Don't waste time (or endure the sticky fingers) peeling a kiwi: Cut the fruit into two halves and use a spoon to scoop out the flesh. A regular spoon will work; a serrated grapefruit spoon is a cut above.

kiwifruit nutrition by the numbers

42

calories per 2-inch kiwi

107

percent of your daily value of vitamin C

2

grams of fiber

POMEGRANATES

The Slimming Story

Pomegranate juice definitely earns its hype as a health booster, but the fruit—actually crunchy, juice-filled sacs called arils—deserves to share the spotlight for its waist-trimming powers. A half cup of the ruby-colored seeds gives you 3½ grams of fiber for only 72 calories. Fiber is the supernutrient with a trifecta of trimming benefits: (a) It fills you up; (b) it keeps blood sugar and insulin levels steady, which controls hunger and discourages your body from packing on excess fat; and (c) it helps move some of the fat and calories you eat through your system before your body absorbs them and stores them on you. (For more info on fiber, check out page 38.)

Pomegranate arils produce scalable results thanks to their high water content, too. That, along with its scant amount of fat, makes the fruit a low-energy-dense food, meaning you get plenty to eat for relatively few calories, helping you stay satiated—so you naturally eat less overall without feeling deprived. Plus, if you crave candy, the tiny sacs' natural sweetness, juicy quality, bright color, and bite-size snackability make them a perfect substitute for nutrient-void sugar bombs (ahem, jelly beans) you might be tempted to binge on.

➡ **Trim-Down Tip:** Keep a small container of preshucked arils at work in the event of a midafternoon candy craving.

The Amazing Proof

- Studies routinely show that increasing your intake of fruits and veggies may help you lose weight. One especially worth noting is from the State University of New York in Buffalo: Two groups of families were similarly counseled on weight loss at regular meetings, with one crucial exception—the first group's sessions focused on eating more fruit (at least two servings per day) and vegetables (at least three servings per day), while the other families were told to concentrate on eating fewer high-fat foods and foods with added sugar (for example, no more than ten servings per week). After a year, the fruit and veggie group lost significantly more weight, ate more produce, and decreased their intake of fatty and sweetened foods more than the second group did.

→ **Trim-Down Tip:** Instead of focusing on the foods you're trying to limit, focus more on all the fresh, mouthwatering fruit such as pomegranates you *can* eat.

- Fiber intake is a key factor in weight loss success, but eating more fruits and veggies can enhance its effects, according to researchers at the University of Navarra in Pamplona, Spain. They analyzed the eating habits and weight gain of more than eleven thousand people and found that those who consumed the most fiber (30 grams or more daily) and the most fruits and vegetables (six servings or more per day) were 31 percent less likely to have gained a significant amount of weight over five years.

WANT TO EAT MORE POMEGRANATES STARTING TODAY?

Pomegranate arils make a tangy, crunchy addition to salads. They balance the flavors and textures of the following salad combos especially well: spinach, Gorgonzola, and pears; or arugula, cherry tomatoes, and goat cheese.

DON'T LIKE POMEGRANATES?

Use the juice to make a refreshing ice pop; you'll still get plenty of pom's fat-fighting vitamin C. Blend $1/2$ cup nonfat vanilla yogurt, $1/2$ cup mixed berries, and $1/2$ cup pomegranate juice. Pour mixture into two ice molds and freeze.

→ **Trim-Down Tip:** Don't spit out the seeds! Each juice-filled pomegranate aril contains a tiny seed that houses much of the fruit's fiber.

Three More Reasons to Eat Pomegranates

1. *They're a red-letter fruit for your heart.* Potent antioxidant polyphenols in pomegranates and their juice may help quell inflammation (a normal immune response in the body that can get out of control and contribute to disease). They also work against atherosclerosis, the buildup of fatty deposits in arteries. People with carotid artery disease, for example, which can lead to stroke, were able to reverse some damage by drinking a little less than 2 ounces of pomegranate juice daily, reports a study in the journal *Clinical Nutrition.*

2. *Poms are promising cancer fighters.* A rash of recent studies also links pomegranate juice, extract, and seed oil and its compounds with anticancer activity; they've been shown to kill off or inhibit the growth of cells related to lung, breast, and colon cancers, among others.

Sip Your Seeds!

Pomegranate arils' ruby shade makes them a beautiful and slimming accessory in cocktails or champagne. Or toss a half cup into a blender with other fruits and skim milk for a hearty, fiber-filled smoothie.

→ **Trim-Down Tip:** If you're tempted to gulp the juice, keep in mind that pom juice, like all fruit juices, is high in calories (134 per cup) and contains none of the slimming fiber you get from whole fruit. A little is okay—try the ice pop recipe, previous page, or mix a splash with seltzer—but limit your intake and look for brands that contain 100 percent juice and no added sugar.

3. *They may help lower your risk for arthritis and Alzheimer's disease.*
Pomegranate's powerful antioxidant compounds could have a
protective effect on joint cartilage and help shield the brain
against damage that contributes to Alzheimer's. In a mouse
model of Alzheimer's, animals that drank the human equivalent
of 1 to 2 cups of pomegranate juice per day had less plaque
buildup in the brain (a symptom of Alzheimer's) and learned
maze tasks more quickly than mice that drank a placebo, according to a study in *Neurobiology of Disease.*

Get the Juicy Goods

If you've never attempted to release pomegranate arils from the fruit's
leathery-skin encasement, the task may seem daunting. Follow these
easy-peasy steps:

1. *Cut off the crown.* Slice half an inch off the top of the pom, where
the skin juts out slightly like a spiky crown.
2. *Score the peel.* Make four shallow cuts from where you've sliced
to the base. Hold the fruit under water in a bowl and gently but
firmly break it into quarters along your score lines. (By keeping
it underwater, you'll prevent renegade squirts from staining
your clothing.) Pat the quarters dry.
3. *Scoop the fruit.* Using a spoon or your fingers, carefully detach the
aril clusters from the peel. Discard the skin and pick out the
spongy white pith. Enjoy on the spot, or transfer to a plastic storage container and refrigerate until you're hungry.

Three Reasons to Buy Whole Pomegranates

Ready-to-eat, preshucked arils are fuss-free, but whole pomegranates
offer plenty of convenience, too.

• They're already ripe. Pomegranates are sold ripe, so there's no
need to wait before you dig in. Pick one with smooth skin that has
some heft—the heavier the fruit, the juicier it is.

- They have a lengthy shelf life. Whole pomegranates last longer than most other fruit; kept in a plastic bag in the fridge, one will stay fresh for up to three months. Spot a sale on poms? Stock up!
- You can store the seeds. Once freed of their protective peel and membrane, the arils will last six months in an airtight container in the freezer or about three days in the fridge.

pomegranate nutrition
by the numbers

840
average number of arils in 1 pomegranate

72
calories per ½ cup of arils

15
percent of your daily value of vitamin C

3.5
grams of fiber

drop *10* inspiration

"I don't miss any of my old binge foods."

NAME: Andela Armand
AGE: 37
OCCUPATION: Restaurant floor manager
FAMILY STATUS: Married
HEIGHT: 5 feet 8 inches
STARTING WEIGHT: 191
DROP 10 WEIGHT: 178
LOST: 13 pounds in seven weeks

My story: "I have always felt heavy, unfit, and low in energy. I got my wake-up call when my doctor told me that my blood sugar was high. The idea of developing diabetes scared me to death. I've tried fad diets before, but they only worked for about two weeks, and then they'd become too hard to maintain. I'd put the weight back on—plus more."

Biggest challenge to losing weight: "My pantry, and getting used to exercising regularly. I needed to rid the pantry of all temptations and stock it up with healthy options. At the beginning of the plan, I also made sure I had access to classes like Zumba, which I knew would be a workout but loads of fun as well."

Why Drop 10 clicked: "I never felt like I was on a diet. I was introduced to new foods that are not only tasty, but healthy. They made me feel good inside and out, and gave me energy to exercise. I also learned how much to eat when I am out to lunch or dinner."

How my body changed: "I lost 3 inches off my waist and one dress size. And my blood sugars are now normal. Woo-hoo! Plus, I have a better sense of who I am and how my body works. As long as I persevere, I can accomplish what I set out to achieve. I want to keep going with the plan!"

Success tips: "I rely on two or three menus for breakfast, lunch, and dinner—so when I'm in a rush, it's easy to grab a tried-and-tested meal that is both satisfying and healthy."

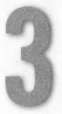 Super Vegetables

. . . .

ARTICHOKES

. . . . .

The Slimming Story

These prickly globes may intimidate novice chefs, but it's fat that should be afraid. Very afraid! Artichokes contain more pound-peeling fiber than any other vegetable; a teeny ½ cup of artichoke hearts serves up 7 grams, all for a mere 45 calories. Snack on the fiber-rich petals as well—don't worry, we'll tell you how to do it—and you'll take in an impressive 10 grams! Fiber ushers some of the fat and calories you eat out of your body before you absorb it all, and it squelches hunger by digesting slooowwwly and adding bulk and weight to food without extra calories.

The fact that your body digests fiber slowly also keeps blood sugar and insulin levels down, discouraging your system from storing excess fat. Artichokes' fiber probably doesn't work alone to prevent insulin spikes, however. Researchers from the Institute of Neuroscience in Cagliari, Italy, find that animals fed a fiber-free artichoke extract prior to eating had lower postmeal blood sugar levels than those who didn't get the vegetable. Although the scientists are not certain why, the results solidify the veggie's spot as a bona fide belly flattener.

To Choose a Tasty Choke, Use Your Senses!

- Look for a globe with a firm stem, which indicates that its flesh is well hydrated.
- Listen while giving the orb a gentle squeeze; if you hear it squeak, you've got a fresh one.
- Grab a globe that's compact in shape and heavy for its size.

But it gets even better. Artichokes contain resistant starch, a type of carbohydrate that research suggests may increase fat burning, shrink fat cells, and stimulate the hormones in your gut that tell your brain, "I'm full. Stop eating." (Want to learn more about resistant starch? We thought so! Turn to page 70.)

→ **Trim-Down Tip:** If you've never eaten a whole artichoke, see the how-to below. Getting at the flesh in the petals and eventually reaching the delicate (and delectable) heart takes time, forcing you to eat slowly and savor the flavor. Doing that may help you consume fewer calories and feel full longer.

The Amazing Proof

- Over the course of twenty months, for every 2 grams of fiber a woman added to her diet, she lost half a pound and 0.25 percent of her body fat without increasing her exercise habits, a study published in *The Journal of Nutrition* reveals.
- Artichokes and other fiber-rich veggies are a staple of the good-for-you-and-your-waistline Mediterranean diet. In a study of more than ten thousand Spanish people, those whose eating habits most closely followed the Med diet were 24 percent less likely to gain significant weight over a four-year period, according to a study published in *The American Journal of Clinical Nutrition*.

WILL THE REAL ARTICHOKE PLEASE STAND UP?

Although similar in taste to the green globe artichoke, a Jerusalem artichoke (also called a sunchoke) actually looks like a hunk of fresh ginger and is part of the sunflower family.

Two More Reasons to Eat Artichokes

1. *They're antioxidant-rich, disease-fighting powerhouses.* With more healthy antioxidants than any other vegetable, artichokes may help you fend off damage from free radicals that could contribute to cancer and other diseases. Research from the Molecular Pathology and Ultrastructure Laboratory in Rome has also found that polyphenols in artichokes induce liver cancer cells to self-destruct.

2. *Eat hearts for the good of your heart.* Aside from artichokes' high concentration of heart-healthy antioxidants, their fiber works to ferry cholesterol out of your arteries. The veggie also delivers a good amount of folate, a nutrient that helps maintain heart function and control blood pressure.

WANT TO EAT MORE ARTICHOKES
STARTING TODAY?

Keep a bag of frozen hearts on hand so you can add them on the fly to homemade or prepared pasta sauces, vegetable soup, and casseroles. Before using, let them sit out for about ten minutes, then squeeze out excess moisture.

DON'T LIKE ARTICHOKES?

Hide them in a veggie-loaded homemade pizza: When they are finely chopped and either mixed into your sauce or spread on top, you'll barely be able to taste them amid the other ingredients.

THREE STEPS TO PREPPING A FRESH ARTICHOKE

A fresh-from-the-market choke supplies bushels of flavor ripe for snacking or serving as a side dish. Follow these tips to get at the soft flesh and tasty heart:

1. Wash and trim. Rinse your choke under cold water, making sure you get it between the open petals. Cut about a half inch from the top and trim off the stem.

2. Steam or microwave. To steam, fill a saucepan with a few inches of water and lemon slices and heat to boiling. Place your choke(s) in a steaming basket in the pot, cover, and cook over a low boil about 45 minutes. If you're in a hurry, place the veggie in a microwave-safe glass container, add half an inch of water, and cover. Cook on high until the petals near the center are soft and pull apart easily, 6 to 8 minutes. (Avoid boiling the artichokes; you'll lose some of their water-soluble nutrients.)

3. Pluck, scoop, and enjoy! Transfer the artichoke to a plate and pluck off the petals one by one, scraping the base between your teeth to squeeze out the soft inside. (Discard the leaf.) Once you've finished the petals, cut the choke in half, scrape out the inedible hairs, and scoop out the heart. You may want to dip the petals or heart in sauce before you dig in. Low-fat mayonnaise and garlic or lemon butter are popular, but this simple, scale-friendly dip will double your superfood intake: Combine ½ cup fat-free Greek yogurt, the juice of 1 lemon, 1 tablespoon each of Dijon mustard and chopped parsley, and salt and pepper to taste.

Artichokes: Slimming at All Sizes

Don't skip over the baby artichokes you see at farmers' markets. They're neither immature nor inferior; their size simply indicates they grew farther down the stem of the plant. You might even prefer them to larger chokes: Because smaller chokes have fewer outer leaves and no inedible, hairy inner portion, it's easier to get at the yummy heart.

RESISTANT STARCH: THE FAT-MELTING, HUNGER-TAMING CARB

Carbs have gotten a bad rap over the years. Sure, refined grains are no friend to your thighs (we're looking at you, bagel), but as a food group, they aren't the enemy. In fact, one type you'll want to meet again and again is resistant starch (RS). Found in artichokes, sweet potatoes, lentils, and the whole-grain superfoods recommended for weight loss in chapter 4, RS may help you burn extra flab and drop weight. Here's how:

- RS helps tame your appetite. Resistant starch acts the same way fiber does in that your body doesn't break it down quickly or digest it in the gastrointestinal tract as it does other carbs. (It's resistant—that's how it got its name.) As with fiber, you digest RS slowly so you feel fuller on fewer calories, and that feeling lasts longer, too. RS eventually is fermented in the colon, where it may increase the production of GLP-1 and PYY, two peptide hormone compounds that function as messengers between gut and brain, sending the signal to stop eating.

- RS ramps up the burning of fat and calories: Other than their appetite-regulating effects, GLP-1 and PYY may turn up the body's furnace, causing it to scorch more fat. After eating a meal containing a modest amount of resistant starch (5 grams, or about the amount in $^3/_4$ cup of lentils), study subjects sizzled 23 percent more fat than after consuming a similar meal without RS, according to a study from the University of Colorado Health Sciences Center, Center for Human Nutrition, in Denver. Animal research from Louisiana State University finds that a diet rich in RS also increases the expression of POMC, a hormone that boosts energy expenditure (calories burned). Both of these effects help explain why rats fed RS lose weight even when they don't eat fewer calories.

- RS may help prevent the production and storage of fat. A diet high in resistant starch seems to shrink fat cells and fat deposits and also reduces the amount of fat the body stores, according to animal and lab research published in *Nutrition Journal.* Experts aren't exactly sure why. Additional research also suggests that consuming foods with RS seems to inhibit enzymes related to fat production.

Although several studies have been done, information on the special fat-burning carb is still relatively limited, including exactly how much of it you get from different foods. One complication is that temperature can alter the amount of RS; cooking with moist heat (for example, steaming or boiling) decreases it, but the resistant starch re-forms as food cools. (Thus, cold lentil, potato, or artichoke salad, for example, has more RS than hot foods do.) Bottom line: The weight-loss-inducing superfoods that contain RS—including artichokes, sweet potatoes, lentils, and whole grains—all have serious slimming benefits going for them already, and RS is one more incentive to eat up. We say, Let them eat (healthy) carbs!

Save Time—Buy Canned or Frozen Artichokes

If you don't want to fuss over a fresh choke, go for canned or frozen ready-to-eat, fully cooked hearts. Tender canned hearts are great for snacking and a diet bargain at 16 calories a pop. Choose those that are packed in water (not oil) and have the least amount of sodium. Even then, rinse thoroughly before using to wash away any residual salty brine. If you buy frozen, you should also watch for added sodium. Before using, thaw by letting them sit out in a bowl, then gently squeeze out excess moisture.

artichoke nutrition by the numbers

64

calories per 1 medium cooked artichoke

10

grams of fiber

3

grams of protein

AVOCADO

The Slimming Story

We aren't going to sugarcoat it. Avocados have a lot of fat (29 grams each). Calories, too (322, to be exact). But here's the honest-to-skinny truth: They're not necessarily fattening. (Avocados are technically a fruit, but most people treat them as a veggie; that's why we put them here in chapter 3.) They are dripping with monounsaturated fat, a healthy type that improves cholesterol and doesn't promote blocked arteries. What this fat does block: hunger, cravings, and the urge to binge.

Compared with carbs and protein, monounsaturated fat takes longer to leave your stomach. This delay triggers your body to produce the appetite-regulating hormones that help you feel satiated and keep cravings at bay. Plenty of research shows that foods high in monounsaturated fat, consumed moderately, won't blow out your scale and can even help you push the needle in the downward direction and stick to a low-calorie eating plan.

An avocado's fat doesn't fight hunger solo; however, half an avocado delivers almost 7 grams of filling fiber. Fiber (and monounsaturated fat,

---

Peel 'n' Eat

Preparing an avocado for noshing is as easy as 1-2-3.

1. **Make the cut**. Slice the avocado in half lengthwise, cutting around the large seed. Gently twist the halves in opposite directions until they separate.
2. **Scoop out the seed.** Using a knife or spoon, carefully pop out the embedded seed. (Yup, what you probably think of as a pit is actually a seed. In fact, you can grow a houseplant from it: For instructions, check out avocado.org/grow-your-own-tree.)
3. **Spoon out the flesh.** Wedge the utensil as close to the peel as possible, gently separating the green fruit from its protective jacket. Remove the entire half; slice or dice as desired.

IT'S EASY STAYING GREEN

If you premake guacamole or eat only a portion of a whole avocado, sprinkle the exposed green areas with lemon or lime juice, and keep in a sealed container in the refrigerator to preserve its vivid hue. You certainly can store a cut avocado with its seed, but it's a myth that doing so prevents browning.

for that matter) helps keep insulin levels steady, preventing the spikes that encourage your body to store fat. Fiber also saves you from fully absorbing all the calories you eat by moving food through your digestive tract. Hello, avocado! Goodbye, fat!

The Amazing Proof

- Over the course of an eighteen-month weight loss trial, a full 80 percent of those in the low-fat-eating group dropped out, whereas only 46 percent of the moderate-fat-eating participants called it quits, according to a study from Harvard University. What's more, when researchers measured everyone at eighteen months, people in the moderate-fat group were down an average of 9 pounds each; those in the other group had gained 6 pounds per person. (The moderate-fat group consisted of those who took in 35 percent of their calories from fat, 15 to 20 percent from monounsaturated sources.)

- In a study published in *The American Journal of Clinical Nutrition,* two groups of dieters ate similar low-calorie meals, except one consumed 18 percent of its calories from fat, and the other took in 33 percent fat, with all the extra coming from unsaturated sources. Members of both groups lost more than 2 pounds per week over the course of six weeks, but the high-fat group maintained lower levels of triglycerides (a type of fat in the blood) four weeks after the diet program ended; the low-fat group's triglyceride levels rebounded immediately.

→ **Trim-Down Tip:** Swap out saturated fat for monounsaturated when possible. Instead of buttering your whole-grain toast, for example, eat it with a few slices of avocado.

Three More Reasons to Eat Avocados

1. *You'll shrink your risk for cardiovascular disease.* Eat more avocados to see changes in your heart health. Diets high in monounsaturated fat may help lower blood pressure, "bad" LDL cholesterol, and triglycerides at the same time that they raise levels of "good" HDL cholesterol, the type that acts like a broom inside arteries, helping to keep them clear. The fiber in avocados, as well as in other fruits and vegetables, also helps carry cholesterol out of the body.

2. *Nutrients in avocados may help thwart diabetes.* Researchers from Rovira i Virgili University in Tarragona, Spain, find that older adults who ate a diet high in monounsaturated fats cut their risk for diabetes by more than half, compared with those who followed a diet lower in fat. Healthy fats help regulate your body's insulin response after a meal, but the plant foods rich in those

→
WANT TO EAT MORE AVOCADOS STARTING TODAY?

Mashed avocado is a perfect waist-whittling, creamy substitute for mayonnaise, cream cheese, butter, margarine, or sour cream. Spread a quarter of an avocado (about 2 ounces) on a sandwich or whole-grain bagel or bread, or spoon it into a bowl of chili.

DON'T LIKE AVOCADO?

Slip it into a smoothie; avocado adds an undeniably creamy texture but a barely detectable taste. In a blender, combine 1/4 avocado (seeded and peeled), 1 banana, 1 cup orange juice, 1 cup berries, and ice.

fats (such as avocado, olive oil, and nuts) also contain phytonutrients that may play a role in preventing the disease.

3. *Eating an avocado is like taking a multivitamin.* An avocado boasts twenty different vitamins and minerals, in addition to other healthy phytochemicals, that all work together to keep your system functioning optimally. You'll get especially high doses of potassium; vitamins C, E, and K; and folate.

→ **Take-Away Tip:** Add avocados to your salad or salsa. Pairing foods rich in fat-soluble vitamins with avocado increases their absorption. For example, if you eat foods such as carrots, kale, broccoli, and tomatoes with avocado, you'll take in fifteen times more immunity-boosting beta-carotene and five times more lutein, both of which promote healthy eyes.

The Ripeness Report

Follow these tips for picking the best avocado. One note: If you're on a budget, don't bother spending extra money on organic. Avocados' thick skin earned them a spot on the Environmental Working Group's "clean 15" list of produce (fruits and veggies that retain low levels of pesticides when conventionally grown).

- Put the squeeze on. A ripe, ready-to-eat avocado feels soft but not mushy. If one gives too much, move on—it could be overly ripe.
- Go to the dark side. The pebbly skin of a Hass avocado, the most popular variety, gets darker the riper it is. Other types may not darken, but they will get softer.
- Ripen rapidly. A hard green avocado ripens in two to five days in a paper bag. Short on time? Drop an apple or banana in the sack; both emit ethylene gas, a ripening agent that speeds up the process.

avocado nutrition by the numbers

90
calories per 2-ounce serving (about ¼ avocado)

9.5
grams of unsaturated fat

4
grams of fiber

BROCCOLI

The Slimming Story

If your mom ever demanded that you finish your broccoli ("before leav-ing the table!"), start channeling her persistence now. The so-called little green giant is a colossal boon for your belly-shrinking efforts, feeding you a considerable dose of vitamins and minerals and more antioxidants than most other common veggies, all for a scant 31 calories per chopped cup—not that you'll feel as if you're eating less. Broccoli is one of the foods lowest in energy density, meaning you can eat a lot of it without worry because the calorie count is so low relative to the volume. So pile it on! The low energy density, combined with its crunch-and-chew fac-tor, fills and satisfies you for only a few calories, helping you lose fat and bypass the hunger pangs that otherwise may come with dieting.

Broccoli's water content (nearly 90 percent!) helps make it low in energy density, and its fiber helps, too, by slowing digestion to keep in-sulin levels low. (When food breaks down quickly, insulin spikes, which can trigger the body to store excess fat.) Broccoli's fiber also demands extra chewing time, which downshifts eating from a sprint to a leisurely stroll; when you're taking your time, you can better detect those "I'm full" signals from your stomach and put down your fork earlier. Plus, by pulling food through your gastrointestinal tract, fiber reduces the amount of fat and number of calories you absorb from your meals.

You'll still take in plenty of the veggie's fat-burning vitamin C, how-ever. Broccoli touts more of the nutrient per ounce than an orange; a single cup contains 135 percent of your daily quota. Your body needs vitamin C to make carnitine, a compound that moves fat into cells to burn for energy. Low levels of the vitamin may stymie your ability to sizzle flab during exercise, but—thankfully—munching C-rich foods can turn things around. Now, go on, finish that broccoli!

→ **Trim-Down Tip:** As with any of the veggies in this chapter, choose fresh or frozen broccoli, depending on which version will get you to

eat more. If you go for frozen, however, check labels for extra sodium, fatty sauces, and other additives.

. . . .

The Amazing Proof

- In a study of 658 dieters, those who increased their intake
  of low-energy-dense produce by about three servings per day
  dropped the most weight—13 pounds on average—after six
  months, according to researchers from Pennsylvania State University in University Park. And get this: Even though people in
  that group took in 500 fewer calories per day, they actually increased the total volume of food they consumed by more than half
  a pound a day.
- When subjects ate a 3-cup, low-energy-dense salad prior to a big
  pasta lunch, a study in the *Journal of the American Dietetic Association* finds, they consumed nearly 100 fewer entrée calories than
  when they ate a salad half the size with the same number of calories (that is, with fewer veggies but more full-fat dressing and
  cheese).

. . . .

→ **Trim-Down Tip:** Whether at home or eating out, start with a
broccoli-loaded veggie plate or toss ½ cup of broccoli florets into an
appetizer salad (and go light on the dressing) to lower its energy
density; you'll take in fewer calories without feeling hungry.

. . . .

Four More Reasons to Eat Broccoli

1. *It could slash your cancer risk.* Cruciferous vegetables such as broccoli contain chemicals that turn on your body's natural detoxify-
   ing enzymes, helping you guard against cancer cells. Multiple
   studies link eating the crunchy veggie with a reduced risk for
   colorectal, lung, and stomach cancers.
2. *Broccoli keeps your heart healthy.* The green bunch is loaded with
   ticker-protecting nutrients, including folate (which lowers blood
   pressure) and antioxidants (which protect against oxidative dam-

> ## WANT TO EAT MORE BROCCOLI STARTING TODAY?
>
> Roast it! Cooking broccoli at a high temp caramelizes its natural sugars, turning it into an irresistibly crispy, tasty snack or side dish. Spread chopped florets on a baking pan, drizzle with 1 tablespoon olive oil (or spray with olive oil cooking spray), and roast at 450 degrees for 20 minutes.
>
> ## DON'T LIKE BROCCOLI?
>
> Puree a cup of raw broccoli (stalks and all), and mix with ground turkey when making turkey burgers or meatballs to give meals a superfood boost with little change to their flavor.

age from the rogue molecules known as "free radicals"). Broccoli also helps fight inflammation. Women who ate broccoli at least four times per month were nearly 50 percent less likely to die of coronary heart disease, a study published in the *American Journal of Epidemiology* reveals.

3. *Your skin may stay younger looking, too.* You need vitamin C for healthy collagen, which acts as skin's scaffolding, essentially propping up what you see in the mirror. The stronger and healthier your collagen is, the smoother your complexion. In fact, women who ate the most C-rich foods (broccoli is a top choice) were 11 percent less likely to have wrinkles than those who consumed fewer, according to a study in *The American Journal of Clinical Nutrition.*

4. *You'll be a vision of eye health.* Fill your plate with broccoli to take in loads of lutein and zeaxanthin, two carotenoids that protect eyes against UV damage that may lead to cataracts. The pigmented vitamins also act like a filter, helping to reduce glare.

The Broccoli Breakdown

Want to get the most out of your veggies? Follow these buying and cooking tips.

- Go green. When picking broccoli at the supermarket, choose the darkest green, most tightly packed bunches you can find. A richer color indicates a higher nutrient value, including more fat-fighting vitamin C.
- Stand firm. Another test of broccoli quality: the firmness of the stalk. Before buying, gently try to bend it; if it's rubbery or gives easily, move on to another.
- Get steamy. Don't like raw broccoli? Steam your stalks just long enough so the veggie is soft when pierced with a fork, but still firm and vivid in color, usually seven to ten minutes. Avoid boiling, as much of broccoli's healthy nutrient content will seep out into the hot water.
- Savor the stems. Yep, the stalks are slimming, too! After chopping the florets, julienne the stems and add to soup, salad, pasta, stir-fry, or pretty much anything else.

broccoli nutrition by the numbers

31

calories per cup of chopped broccoli

135

percent of your daily value of vitamin C

2

grams of fiber

EDAMAME

The Slimming Story

Ta-ta, tofu! Edamame (pronounced "ed-ah-MAH-may") is a better bet when it comes to the get-lean soybean. The lightly cooked, crunchy green soybeans, which you'll find either in or out of their pods, supply all the cholesterol-free protein of the standard soy staple (17 grams per cup), but you'll take in four times the stomach-filling fiber (8 grams) and two times the bloat-busting potassium!

Think of those three nutrients—protein, fiber, and potassium— as gold, silver, and bronze in the race to whittle your middle. Your body burns double the calories simply to digest protein, compared with carbs and fat. Protein is also the most satiating of all nutrients, helping to stamp out hunger for hours, and it keeps blood sugar and insulin levels steady, which discourages your body from storing extra calories as fat. What's more, you need protein to build and maintain lean muscle mass—and adding lean muscle is one secret to a speedy metabolism.

Like protein, fiber fills you up and regulates your body's insulin re-sponse after eating. It also prompts you to shed weight effortlessly by pushing some of the calories you eat out of your body before they turn into pounds. Potassium slims by grabbing hold of sodium and pulling it out of your body—so no puffy face or rounder belly.

Edamame has a few other tricks that may help make fat disappear. It's rich in choline, a compound that blocks fat absorption and breaks down fatty deposits; plus, it contains nutrients that animal studies sug-gest promote weight and fat loss. Although we need more research, we already know enough good stuff about the mod pods to give clear ad-vice: Start popping them, pronto!

→ **Trim-Down Tip:** Edamame beans are crisp and usually served with a sprinkling of salt. Sound like any other snack food you know? Next time you crave potato chips or pretzels, munch on slimming soybeans instead.

The Amazing Proof

- It's a fact that your body torches more calories digesting protein than it does processing carbs and fat, but researchers from the Federal University of Viçosa in Brazil discovered that study subjects burned about 70 more calories per day breaking down meals when they ate breakfasts containing soy protein, as opposed to when their a.m. meal contained other types of protein.
- Another study published in the *British Journal of Nutrition* indicates that the more plant protein you eat, the slimmer your waistline and the lower your body mass index (BMI), a measure of body fat.

→ **Trim-Down Tip:** You don't need to give up meat to ditch extra fat (steak is a superfood for weight loss, after all); simply eat plant protein a few times a week instead. For example, add ½ cup of shelled edamame to your salad in lieu of grilled chicken.

- Edamame is rich in both fiber and protein, two important nutrients for successful weight loss. (Quinoa, another superfood for weight

WANT TO EAT MORE EDAMAME STARTING TODAY?

Whip up a batch of edamame hummus using soybeans in place of chickpeas. Pair with crudités or serve with whole-grain pita. In a food processor, blend 1½ cups cooked, shelled edamame, 2 tablespoons tahini paste, 1 teaspoon lemon zest, the juice of 1 lemon, 1 crushed garlic clove, and 2 teaspoons olive oil. Add water if needed for a smoother consistency.

DON'T LIKE EDAMAME?

Puree equal amounts cooked edamame and either chickpeas or white beans to make a tasty sandwich spread. Smear 3 tablespoons of the mixture on a whole-wheat tortilla, top with 3 ounces grilled chicken, a dollop of salsa, and a few slices of avocado.

loss, supplies hearty amounts of both, too.) In one ten-week trial, according to a study from the University of Otago in Dunedin, New Zealand, people who followed a diet rich in protein (about 25 percent of their daily calories) and fiber (30 grams per day) lost about 2½ more pounds than those whose diet was lower in the two nutrients, even though they didn't consciously cut calories or diet. Even better, the high-protein, high-fiber group's weight loss was composed of 2 more pounds of fat and 1½ pounds more belly fat.

→ **Trim-Down Tip:** Headed out for sushi or noodles? You'll almost always find edamame on the menu. Make it a rule to order it as an appetizer instead of, say, fried tempura, dumplings, or fatty pork ribs.

EDA-WHAT?

Not familiar with this versatile form of soy? Here's the 411:

- What it is: *Edamame* is a Japanese word that roughly translates to "beans on branches." Although the same species as traditional grain soybeans, edamame are sometimes called vegetable soybeans because the seeds are bigger, sweeter, and eaten as a veggie.
- Where to buy it: You can find fresh edamame at farmers' markets, but the crop spoils in only a few days, so it's easier to grab the frozen bagged edamame stocked year-round at grocery stores.
- How to prepare it: Boil a small amount of water, place the pods in a steaming basket, and cook for 3 to 5 minutes. Sprinkle with sea salt and serve. If you buy frozen, preshelled, cooked edamame, set the beans out to thaw or steam them for a few minutes.
- When to eat it: Anytime! Edamame pods make a perfect snack; use your teeth to squeeze out the seeds and lick up the salt, then discard the pod. Or toss shelled edamame into salads, soups, pasta, stir-fries, scrambled eggs—anything!

A Note About Soy and Breast Cancer

For most women, eating edamame and other soy foods can benefit overall health, but researchers are still investigating soy and its phytoestrogens' exact relationship with breast cancer risk. Studies in the lab, for example, show that breast cancer cells proliferate when exposed to isolated soy compounds; yet in the body, dietary soy may reduce or not affect risk.

The good news: Research suggests that eating soy during childhood and adolescence actually lowers the chance of getting breast cancer later in life. Although women who start consuming soy as adults may not reduce their cancer risk, two to four servings per week is part of a healthy diet, and studies suggest that soy may reduce mortality from all causes. Breast cancer survivors or those with a family history of the disease who have not been eating soy regularly, however, may still want to consult their doctor before suddenly adding edamame to their diet.

Three More Reasons to Eat Edamame

1. *It's soy good for your heart.* If you trade protein sources high in saturated fat and cholesterol (such as fatty red meat) for edamame, you'll do your heart a favor; the beans' load of fiber, vitamins, minerals, phytonutrients, and ticker-friendly unsaturated fats may help control your cholesterol levels and reduce your risk for heart problems. Researchers from Yao Municipal Hospital in Osaka, Japan, also discovered that premenopausal women who consumed soy isoflavones daily showed reduced artery stiffness; plus, nonsmokers saw improved blood vessel dilation regardless of age.

2. *The beans are a boon for bones.* Eating edamame could protect you from bone loss and reduce your risk for fractures as you get older. Soy's isoflavones seem to jump-start cells responsible for forming bone and offset the loss of bone density that comes with age, especially after menopause.

3. *PMS won't be such a pain.* The phytoestrogens in edamame may help regulate estrogen and ease symptoms of PMS. Women who ate 30 grams of soy daily (a little over an ounce of edamame) had reductions in period-related breast tenderness, headaches, and cramps, a study in the *British Journal of Nutrition* reveals.

→ **Trim-Down Tip:** When a casserole or other recipe calls for peas, lima beans, or chickpeas, swap in shucked edamame to get more filling protein.

edamame nutrition

by the numbers

189
calories per cup of shelled beans

8
grams of fiber

17
grams of protein

19
percent of your daily recommended intake of potassium

KALE

The Slimming Story

All hail kale! The veggie is a king among leafy greens, thanks to all the weight-trimming power it wields. Chief among them is its status as a low-energy-dense food that satisfies you for few calories, so you can shed pounds without going hungry. That's right, the amount of food you eat seems to count more in filling you up than its calorie content does, so go ahead, load your plate with kale; a single cup of raw kale contains a mere 34 calories. Kale's hardiness—the amount you have to chew—adds to the sensation that you're eating a lot, which makes you less apt to over-indulge at the dinner table.

Kale also packs a trio of fat-obliterating nutrients in its ruffled leaves. Here's the breakdown:

Fiber: Because your body doesn't digest fiber, it takes longer to break down the leafy green and any food you eat with it. This process keeps your stomach full and blood sugar and insulin levels stable, which quells hunger and the craving for excess fat. You also absorb fewer calories from kale-containing meals because fiber packs up a portion of what you eat and ships it out, lickety-split.

Vitamin C: A single cup gives you an off-the-chart 134 percent of your daily intake of C, which triggers the production of carnitine, a compound that is necessary for your body to burn fat for fuel.

Flavonoids: Kale is chockablock with these health-promoting, anti-oxidant phytochemicals, including kaempferol. Lab research from the Harvard Medical School suggests that flavonoids increase calorie burning in cells and power up the gene responsible for activating the thyroid hormone, which plays an important role in your metabolism.

The Amazing Proof

- Researchers at Japan's National Institute of Health and Nutrition find that women whose diet consisted of heartier foods that re-

KALE: COOKING CHAMELEON

Cabbage's cousin is as versatile a veggie as they come—it tastes delicious any way you eat it. Before trying any of the following tips, thoroughly wash and dry the large leaves and remove them from their thick stems with a knife. Then slice the leaves into long ribbons or chop or tear into smaller pieces.

Raw: Use raw kale to make a healthy, slimming green smoothie. Blend 1 cup raw kale, 1½ cups soymilk, ¼ cup orange juice, ½ banana, 2½ tablespoons ground flaxseed, and 1 teaspoon vanilla extract. Other ideas: Swap it for lettuce on a sandwich, or eat it in a salad with cubed avocado, apple, pine nuts, and vinaigrette dressing.

Bake: If you love potato chips, get ready to meet a new favorite— kale chips! Chop the veggie into bite-size pieces, spread evenly on a cookie sheet, drizzle with olive oil, and sprinkle with sea salt. Bake at 350 degrees until crisp and slightly brown at the edges, 10 to 15 minutes.

Steam: Boil about 2 inches of water, then place kale in a steaming basket and cook 5 minutes. Remove and toss with sesame seeds, sesame oil, and fresh lemon juice. Or stir ½ cup steamed kale into a serving of whole-wheat boxed mac 'n' cheese.

Sauté or stir-fry: Heat a small amount of olive oil in a skillet, add chopped garlic, and cook for 1 to 2 minutes. Add kale; cook until slightly soft, 6 to 8 minutes. Or simply toss kale into the pan when following a stir-fry or sauté recipe. (Keep in mind that a huge amount of raw kale will cook down significantly—that is, like spinach, starting with several cups of the raw veggies may yield you only a cup or less.)

quire a lot of chewing—including leafy greens such as kale—had a slimmer waistline than those who filled their plate with softer fare.

- Eating flavonoid-containing fruits and veggies, such as kale, could put the brakes on weight creep. Women with the highest intake of the phytonutrients gained 58 percent less body mass over the course of fourteen years than those with the lowest intake, according to a study from Maastricht University in the Netherlands.

- Kale is bursting with the antioxidant beta-carotene and other carotenoids; a study in *The Journal of Nutrition* finds that people with the highest levels of carotenoids in their blood have a 45 percent lower risk for metabolic syndrome, a cluster of symptoms that includes a tubbier tummy. It's possible that the vitamins offer protection, although research is thus far inconclusive.

Four More Reasons to Eat Kale

1. *Kale and cancer don't mix.* Like broccoli, kale is a cruciferous vegetable and contains the same phytochemicals that ramp up your system's natural defenses against cancer cells. It's also rich in other potentially cancer-fighting antioxidant compounds, including glucosinolate and sulforaphane. People with a history of skin cancer who ate a daily serving of leafy greens (such as kale or spinach) reduced their risk of developing subsequent tumors by more than 50 percent, according to a study in *The International Journal of Cancer.*

→ **Take-Away Tip:** Sauté kale with mushrooms (another superfood for weight loss!) and garlic for a quick, cancer-fighting side dish. Sulforaphane, a main antioxidant in kale, is up to thirteen times more effective at fighting cancer-causing free radicals when eaten with the selenium in mushrooms.

2. *Your heart and peepers vote aye on kale.* Kale's multitude of antioxidant vitamins and phytochemicals may help reduce risk factors for heart disease. The veggie is also one of the top sources of lutein and zeaxanthin, two carotenoids your eyes rely on for protection against sun damage, cataracts, and glare.

3. *You'll help preserve skin's youthful glow.* Think of kale as a superfood for your skin, too. The leafy green is brimming with beauty-

WANT TO EAT MORE KALE STARTING TODAY?

Coarsely cut, raw kale is a welcome and easy addition to bean, lentil, and minestrone soups. Add ¼ cup of raw kale per cup of hot soup right before serving. Stir until kale is wilted.

DON'T LIKE KALE?

Sautéing kale helps mellow its peppery flavor. Try finely chopping the green, then sauté it lightly and mix into a casserole, lasagna, or stew.

full doses of wrinkle-fighting vitamin C and skin-smoothing beta-carotene (which your body converts to vitamin A). It also delivers iron, which blood cells use to carry oxygen to skin, helping increase its radiance.

4. *You'll maintain a youthful brain.* Older women who ate the most leafy green veggies showed a significantly slower rate of cognitive decline—on a par with women one to two years younger—than those who consumed the least, according to research in the *Annals of Neurology.*

You've Got Kale

Check out these quick tips for picking and storing the leafy green.

Know the different types. You'll typically find two different varieties: Curly kale has more rigid, ruffled leaves that curl inward; it's dark green with a thick, hard stem and has a stronger flavor. Tuscan kale, aka lacinato or dinosaur kale, has flat, textured leaves and may taste milder. You might want to try both to see which you prefer. Either way, you'll start slimming!

Find the best bunch. Before tossing kale into your basket, scope out its leaves and stems. A tasty bunch will be dark green and look crisp and firm. Skip over those that seem wilted or yellow. Also consider buying organic; kale is on the Environmental Working Group's "dirty dozen" list, as conventionally grown kale tends to hold on to more pesticides than other produce does.

Keep it fresh. Store kale in an open plastic bag in the crisper drawer of your refrigerator. Don't wait more than a few days to eat it; the longer kale sits, the more bitter it can become.

kale nutrition by the numbers

34
calories per cup of raw, chopped kale

134
percent of your daily value of vitamin C

1.3
grams of fiber

MUSHROOMS

The Slimming Story

Brightly colored veggies tend to steal the healthy-diet spotlight, but mushrooms are the dark horses. The veggies' blue-ribbon weight loss benefits lie in their dense and meaty texture, unique savory taste, and ridiculously low calorie content. Just how low are we talking? A cup of sliced button mushrooms, the most common type eaten in the United States, contains a barely-there 15 calories.

Mushrooms maintain such a low calorie profile partly because they're so high in water (92 percent H_2O!) and contain some fiber, both of which add lots of weight and volume to 'shrooms but little else. That means you can devour a linebacker's portion yet take in only a Lilliputian number of calories. Compare that with a high-energy-dense food such as French fries: A small serving feeds you tons of calories but leaves you hungry for more. Indeed, when it comes to feeling full, the quantity of food may count more than the calorie haul, and mushrooms effectively bulk up any meal.

The vegetable's unique texture and taste give it a slight edge over other low-energy-dense veggies, too. Mushrooms feel soft yet meaty and substantial as you chew—a bit different from other veggies—which may dupe your brain into thinking you're getting meat, something many of us equate with being well fed. Fungi also contain compounds that confer natural umami flavor, a savory taste that experts say may contribute to mushrooms' incredibly satiating quality.

The Amazing Proof

- When researchers at Johns Hopkins Bloomberg School of Public Health in Baltimore substituted chopped button mushrooms for beef in a prepared lunch and told study subjects to eat as much as they wanted, the testers consumed an incredible 444 fewer calories, yet they didn't feel hungrier or any less satisfied than after they ate the same dish with beef replacing the 'shrooms. Even better, they didn't gobble up hundreds of calories later in the day to compensate.

- The more water-rich foods (such as mushrooms) that women consumed as part of their diet, the more likely they were to have a lower BMI (a measure of body fat) and a slimmer waist than those who took in less, according to a study of 1,136 young women published in the journal *Nutrition*. Intake of water from beverages, on the other hand, didn't make a difference.

→ **Trim-Down Tip:** You can buy dried mushrooms for cooking, but the fresh ones contain water, making them lower in energy density and better able to fill you up.

Three More Reasons to Eat Mushrooms

1. *You'll boost your immunity.* Adding mushrooms to your regular diet may stimulate your immune system in a way that could help ward off infections. Animal studies indicate that good-for-you bacteria or nutrients within fungi's cell walls seem to strengthen the body's defenses against disease.

2. *Mushrooms could put a cap on cancer risk.* Their immune-strengthening properties may also help fend off cancer; plus, fungi are a top plant source of selenium, an antioxidant mineral that may protect against certain forms of cancer. Case in point: Women in China who ate less than a tablespoon of mushrooms daily had a 64 percent lower risk for breast cancer than those who didn't eat the spongy veggies, according to a study in the *International Journal of Cancer*.

3. *Fungi are fun foods for your heart and skin.* Lab studies conducted at Arizona State University in Mesa suggest compounds in mushrooms may make the lining of endothelial cells less sticky, which could help inhibit the plaque buildup that compromises blood flow and ups the chance of heart attack. Fungi also contain beta-glucan and chitin, two types of fiber that absorb fat and

MAKE ROOM FOR 'SHROOMS

No one type of mushroom is necessarily better for your waistline than another; all are similarly low in calories and highly tasty. Use this chart to learn about the most common varieties and to pick one that best suits your palate.

Mushroom Type	Flavor and Texture	In Case You Didn't Know	Calories per Chopped or Sliced Cup
Button or white	Mild and smooth, they can go with, in, or on pretty much anything. They're also one of only a few types you'd want to eat raw. (Cremini, enoki, and porto-bello are the others.)	Buttons are the type that usually show up on mush-room pizza; they make up more than 90 percent of the fungi consumed in the United States.	15
Chanterelle	Thanks to their somewhat tough texture, these delicate-tasting, spongy-capped 'shrooms may re-quire longer cook-ing than some of the other varieties.	Chanterelles are golden in color and shaped like a trum-pet, and you don't want to eat them raw—yuck!	20
Cremini, aka baby bella	They're similar to buttons but slightly stronger and earth-ier in flavor.	Creminis look like buttons but are a bit firmer and look more brown or beige.	19
Enoki	These beauties are mild-tasting and somewhat crunchy.	An enoki 'shroom is a cluster of slender, long stems tipped with small, button-shaped caps. Trim off an enoki's base before using.	29
Maitake, aka hen of the woods	They're notably strong, rich, and woodsy.	These capless, ruf-fled 'shrooms look more like flowers than fungi.	26

Oyster	Light and delicate-tasting, these have a velvety, somewhat chewy texture.	Shaped like a funnel, oysters may look gray, pale yellow, or brown.	37
Portobello	They're earthy and meaty.	You can grill and eat these burger-sized caps the way you would a meat patty. Try it—you'll save an incredible 177 calories and nearly 13 grams of fat. If you make the swap once per week, you could drop more than 2 pounds and save about 660 grams of fat in a year.	22
Shiitake	They're smaller than portobellos but have the same rich and meaty taste.	Ditch shiitake's stems; unlike the cap, they're tough and rubbery.	78 (cooked)

carry it out of the blood, lowering your risk for heart disease. You'll also take in niacin, a B vitamin that helps fight wrinkles and contributes to a healthy complexion.

Magic Mushrooms, Vitamin D, and Your Waistline

It sounds like something out of a sci-fi flick: Exposing mushrooms to ultraviolet-B light (the same type of rays that can give you a sunburn) causes the veggies' usually scant vitamin D content to skyrocket. What's more, researchers from University Medical Center Freiburg in Germany discovered that eating the irradiated 'shrooms can boost levels of vitamin D as much as taking a supplement containing the same amount of the vitamin.

That's exciting news, considering that up to 77 percent of Americans

WANT TO EAT MORE MUSHROOMS
STARTING TODAY?

Instead of meat, make 'shrooms the mainstay of a meal or dish. Swap a ground beef burger patty for a grilled portobello cap. Or slice the large mushroom and stir-fry it with other veggies instead of chicken. Chopped mushrooms can also mimic meat in pasta sauce, lasagna, and casseroles.

DON'T LIKE MUSHROOMS?

Bury them in a tasty turkey meat loaf; finely chopped mushrooms will get lost amid the ground turkey, onions, and other ingredients. Try the Vegetable Meat Loaf on page 282.

may not have beneficial levels of vitamin D in their blood. Aside from promoting healthy bones and a strong immune system and potentially reducing your risk for heart disease and other illnesses, such as cancer, higher levels of D may make it easier for you to lose fat. Not all mushroom packagers are setting their fungi under sunlamps just yet, but there are a few, including Dole and Monterey Mushrooms, that sell mushrooms with 100 percent of your daily D quota per serving. Check out nutrition labels to see if your mushrooms contain extra D.

→ **Trim-Down Tip:** Feeling bloated? Lunch on a portobello burger, or chop one up and toss with a salad. The coaster-size caps are high in sodium-sacking potassium.

Selecting and Storing Mushrooms

At the store: Regardless of type, mushrooms should be firm, smooth, and without slimy areas.

At home: Keep fungi in their original plastic packaging or in a paper bag in the refrigerator; they'll last about a week. Avoid airtight containers, which may allow moisture to build up, spoiling them fast. Also, don't soak mushrooms; rinse or wipe them with a damp cloth before using to preserve their flavor.

mushroom nutrition by

the numbers

15

calories per cup of sliced white 'shrooms,
the most common type

92

percent of water in most types of mushrooms, which
helps make them filling

9

percent of daily intake of bloat-ridding potassium per
1 portobello cap

1

gram of fiber

SWEET POTATOES

The Slimming Story

How sweet it is! Adding these orange veggies to your plate helps subtract pounds from the scale. The first thing a sweet potato has going for it: about 4 grams of fat-fighting fiber, which slows digestion, staves off hunger, and helps move food through the digestive track so you end up absorbing fewer of the calories you eat. Fiber also helps prevent the spikes in blood glucose and insulin that can lead to the production of fat. Yep, even though it's called a sweet potato, eating the spud won't cause blood sugar to rise as much as its white cousin does.

Sweet potatoes also contain resistant-starch carbohydrates, which are similar to fiber in that they don't flood your blood with glucose the way other starches do; instead, they may actually increase fat burning—research shows that RS encourages cells to oxidize fat and increase energy expenditure. It also helps boost satiety, so you feel fuller on fewer calories. (Want to know more about this magic "skinny" carb? Turn to page 70.)

Eat one medium-size spud and you take in 37 percent of your day's quota of vitamin C (which may also help rev up fat burning—you need vitamin C to make carnitine, a compound that transports fat into cell furnaces), as well as 15 percent of your bloat-fighting potassium needs. In addition, sweet potatoes contain significant doses of several other health-promoting vitamins and nutrients, all for around 100 calories per spud. Bottom line: This veggie is one hot potato for dieters.

→ **Trim-Down Tip:** Sweet potato mash is the perfect skinny side dish. Avoid boiling your spuds, though; it can cause them to lose some of their nutritional punch. Instead, bake or steam the potatoes, and keep the skin on—you'll take in 1 or more grams of fiber and more nutrients.

The Amazing Proof

- Research repeatedly finds that people lose more weight on high-fiber diets than they do on low-fiber regimes. And when researchers at Tufts University reviewed several of the studies, the results were eye-opening: In the trials in which subjects could eat as much as they wanted as long as they met their fiber requirements, increasing fiber intake by 14 grams per day led people to consume about 10 percent fewer calories and lose an average of more than 4 pounds in about four months. What's more, in studies of low-calorie diets, fiber reduced hunger.

- After eating both a breakfast and a lunch containing resistant starch, study subjects consumed about 10 percent fewer calories over the next twenty-four hours compared with when they ate similar meals with a placebo, according to research from the University of Surrey in England. Following the RS meals, testers' insulin levels were also lower.

Four More Reasons to Eat Sweet Potatoes

1. *They're nutrition all-stars.* Sweet potatoes may be relatively inexpensive, but they're seriously loaded when it comes to nutrients you need to stay healthy. Sweet potatoes are so rich, in fact, that the Center for Science in the Public Interest's *Nutrition Action Healthletter* named them the number one healthiest food. (Plain Greek yogurt, broccoli, wild salmon, and leafy greens such as kale are the other superfoods for weight loss that cracked the top ten.)

2. *Sweet spuds are heart studs.* One potato packs more antioxidant beta-carotene than nearly any other fruit or vegetable. It hooks up with lipoproteins in the blood, where it helps prevent damage that can lead to clogged arteries. Studies show that regularly eating foods rich in beta-carotene help safeguard your ticker.

3. *You could cut your chances of getting cancer.* Researchers from Harvard University found that premenopausal women who consumed the most beta-carotene from food (sweet potatoes are

WANT TO EAT MORE SWEET POTATOES STARTING TODAY?

Homemade baked sweet potato fries are a giant, fat-fighting step above the white-potato fries you find in the freezer section of the market. To make, scrub a whole sweet potato and cut into French fry–size pieces. Spread on a baking sheet, drizzle with olive oil, sprinkle on your favorite spices (try garlic powder, dill, cayenne), and bake at 400 degrees for about 20 minutes.

DON'T LIKE SWEET POTATOES?

Homemade muffins and quick breads are the perfect hiding spot for mashed or canned sweet potatoes, and—bonus!—they'll bestow a supermoist texture.

tops) had the lowest risk for breast cancer. (For those with a family history of the disease, the risk was even lower.) A diet rich in vitamin C–filled fruits and veggies may reduce the likelihood of oral, esophageal, pancreatic, and colon cancers, too.

4. *Your skin will thank you every time you look in the mirror.* In skin, sweet potatoes' beta-carotene converts to vitamin A, which encourages the cell turnover that keeps your complexion smooth and clear. Carotenoids may also decrease skin's sensitivity to the sun—another plus for warding off wrinkles.

You Say Potato, I Say—Yam?

What's the difference between a sweet potato and a yam? Not much, if you're talking about what your local supermarket sells—both will help you drop pounds. In the United States, orange root vegetables called yams or yam sweet potatoes are actually a variety of sweet potato that may have a softer, moister consistency after cooking. True yams are a different species altogether; native to Africa and Asia, they're much bigger, starchier roots with rough skin and white flesh.

The Four S's of Buying and Keeping Sweet Potatoes

- Skin: Look for a smooth, clean, deep orange outer jacket. If there's a bruise or sprouted spot, move on; even if you cut away a damaged part, the potato may still have an off taste.
- Shape: Plump sweet potatoes that are evenly shaped tend to taste the best.
- Size: Counting calories? A medium-size potato is about 5 inches long and 2 inches in diameter and weighs in at 103 calories.
- Storage: Keep sweet potatoes in a cool, dry spot in your kitchen or pantry. Avoid the fridge, where they develop a hardened core.

→ **Trim-Down Tip:** Fresh sweet potatoes have the most fiber, thanks to their skin, but they aren't your only option. Canned versions make a filling, nutritious addition to soups, purees, muffins, and other dishes. Look for brands that contain only potatoes—no added sugar, salt, butter, or anything else.

sweet potato nutrition by the numbers

103
calories per medium baked sweet potato

438
percent of your daily value of vitamin A/beta-carotene per medium-size spud

37
percent of your daily value of vitamin C

15
percent of bloat-fighting potassium

4
grams of fiber

drop 10 inspiration

"I worked out less and lost weight!"

NAME: Rachel Roberts

AGE: 30

OCCUPATION: Second-grade teacher

FAMILY STATUS: Single

HEIGHT: 5 feet 6 inches

STARTING WEIGHT: 172

DROP 10 WEIGHT: 162

LOST: 10 pounds in five weeks

My story: "I gained about 100 pounds in college, and I was very unhappy. I'm an emotional eater and used food to comfort me. When I graduated, I started eating healthier and working out—and lost 90 pounds. I've kept it off for five years but was stuck at that weight. One of my major motivators to lose was my mother: She has diabetes and kidney disease. Watching her live with these life-threatening illnesses made me determined to change my lifestyle so I wouldn't face the same struggles."

Biggest challenge to losing weight: "Feeling starved all the time. I'd just reach for fast food."

Why Drop 10 clicked: "The first week helped me see how important it is to eat only when I feel hungry and not because I am bored or feeling down. And this diet taught me to plan healthy meals. I scanned the meal options in advance and highlighted the ones I wanted to try each week; over the weekend, I would prepare all my lunches and dinners. And the balance of carbs, protein, and fiber in these foods helped me feel fuller longer, so I didn't have hunger pangs."

How my body changed: "Aside from looking more toned, the biggest change is that I don't feel hungry in the morning. I used to always wake up starving."

Success tip: "I realized that when I am eating the right foods, I can cut my time in the gym. I used to try to work off the extra fries or a fast-food meal I'd eaten. It's nice to see that I can lose weight without all the work. I'm not going to stop now!"

4   Super Legumes and Grains

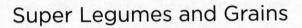

LENTILS

The Slimming Story

Compared with other diet-friendly legumes, lentils have a slimmer shape and smaller size that hint at their fat-trimming edge. Lentils contain more tummy-flattening fiber than almost any other food the USDA has analyzed: an extraordinary 16 grams per cooked cup. That keeps your stomach full and hunger at bay for hours; plus, it helps cut the amount of fat and number of calories you absorb from meals. Lentils' sky-high fiber content also directs your body to dole out glucose a little at a time, providing you with fuel for the slow, steady burn that will help you lose weight; quick-digesting carbs (such as cookies), on the other hand, flood your system with glucose and cause sharp spikes in insulin that may mess with your metabolism over time and cue your body to store fat.

Lentils are also rich in resistant starch, a type of carbohydrate that may encourage fat burning and shrink fat cells. (To learn more, turn to page 70.) Meanwhile, you'll torch extra calories simply digesting lentils' protein, which also provides the raw material needed to build metabolism-stoking muscle.

QUICK COOKING TIPS

Lentil novice? Follow these tricks and lentil prep will be a snap.

- Skip the soak. Unlike other dried legumes, you don't need to soak lentils before cooking. Discard any damaged or shriveled lentils, then rinse under cool water to remove dust or other debris.
- Boil and simmer. For the best water-to-lentil ratio, follow the directions on the package. Then bring the mixture to a boil, reduce heat, and simmer 15 to 25 minutes.
- Add some salt. Sprinkling $1/4$ teaspoon salt into the water before it boils helps lentils better retain their shape.
- Taste test. Because different types of lentils have different cooking times—and the older your lentils, the slower they cook—taste frequently after about fifteen minutes until you get the texture you want. When it's just right, drain the water and enjoy!

➡ **Trim-Down Tip:** If you'd rather not hassle with cooking lentils, some stores now stock precooked, ready-to-eat versions in the refrigerated section near the vegetables.

The Amazing Proof

- People who ate a balanced meal containing 5 grams of resistant starch—about what you get from ¾ cup cooked lentils—burned 23 percent more fat over twenty-four hours than when they tucked into a meal with no resistant starch, researchers at the University of Colorado in Denver find.
- After eight weeks, dieters who ate lentils and other legumes four times per week lost 54 percent more weight than those who followed a similar low-cal meal plan without the fiber-rich foods, according to a study from the University of Navarra in Pamplona, Spain.

- Overweight subjects who swapped out refined bread and cereal for two servings of lentils or other legumes per day (and consumed four servings of whole grains daily) lost nearly 14 pounds after six months and dropped more total belly fat after eighteen months than subjects who followed a low-cal diet with more refined-grain bread and cereal, a study from the *Journal of the American College of Nutrition* reports.

Four More Reasons to Eat Lentils

1. *Legumes keep your heart healthy.* A serving of lentils has loads of soluble fiber, which ferries cholesterol out of your body, plus significant amounts of folate and magnesium, two nutrients that promote healthy heart functioning. In the weight loss study from the University of Navarra mentioned on the previous page, the legume group also saw improvements in cholesterol and other factors that contribute to cardiovascular problems.

2. *A lentil-rich diet could protect you from diabetes and certain cancers.* Fiber and other compounds in legumes may play a role in warding off colon and breast cancers, as well as blood sugar problems. For example, eating roughly 1 cup of legumes a week reduces the risk of developing diabetes by as much as 40 percent, according to research from Vanderbilt University in Nashville, Tennessee.

3. *Eating lentils helps you look and feel energized.* Lentils are a top plant source of iron, which your red blood cells use to transport revitalizing oxygen to organs and tissues, including your skin. (Fatigue and a pale complexion can signal that you need to up your intake.) Pair lentils with vitamin C–rich broccoli or kale: C helps your body absorb more iron from plants.

4. *Choose lentils for a healthy digestive system.* Lentils contain a hefty dose of resistant starch. Aside from its slimming abilities, RS may act as a prebiotic, helping to feed the healthy bacteria in your intestines, which helps keep your system running smoothly.

WANT TO EAT MORE LENTILS STARTING TODAY?

Instead of a beef burger or cold-cut sandwich, lunch on a lentil burger. (See recipe on page 282.) You can make a large batch of the patties and freeze the extras to have on hand for a quick meal. When they're frozen, simply nuke for one to two minutes until warm, then serve on a whole-wheat bun piled high with veggies (try tomato, onion, avocado, and kale) and your favorite condiments.

DON'T LIKE LENTILS?

Puree $1/2$ cup cooked lentils and stir into a serving of mashed potatoes or sweet potatoes, pasta sauce, or homemade or canned soup.

The Lentil Rainbow

Lentils are sold dry and come in an array of colors including brown, red, and green. All are high in fiber, resistant starch, and protein, and they all taste similar and are incredibly versatile. The only significant difference: postcooking texture. Here's what to expect:

Brown: Easy to find and inexpensive, brown lentils stay firm and hold their shape pretty well if cooked for about twenty minutes. They will, however, get softer, even slightly mushy, the longer they're on the stove.

Best for: Anything! Add them cooked to green salads, soup, or chili, or make this simple, slimming side dish: Toss lentils with grilled veggies and a small amount of olive oil and Dijon mustard.

Red: The name is a little deceiving—these lentils actually look salmon pink or orange in the bag, then turn gold or yellow after cooking. Nonetheless, they cook more quickly than other types (in twelve to fifteen minutes) and lose their shape easily. That's not necessarily a bad thing, depending on what you're making.

Best for: Lentil soup or thickening other hearty soups and stews, or a fiber-rich puree as a side dish.

Green: Sometimes called French green lentils, these legumes tend to hold their shape better than the other varieties and typically turn brown during cooking.

Best for: Salads and side dishes, as they don't turn mushy when cooked.

lentil nutrition
by the numbers

230
calories per cup of cooked lentils

18
grams of protein

16
grams of fiber

7
milligrams of iron
(about 40 percent of your daily quota)

OATS .

The Slimming Story

That old saying "feeling your oats" is a lot more literal than you think. Oatmeal is one of the most satiating foods you can eat; have a bowl and it will stick with you, keeping your belly full with slimming, fiber-rich whole grains for hours. A 1-cup serving contains 4 grams of fiber, including an especially filling form called beta-glucan. Not only does oatmeal take its time digesting and promotes satiety, but research suggests its beta-glucan may trigger the release of appetite-controlling hormones. In other words, spoon up a bowl for breakfast and you'll be able to breeze right past that plate of doughnuts at your ten a.m. meeting.

Adding oatmeal to your diet gives you all the other benefits of fiber, too. You'll absorb fewer calories from the food you eat, and because your body digests oatmeal slowly, it prevents the rush of glucose and the corresponding insulin spike you get from many other carbs that can result in excess fat. Plus, fiber from oats may increase sensitivity to insulin and help fight inflammation, which could help prevent belly-fattening metabolic syndrome. Bet your cornflakes can't do all that!

→ **Trim-Down Tip:** Oatmeal isn't just for breakfast. At 83 calories per half-cup serving, it makes a tasty, filling afternoon snack. Add a dollop of fat-free yogurt and a few nuts or pumpkin seeds for an extra hit of protein and healthy monounsaturated fat.

The Amazing Proof

- Dieters who ate 3 cups per day of a whole-grain oat cereal saw a 43 percent greater reduction in waist size, indicating less belly fat, after twelve weeks than people following a similar low-cal diet who consumed corn cereal and other refined grains instead, according to a study in the *Journal of the American Dietetic Association*.
- Researchers from Maastricht University found that for every ad-

ditional gram of whole grains women consumed, the risk of being obese dropped by 4 percent—impressive, considering there's about 16 grams of whole grains in a half-cup serving of oatmeal.

Four More Reasons to Eat Oats

1. *Their heart-healthy benefits are undeniable.* The evidence of oatmeal's protection against heart disease is so convincing that products made with whole-grain oats were given permission by the FDA back in 1997 to make heart-healthy claims on packaging. The benefits aren't necessarily all fiber's doing, however; oats are also rich in unique antioxidants called avenanthramides, which also protect arteries against atherosclerosis.

→ **Take-Away Tip:** Top oatmeal with other superfoods for weight loss—vitamin C–rich fruit such as kiwi and some vitamin E–packed peanuts. Research from Tufts University suggests that oatmeal's avenanthramides work better at protecting against damage that can lead to heart problems when paired with the vitamins.

2. *Oats help your immune system do its job.* The next time you've got a cold, skip the chicken soup and try oatmeal. The soluble fiber in oats and other foods boosts your levels of a healing protein. Mice fed soluble fiber recovered faster from an infection and had fewer symptoms than those getting insoluble fiber, according to researchers from the University of Illinois at Urbana-Champaign. Oats may also help protect you from certain cancers, including pancreatic cancer.

3. *Your risk for diabetes could plummet.* Women who consumed two servings of whole grains daily were 21 percent less likely to develop type 2 diabetes, according to researchers at Harvard University. Oats, like other whole grains, are rich in magnesium, a mineral essential to sugar metabolism, as well as other nutrients that may play a role.

4. *Oatmeal provides spoonfuls of serenity.* Feeling stressed? The B vitamins you'll take in from oatmeal help stimulate the production

of serotonin, a key neurotransmitter that tells your brain to chill out. And because your body digests oatmeal slowly, you get a steady dose of the relaxing nutrients.

Know Your Oats

Any way you eat 'em, oats are a waist-trimming whole grain. They're not all created equal, however. Here's a guide to what you'll find on store shelves:

Good: Instant oats. Rolled superthin, this version cooks in a flash—you need only add hot water and stir. You can't beat the convenience, but because they go through an extra step of processing, instant oats may not contain as many healthy nutrients or as much fiber.

→ **Trim-Down Tip:** Flavored instant oatmeal can contain loads of diet-busting sugar; avoid those that list sugar as an ingredient and instead add your own hint of sweet from fruit, 100 percent maple syrup, or honey.

Better: Old-fashioned oats. Although still rolled flat, these oats may hang on to more nutrients and fiber than instant does, and they take only about five minutes to prepare. If you like your oatmeal on the chewier

WANT TO EAT MORE OATS STARTING TODAY?

Oatmeal isn't the only way to get your oats: Whip up a batch of homemade granola (see page 261 for recipe), and store in an airtight container at room temperature for up to two weeks. Pair with low-fat milk, top with yogurt or low-fat ice cream, or snack on it plain.

DON'T LIKE OATMEAL?

Swap equal amounts of raw oats for bread crumbs in turkey meat loaf or meatball recipes. We've got one you'll love on page 285.

side, boil water first, then add the oats. For a creamier consistency, combine oats and water, then bring to a boil.

Best: Steel-cut oats. Also known as Scotch oats or Irish oatmeal, these oats are cut into small pieces rather than rolled. Minimally processed, they have a heartier texture and nuttier taste but take longer to cook—about thirty minutes on the stove or ten minutes in the microwave. You can also prepare them in a slow cooker. Check out the instructions below.

Wake Up to Middle-Whittling Steel-Cut Oatmeal

Don't let a hectic morning schedule come between you and a fat-fighting breakfast or snack. Before going to bed, combine 1 cup steel-cut oats, 4 cups water, and ½ cup skim milk in your slow cooker. Cover and cook on low for 6 to 7 hours. When you wake, breakfast will be waiting! Simply top with your favorite fruit and nuts. (This amount nets four ¾- to 1-cup servings; store the extras in the fridge and eat them all week—simply nuke for 2 to 3 minutes.)

oatmeal nutrition by the numbers

166
calories per cup of cooked oatmeal, regular or instant

4
grams of fiber

6
grams of protein

WHOLE GRAINS: SUPERCARBS FOR SUPER SLIMMING

The low-carb craze is, thankfully, behind us, but there are two things about the philosophy worth remembering: Refined, highly processed carbs such as squishy white bread could make you squishy, too, and eliminating them from your diet is one of the easiest ways to jump-start weight loss. What low-carb diets didn't seem to get (and one reason they ultimately fail) is that whole grains (like the foods in this chapter) are extremely healthy, make dieting easier, and can help you shed weight and keep it off.

Think of whole grains as supercarbs. As their name implies, they contain the grain's entire seed: the outer bran coating, the inner germ, and the starchy endosperm. Most of a grain's fiber lives in the bran; the germ holds some protein and a small amount of healthy fats; and both parts are rich in vitamins, minerals, and disease-fighting phytochemicals. Refined grains are stripped of all that good stuff, leaving behind mostly the quick-digesting starch. That's why whole grains take a lot longer to digest. And instead of rushing a gusher of glucose into your blood all at once, causing a fat-promoting spike and a drop in insulin, your body gets a little bit of glucose at a time. That keeps insulin levels steady, which encourages the breakdown and burning of fat rather than fat storage. Plus, you feel full, satiated, and craving-free.

Whole grains' slow release of glucose and steadying effects on insulin place them lower on the glycemic index (or GI, a measure of a food's effect on blood sugar) than most refined carbs. Aside from preventing fat storage, low-GI carbs may also steer your body to burn more fat. Women who ate low-GI carbs torched 55 percent more fat during exercise than those who ate high-GI carbs, according to a study in *The Journal of Nutrition*.

It's worth knowing what GI means, but you needn't bother tracking down and monitoring the GI ratings of different foods. If you start eating more fiber-rich, whole-grain items such as the superfoods for weight loss in this chapter, and other whole-grain carbs, you'll be doing great: Research suggests that swapping refined grains for whole-grain foods could help you lose fat around the middle and that people who eat two to three servings of whole grains a day are lighter and have a trimmer waistline than those who consume less. Experts haven't put the puzzle pieces together yet, but they think whole grains' positive effects on blood glucose and insulin levels, as well as on inflammation, may play a role. (To read more about fiber's superpowers, turn to page 38.) By helping to steady insulin levels, whole grains may also help you feel less hungry and potentially curb cravings.

Three servings of whole grains per day is the least amount to aim for, but eating mostly whole-grain carbs instead of refined carbs could lead to even better results on the scale. Here's what counts as a serving:

- ½ cup cooked oatmeal, whole-grain pasta, quinoa, or other whole grain (see the full list below), or 1 ounce dry (if you measure before preparing)
- 1 slice 100 percent whole-grain bread
- 1 cup 100 percent whole-grain, ready-to-eat cereal
- 3 cups popcorn

Hunting for Whole Grains? Arm Yourself with These Tips

- Know your wholes. The following foods and ingredients are all whole grains: oats and oatmeal, popcorn, quinoa, and whole-wheat and whole-grain pasta—the four whole-grain superfoods for weight loss—plus amaranth, barley, brown and wild rice, buckwheat, bulgur wheat, millet, spelt, wheat berries, and whole-wheat flour.
- Be a label sleuth. Finding 100 percent whole-grain prepared foods such as bread, crackers, and ready-to-eat cereal can be tricky. Manufacturers stamp packages with phrases like "made with whole grains" or "an excellent source of whole grains"

and terms such as "multigrain"—which can make products sound healthier than they are. The only way to know you're getting a 100 percent whole-grain food is if it says exactly that on the packaging or if all the grains or flours listed as ingredients are either whole grains themselves (such as oats and quinoa) or contain the word *whole* in front of their name (for example, whole-wheat flour). Enriched wheat and semolina flours, for example, are refined.

- Pay attention to whole-grain grams. Eating 100 percent whole-grain foods benefits your waistline most, but if you choose a product made partially of whole grains, the more grams you get the better. There are 16 grams of whole grains in a serving, so a food boasting, say, 5 grams isn't doing you much good.
- Look for the yellow stamp from the Whole Grains Council. You'll find two versions of the voluntary label: one for foods made with 100 percent whole grains and one for foods that contain at least a half serving (8 grams) of whole grains.

POPCORN

The Slimming Story

Pop go extra pounds! Despite the diet-busting company popcorn keeps—chips, cheese curls, and the like—it's an angel among snack foods. Unlike its counterparts, popcorn is a bona fide whole grain, contains no saturated fat (when air-popped), and delivers a gram of fiber per cup. Not that you need to limit yourself to just one—a single cup contains a mere 31 calories. You can guiltlessly have 2 cups; go for a third and you've got an entire serving of whole grains and 3 grams of fiber under your belt for under 100 calories.

And you'll be tightening that belt in no time if you snack on popcorn regularly. Fiber fills you up and slows the digestion of starch, keeping insulin levels low, which silences hunger and discourages fat storage. Eating plenty of fiber also means you absorb fewer calories and fat from the food you eat, while popcorn's resistant starch could turn up your body's fat-burning furnace. (To read more about resistant starch, check out page 70.)

All whole grains benefit your waistline in a similar way, but popcorn has something else going for it that most others don't: air. It sounds far-fetched, but there's a kernel of truth to the idea that you can fill up on air, at least in popcorn's case. Just as low-energy-dense fruits and veggies count on water and fiber to add calorie-free and filling weight, popcorn derives similar benefits from air. You get to eat a large portion, which helps you feel fuller, yet it all tallies up to a minor blip in your day's calorie haul.

→ **Trim-Down Tip:** Although air-popped popcorn is lowest in calories and fat, the oil-popped version, which clocks in at a still diet-friendly 55 calories per cup, isn't off-limits. Use olive oil, another superfood for weight loss, instead of vegetable oil to prepare it.

The Amazing Proof

- Three cups of popcorn is equal to about an ounce, or 1 serving, of whole grains, and eating the kernels will put you well on your way to a skinnier middle. Dieters who ate five servings of whole grains a day lost more stomach fat than those who merely cut calories and ate refined grains, a study in *The American Journal of Clinical Nutrition* reveals.
- Study subjects who were told to eat as much as they liked of two similar snack foods—one more aerated than the other—consumed 70 fewer calories on the days they were given the puffed-up snack yet took in a portion that was 70 percent larger by volume, report researchers at Pennsylvania State University in University Park.

➡ **Trim-Down Tip:** No air popper? No problem! Place ¼ cup kernels in a paper bag, fold the top over a few times for a loose seal, then microwave for 2 to 3 minutes.

Three More Reasons to Eat Popcorn

1. *It's one of the best things you can do for your heart.* Numerous studies using data from hundreds of thousands of people show that eating whole grains is associated with heart health in all sorts of good ways, including improved blood pressure, cholesterol, and markers of inflammation.
2. *Popcorn is an anticancer, antidiabetes snack.* Women who ate 4½ servings of whole grains a day slashed their risk for colon cancer by 35 percent, researchers in Sweden found. A diet rich in whole grains has also been linked to a lower risk for breast and pancreatic cancers, as well as diabetes.
3. *Popcorn helps zap zits.* Swapping chips and other processed snacks for whole grains like popcorn may help lessen acne. When people cut refined carbs from their diet and instead ate more high-fiber grains, they had half as many pimples after twelve weeks, reports a study in *The American Journal of Clinical Nutrition*.

The Corny Awards

Movies have the Oscars, TV has the Emmys, now meet the best of the best in popcorn:

- Best cooking method: air popping. It's fast and easy, and it requires no oil, which makes it a fat-free snack. Buying a bag of kernels is also significantly cheaper than a box of microwavable corn.

  Runner-up: microwave. If you're willing to pay for convenience, go for it. Not all boxes are equally slimming, however. Choose those with the fewest grams of total fat and sodium. Three cups of a 94 percent fat-free version have only 114 calories, for example. You might also like the new portion-controlled, 100-calorie bags. Just avoid terms like "butter," which is usually synonymous with fattening.

- Best topping: extra-virgin olive oil. Pour this superfood for weight loss into a stainless-steel spray bottle and mist—two pumps adds only about 40 calories and tons of slimming benefits. (Read all about it, starting on page 140.) Sprinkle other spices and flavorings such as garlic and cayenne as well; the oil helps them cling better to your corn.

  Runner-up: buttery spray. When you crave a buttery flavor, this fine mist controls calories and coats your snack evenly. Look for brands that have zero saturated fat, are made with natural ingredients, and are low in sodium. Our favorite: Smart Balance Buttery Burst.

SKIP THE FAT, KEEP THE FLAVOR

Don't get stuck in a butter rut; popcorn pairs well with tons of different flavors. Be creative! Try sprinkling on garlic, onion, curry powder, cayenne pepper, or any other favorite spice. (If you decide to oil-pop, season the oil first.) Or, if you're in the mood for a sweet rather than savory snack, melt an ounce of dark chocolate (another superfood for weight loss!) and drizzle it over your bowl.

- Best serving container: a small bag. Researchers at Cornell University find that people ate significantly more popcorn when it was served in a large container versus a medium one—even when they were given stale corn! If you make a large amount, store it in individual bags of 3-cup servings.

  Runner-up: a small bowl. Doling out a 3-cup portion will help ensure you don't overdo it. Leave some popcorn for tomorrow's snack.

Popcorn at the Theater

Ahhh, the magic of the movies . . . where popcorn can go from fat-fighting snack to fat-making foe faster than you can say supercombo. Good news, though: You can indulge without disaster. Before bellying up to the concessions bar, remember these ordering tricks:

- Do more than downsize. You're right to think that a small bucket is better than a large one. After all, movie corn isn't that high in

WANT TO EAT MORE POPCORN STARTING TODAY?

Trade in fatty chips or pretzels for popcorn, and upgrade your kernels with the superfood power of Parmesan cheese. Lightly mist popcorn with olive oil or buttery spray, and sprinkle on 2 tablespoons of finely grated Parmesan.

DON'T LIKE POPCORN?

If you'd rather not eat your kernels popped, munch on regular corn. Whether fresh (on the cob or off), frozen, or canned, it contains fiber and resistant starch, providing healthy, slimming benefits. If you go for canned or frozen, choose varieties without sauce and added salt. Keep in mind that, cup for cup, regular corn is higher in calories than popped corn, although it is on a par with other grains—143 for a cup (or 99 for a medium-size ear).

calories; a cup without butter runs between 52 and 61 calories, according to an analysis by the Center for Science in the Public Interest. The problem is that your "small" size can mean 6, 8, or even 11 cups, depending on the theater. If you eat the whole thing, that's up to 670 calories! A better plan: Split a small with a friend and put three or four large fistfuls (each is about ½ cup) into an empty soda cup to help you limit mindless munching.

- BYOB (bring your own butter). Who says you can't stash butter spray or other flavorings in your purse? Sprinkling your own is less embarrassing when you consider that 1 tablespoon of movie theater topping adds about 130 calories, and even less so when you picture how much topping you might actually get if you ask for butter. (Last time we saw a flick, it seemed like a heck of a lot more than 1 tablespoon.)

popcorn nutrition by the numbers

31
calories per cup of plain, air-popped corn

1
gram of fiber

1
gram of protein

1
gram of fat

QUINOA

The Slimming Story

Go with this grain, pronounced "KEEN-wah," and you'll see just how smooth the path to your dream body can be. Soft and fluffy like rice but with an extraordinary nutrient profile, quinoa is a hunger-curbing, fat-foiling heavyweight. One cup cooked contains 8 grams of protein, more than any other commonly consumed grain. Plus, unlike its carb cohort, it's a complete protein, delivering all the essential amino acids for fewer calories and less fat than animal sources, the only other foods that can make the same claim. Protein, the most satiating of all nutrients, fills your belly to prevent overeating; it simultaneously chips away at your weight, because it burns through more calories during digestion than carbs and fat do. You also need plenty of protein to build and maintain the lean muscle that gives your metabolism a slenderizing kick.

Quinoa's protein, along with its hefty helping of fiber (5 grams per cup), helps your body digest it slowly, which keeps blood sugar and insulin levels steady, averting the spikes that can throw off metabolism and may lead to extra fat over time. But fiber is a star in its own right. In addition to filling you up, it can reduce the number of total calories you absorb from meals. Protein and fiber aside, quinoa also contains significant doses of multiple vitamins and minerals, including energizing iron.

The Amazing Proof

- In a study of middle-aged adults, those who ate the most whole grains (about three servings per day) had a significantly smaller

GOING GLUTEN-FREE?

Quinoa is a saving grace for those with celiac disease or gluten sensitivity. You can cook and eat the grain itself (which is actually a seed) or look for bread and pasta made out of quinoa.

. . . .
QUINOA Q&A
. . . .

Although quinoa is often referred to as an ancient grain, it's relatively new to the American diet.

Where Do I Buy It?

Supermarkets usually stock boxes in the same aisle as pasta and rice or sometimes in the health food section. Your store may carry only one or two brands, so ask if you don't see it right away.

How Do I Cook It?

The same way you would rice—either on the stove (it takes about fifteen minutes) or in a rice cooker. Before putting it in your pot, rinse quinoa in water to shed its bitter coating and let the delicious, nutty flavor shine through.

What Do I Eat It With?

Anything! Quinoa is incredibly versatile, so don't be afraid to experiment. Try it in the morning as a cereal alternative, or make a filling pilaf by tossing with vegetables, lentils or beans, olive oil and flavored vinegar, or salsa and your favorite spices or hot sauce. It also pairs well with kebabs or other grilled meat and fish.

waist and less visceral abdominal fat (a type of fat deep in the belly that hugs organs and may increase your risk for metabolic disorders) than those who consumed the least, researchers from Tufts University report. What's more, those who munched the most refined grains had a higher body mass index (a common measure of body fat).

→ **Trim-Down Tip:** Two whole-grain superfoods are better than one! Combine ½ cup cooked quinoa and ½ cup oatmeal for a power-packed, supersatiating breakfast. (Precook several servings of quinoa and store in the fridge so you can eat it all week.) Dress it up any way you like: with fruit, nuts, raisins, maple syrup, or skim milk.

. . . .

- Subjects following a reduced-calorie diet consisting of about 115 grams of protein per day (roughly 30 percent of their calories) lost 22 percent more fat mass after four months than those consuming the same number of calories but only 70 grams of protein per day, according to a study in *The Journal of Nutrition*.
- Researchers in Sydney, Australia, tested the effects of four different high-fiber diet plans. Subjects in all four groups lost weight, but dieters who ate more low-GI foods (with 55 percent of their calories from carbs) and those on the high-protein diet (25 percent from protein, but higher-GI foods) lost as much as 80 percent more fat mass than subjects who ate higher-GI foods and less protein.

Three More Reasons to Eat Quinoa

1. *Quinoa is a hearty, disease-fighting grain.* The fiber in quinoa may help lower cholesterol, and the whole grain is high in antioxidants and other nutrients that help protect your ticker by regulating blood pressure. A diet rich in whole grains may also lower your risk for breast and colon cancer, as well as diabetes. For

WANT TO EAT MORE QUINOA STARTING TODAY?

Quinoa makes for a tasty hot breakfast that will help stave off hunger until lunch. Combine $1/2$ cup quinoa, $2/3$ cup water, and $1/3$ cup orange juice in a saucepan, and cook for 15 minutes. Top with your favorite fruit and 1 tablespoon nuts.

DON'T LIKE QUINOA?

Swap quinoa for rice when making a stir-fry or pilaf; it has a similarly mild flavor and texture. You probably won't notice the change—until your too-tight pair of jeans starts fitting perfectly, that is.

example, when obese, prediabetic people exercised and consumed low-GI foods, they regulated their blood sugar and pancreas function better than those who worked out but ate a high-GI diet, according to researchers from the Cleveland Clinic.

2. *You'll up your vitamin and mineral intake.* Quinoa touts a potent mix of vitamins, minerals, and healthy phytochemicals that could put your multi out of business. One cup gives you more than 10 percent of your daily value of ten different nutrients, including 58 percent of your day's manganese, an important mineral for healthy bones, and significant amounts of iron and potassium.

3. *Quinoa promotes a healthy complexion and digestive system.* Trading refined grains and other processed foods for whole grains may help lessen breakouts. Meanwhile, quinoa's fiber helps keep you regular, and its resistant starch feeds the healthy bacteria in your GI tract, which help fight off bugs that may cause stomach trouble.

quinoa nutrition by the numbers

222
calories per cup of cooked quinoa

5
grams of fiber

8
grams of protein

100 PERCENT WHOLE-GRAIN PASTA

The Slimming Story

Craving carb-errific comfort food? We can't vouch for what you might pour over your pasta, but if your noodles are made of 100 percent whole wheat or other whole grains (see page 128 for a full list), you're on your way to becoming as lean as linguine. Multiple studies link eating more whole grains—foods such as pasta made from the entire kernel, the outer bran and inner germ along with the starchy endosperm—with improved weight loss and a lower risk for obesity.

The secret is in the bran and germ, which usually get discarded during the refining process. Not only do they hold much of the grain's healthy vitamins, minerals, and phytonutrients, but they also contain two pound-peeling standouts—protein and fiber. In fact, the bran and the germ hold about 25 percent of a grain's protein, a nutrient that increases the number of calories you burn after eating. It's supremely satiating, too, helping you resist the urge to munch. Whole-grain pasta also touts double to triple the fiber of refined noodles. In addition to working with protein to make your meal more filling, fiber holds on to a portion of the calories you eat so you ultimately absorb fewer. You'll also get resistant starch, a fiber-mimicking carbohydrate that may stimulate fat burning, tame your appetite, and shrink fat cells.

All three of these nutrients work together to slow the digestion of whole-grain pasta and place it lower on the glycemic index, meaning its glucose won't flood your blood or cause the resulting spike in insulin—

A TIP FOR THE PASTA COOK

The whole-grain pasta you choose may require a longer or shorter cooking time than you're used to. If it's your first time, follow the directions on the box and taste-test frequently. Keep in mind that most whole-grain pasta is naturally more al dente when done than traditional pasta, and overcooking will only turn it gummy.

a chain reaction that promotes fat storage. In fact, a diet rich in whole grains may make you more sensitive to insulin's effects. This is a good thing, as it could lower your risk for diabetes and metabolic syndrome, two conditions that go hand in hand with obesity and belly fat.

The Amazing Proof

- In a study of nearly forty-five hundred adults, those who consumed between 47 percent and 64 percent of their calories from carbohydrates had a lower BMI than those who ate fewer carbs, according to the *Journal of the American Dietetic Association.* Unsurprisingly, this group also consumed more slimming fiber than those who ate fewer carbs.

→ **Trim-Down Tip:** Aim to eat the majority of your diet's carbohydrates as whole grains, fruits, and vegetables like the superfoods in this book. Refined and processed carbs aren't banned—nothing is with the Drop 10 diet!—but try keeping your intake to a minimum to help you control hunger, shed fat, and stay healthy. (The Drop 10 meal plan in chapter 10 shows you how you can eat all your favorite treats and still lose.)

- Whole-grain pasta puts the kibosh on weight creep: Increasing one's intake of whole grains was inversely related to weight gain over an eight-year period; for every additional 2½ servings of whole grains chewed per day, weight gain was reduced by more than a pound, according to a study in *The American Journal of Clinical Nutrition.* (See page 113 for what counts as a serving.)

Three More Reasons to Eat Whole-Grain Pasta

1. *You'll help your body fend off heart disease, diabetes, and cancer.* Whole-grain pasta is packed with fiber, vitamins, minerals, and antioxidants that help keep you healthy and fight disease. Researchers at Wake Forest University in Winston-Salem, North Carolina, for example, find that for women, eating 2½ servings

The Soba Story

Soba noodles are a form of buckwheat pasta commonly used in Asian dishes. As with other types of noodles, check ingredients lists to see if they're made with 100 percent whole-grain flour; some brands combine refined wheat and buckwheat flours. The noodle's fiber content is usually a good tip-off. If it's low—around 1 gram per serving—you can bet it's not 100 percent whole grain. Look for brands with at least 3 grams of fiber per serving.

of whole grains per day cuts the risk of cardiovascular disease by 21 percent.

2. *It can put a smile on your face.* Healthy pasta feeds your noodle, too! Carbs increase concentrations of serotonin, low levels of which are linked to depression. A study in the *Archives of Internal Medicine* finds that people on a carb-rich diet (46 percent of their calories) were less depressed and angry after the year-long trial than those following a low-carb plan.

3. *Whole grains banish breakouts.* Trade refined-flour noodles for whole grain and you could see clearer skin. The insulin spikes associated with processed carbs may increase the production of androgens, hormones that, when elevated, can lead to zits.

Oodles of Slimming Noodles!

Your supermarket likely stocks at least a dozen different whole-grain pastas. Finding them can be a macaroni-in-a-haystack expedition, however. (Have you been down the pasta aisle lately?) These tricks will help you suss out the most slenderizing picks.

- Seek the "whole" truth. Your best bet is to look first for packages with the word *whole* in the description—for example, "whole-wheat linguine." Then check the ingredients. Every grain listed should have the word *whole* in front of it. You might also see the phrase *100 percent whole [type of grain or flour]* or the Whole Grains

> ### WANT TO EAT MORE WHOLE-GRAIN PASTA STARTING TODAY?
>
> Add bite-size whole-grain pasta (think macaroni, orecchiette, or mini-shells) to your favorite canned or homemade soup. Add cooked pasta directly before serving; or, for dry pasta, simmer the soup until the pasta is fully cooked, eight to ten minutes more.
>
> ### DON'T LIKE WHOLE-GRAIN PASTA?
>
> If you're not a fan of the chewier texture at first, mix it with regular pasta and shift the ratio each time you make a noodle dish. Or look for whole-grain pasta blends; those made with spelt or quinoa may be less dense.

Council's "100 percent whole-grain" yellow stamp somewhere on the package.

- Watch for confusing language. Pastas made with at least 51 percent whole-grain flour may carry a "made with whole grains" claim. Although they're better than noodles made entirely of refined flour, you'll still lose some whole-grain goodness. The term *whole semolina* is deceiving, too. Semolina isn't a grain, but a type of refined wheat.

- Know your grains. Although a yummy pick, whole wheat isn't your only option. Plenty of noodles are made from various other single grains or whole-grain blends. Taste and texture tend to differ among pastas, so experiment with a few different brands and shapes to find your favorite. Don't like your first choice? Try again! Following are eight slimming whole grains you may find on pasta ingredients lists:

• Barley	• Brown rice
• Buckwheat	• Durum wheat
• Kamut	• Quinoa
• Rye	• Spelt

*whole-grain pasta nutrition
by the numbers**

174

calories per cup of cooked whole-wheat spaghetti

6

grams of fiber

7

grams of protein

*Because nutrient information varies slightly among grains and noodles, we used whole-wheat spaghetti as an example.

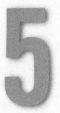 Super Nuts, Seeds, and Oil

....

ALMOND BUTTER

....

The Slimming Story

Spread the news! Once you start dipping into a jar of this delectable, creamy superfood—made only of ground-up almonds—you'll soon be dipping into your wallet for a new, smaller-size wardrobe. Research shows that replacing less healthful foods with almonds and almond butter results in more weight loss and a trimmer waistline, even though the nuts may have more total fat. The nut butter boasts a unique combination of healthy fats, protein, and fiber, which together do a number on hunger and cravings even as they rev your metabolism.

The good-for-you monounsaturated fat in almond butter takes longer to work its way through your stomach than carb- or protein-rich foods, helping you stay full and munchie-free. And the fats blunt the effects of carbohydrates on blood sugar and insulin. A surge in blood sugar followed by a drop can trigger your appetite, while insulin spikes encourage your body to store fat. Almond butter is also high in alpha-linolenic acid, which may speed the metabolism of fats.

The fiber and protein in almond butter help your weight loss efforts,

What About Whole Almonds?

Sure, almonds could have made our superfood list instead of their spreadable sister; after all, the research touting almonds' weight loss effects focuses on the whole nuts. (See below: It's impressive.) But the butter nudged out the nut and took top superfood billing for a few different reasons. For starters, you reap the same slimming and health-promoting benefits from the butter as you do from the whole nut. But nut butters are more versatile, not to mention satisfyingly creamy and delicious. And compared with the old standby peanut butter, almond butter touts higher levels of energizing iron and more calcium, which can help trigger fat burning. It also has a milder, more grown-up taste, giving you the sensation that you're indulging in something special, not simply raiding your kid's lunch box. If you can't find almond butter, however, or just plain don't like it, feel free to munch on whole almonds or enjoy peanut butter instead. You'll still take in plenty of filling, healthy fats, protein, and fiber.

too, by working with fat to fill you up, squash hunger, and keep blood sugar levels steady. But both nutrients also have unique superpowers: Fiber lowers the number of calories you absorb from meals; and you'll sizzle extra calories digesting the protein. Plus, the butter is a good source of magnesium, a mineral that helps regulate blood sugar and insulin function, helping your body efficiently burn glucose for energy. Almond joy indeed!

→ **Trim-down tip:** Opt for chunky almond butter rather than smooth. Although you still take in plenty of the nuts' healthy, slimming fat, a portion will stay trapped in the cell walls of the chunky variety, even after chewing, and pass through your digestive system without your body absorbing it, ultimately saving you some calories.

The Amazing Proof

- Dieters who ate almonds daily shed 62 percent more weight and 56 percent more fat than those who ate about the same number of

ALMOND BUTTER: NOT JUST FOR SANDWICHES

The nutty spread shines between two slices of whole-grain bread, but it buddies up well with a number of other foods, too. Try one of these power couples:

- Breakfast: almond butter + oatmeal. Two supersatiating superfoods for weight loss unite to stomp out hunger and excite your taste buds! Simply stir a tablespoon into your morning bowl.
- Snack: almond butter + nonfat plain Greek yogurt. This combo makes the perfect veggie dip. Two tablespoons of yogurt beef up an otherwise small 1-tablespoon serving of almond butter but add a mere 26 calories. The spread has a smooth, creamy texture and a tart, yummy flavor, as well as fat-fighting protein and calcium.
- Dinner: almond butter + soy sauce. Whisk 2 tablespoons almond butter with 1 tablespoon each low-sodium soy sauce, fresh lime juice, and sesame oil; 1 clove chopped garlic; and honey and rice vinegar to taste, and you've got a yummy, nutty Asian-inspired salad dressing.
- Dessert: almond butter + chocolate. Stir a teaspoon into a low-fat chocolate pudding cup, or spread on a piece of dark chocolate.

calories but no nuts, reports a study from Loma Linda University in California. Nut noshers also saw a greater reduction in their waistline.

- Don't fear the fat! Women who added 344 calories' worth of almonds to their regular diet every day (the equivalent of about 3 tablespoons of almond butter) gained no extra weight or body fat at the end of a ten-week trial, a study in the *British Journal of Nutrition* reveals. The reason: The almonds were filling, causing the women to naturally scale back the amount of other food they would have otherwise consumed. A portion of almonds' fat content also goes unabsorbed.

- Eating a slice of white bread normally causes a surge in blood sugar, but when people ate almonds with the quick-digesting, refined carb, they didn't get the same spike as when they consumed the bread alone, according to a study from the University of Toronto.

Four More Reasons to Eat Almond Butter

1. *Your heart goes nuts for it.* Almond butter is bursting with nutrients that help your ticker stay in top form, including mono-unsaturated fat, which lowers levels of LDL cholesterol (the "bad" type) and reduces blood pressure. Research suggests almonds may improve risk factors for chronic conditions including cardiovascular disease and type 2 diabetes.
2. *It gives your immune system a boost and your skin a lift.* Almond butter may function as a prebiotic, meaning it helps the healthy bacteria in the body flourish, allowing them to better fight off harmful bugs that can make you sick. (Probiotics are the healthy bacteria themselves; prebiotics act as fuel for the germs.) Skin cells, meanwhile, stockpile almond butter's vitamin E, which helps increase hydration and defends against wrinkle-causing free radicals.
3. *You'll help your body bounce back postworkout.* Almond butter is a top source of the antioxidant vitamin E. People with high levels

WANT TO EAT MORE ALMOND BUTTER STARTING TODAY?

Any time you're snacking on fruits or veggies—especially apples, bananas, or celery—add a hearty smear of almond butter and your snack will be supersatisfying. Or swap your usual PB for AB and add a few slices of banana for an extra-filling, extra-slimming sandwich.

DON'T LIKE ALMOND BUTTER?

Almond butter has a milder taste than peanut butter, so you can slip a tablespoon into smoothies or fruit shakes.

of the vitamin in their blood endured less muscle damage after exercising than did those with lower amounts, according to research from Ball State University in Muncie, Indiana.

4. *Almond butter could protect your brain.* Animal research shows that an almond-rich diet improves memory and reduces the buildup of debris in the brain associated with Alzheimer's disease; compounds in the nuts actually seem to work in a similar way as drugs that treat the disease.

Select a Slimming Jar

When it comes to ingredients in almond butter, less is more (slimming). Choose brands that list only almonds and nothing else. Your butter will be just as tasty sans added sugar (which may show up on ingredients lists as "evaporated cane juice") and belly-bloating salt. Also avoid added palm fruit oil, which some makers use as a substitute for heart-harming trans fats; it's not much better for your health or heart.

Keep Your Almond Butter Together

Got separation anxiety? You know, that feeling of unease after finding all of the oil in your jar of natural nut butter floating on top and the solids packed on the bottom? It's actually a good sign. If the separation didn't occur, you can bet your butter the jar contains saturated fat–laden palm oil or trans fat–containing hydrogenated oils. (Not only do evil trans fats raise levels of "bad" LDL cholesterol, but they also lower levels of the "good" HDL type. Plus, if you eat too much, they could cause you to pack on pounds.)

Stirring isn't such a bad trade-off for the missing fats. Do stir regularly, though; the longer the butter sits separated, the harder it is to reintegrate. If things get tough, set the jar in a bowl of warm water for ten to fifteen minutes before stirring, or consider buying a natural nut butter hand mixer. (Check them out at WitmerProducts.com.) They cost about $10, attach right to your jar, and make mixing a snap. Whatever you do, don't drain off the oil—it's the healthy monounsaturated fat that keeps your butter moist, spreadable, and able to ward off hunger.

DIETARY FATS: THE GOOD, THE BAD, AND THE UGLY

Fat fact: You've got to eat it to lose it. It sounds counterintuitive, but like carbs, all fats are not created equal—nor are they evil. Think of the three main types, unsaturated, saturated, and trans fats, like clothes. Unsaturated fats are your ultra-flattering jeans—a staple that can do amazing things for your body, helping you look slim and feel incredible. Saturated fats are a bit like sweats: They're not great for your shape, but you can't avoid them entirely. Then there are trans fats—the hideous holiday sweaters of nutrition. Avoid at all costs. Want to know more? Here's a breakdown:

The Good: Monounsaturated and Polyunsaturated Fats, Omega-3 Fatty Acids

Plentiful in: avocado, olive oil, nuts, seeds, fish

Anything you eat that contains fat likely has both unsaturated and saturated fat, but what counts is the ratio, or how much you're getting of both. If the majority of the fat on your plate comes from the food sources above, you're playing your lards right. Here's why:

- Unsaturated fats help tame your appetite. These same fats, which lower "bad" LDL cholesterol levels while raising "good" HDL levels, are slower to leave your stomach than are carbs or protein, so they fill you up. They also stimulate the release of satiety hormones, which may help curb hunger.
- Cutting calories will be easier. Your body needs fat to stay healthy, and you'll likely crave it if you limit your intake too much. Research shows that dieters on a higher-fat plan were more likely to stick with it than those on a low-fat program.
- You could burn more fat. When you consume fat, your body has two choices: Burn it or store it. Unsaturated fat oxidizes more readily than the saturated type. Although experts aren't exactly sure why, one theory is that monounsaturated fat, specifically, may switch on genes that trigger fat burning and suppress fat storage. Omega-3s, a type of polyunsaturated

fat found in fish, also seem to steer your body toward using fat as energy during exercise rather than keeping it for extra padding.

- Blood sugar and insulin levels stay steady. Healthy fat helps slow digestion, preventing the spikes in blood glucose and insulin that promote the storage of flab. Omega-3s may also directly improve insulin sensitivity, which could help trim your tummy.
- Healthy fats extinguish inflammation. Inflammation is your body's normal response to injury—it flares up to help you heal, then goes away. Or it's supposed to, anyway. A diet low in omega-3s but high in omega-6 fatty acids and trans fats may contribute to chronic inflammation, which is linked to metabolic syndrome, a condition marked by excess belly fat. Eating more omega-3-rich foods helps balance the activities of fats in your body, allowing them to aid in healing without contributing to lasting inflammation.

The Bad: Saturated Fat

Plentiful in: fatty red meat, full-fat dairy, butter

Just as you wouldn't wear a bridesmaid's dress to the office, you should relegate saturated fats to a similar only-as-needed role in your diet. You can't banish them altogether because they pop up in foods that help you lose weight—namely, protein-packed lean beef and calcium-rich cheese—as well as in tasty indulgences like dark chocolate that keep you from falling off the weight loss wagon. You also get a small amount in foods rich in healthy unsaturated fats, such as olive oil. So focus on limiting your intake to about 7 percent of your total calories, or 12 grams per day if you're following the 1,600-calorie Drop 10 plan. (Our menus do this for you automatically.)

Saturated fats are most notorious for raising cholesterol levels; overdo it and you might also pack on pounds. For example, a diet heavy in palmitic acid, a specific type of fat in butter, full-fat dairy, and meat, may cause your brain to ignore hormones that send the "I'm full" signal, a study in *The Journal of Clinical Investigation* reveals. The changes could take effect after three days of a sat-fat overload, so if you indulge at, say, a barbecue one day, try to get back on track the next.

The Ugly: Trans Fat

Plentiful in: processed items (especially baked goods), some fried foods, shortening, margarine

Trans fat can occur naturally in small amounts, but most of what you encounter—and want to avoid—is man-made and added to food. These are unsaturated oils that have been partially hydrogenated by manufacturers to extend a product's shelf life. Look out for the amount of trans fat listed on nutrition labels, and check ingredients for hidden sources—the term *partially hydrogenated* is a dead giveaway that trans fats are present.

Not only is trans fat extra dangerous for your heart because it both raises "bad" LDL cholesterol and lowers your "good" HDL levels, but it also may be extra fattening. A study from Harvard University found that among overweight women, for every 1 percent increase in daily calories consumed as trans fats, they gained an additional 2.3 pounds over eight years. There was no link between weight and intake of unsaturated fats, however. Research also shows that trans fats are the most significant dietary factor related to abdominal fat. What's worse, the fats may increase your risk for depression, too. Makes you think twice about biting into that packaged doughnut, doesn't it?

Want to Trim the Fat? Follow These Tips

- Know your limits. All fats are high in calories, so keep an eye on your intake of even the good stuff; roughly a quarter to a third of your daily calories should come from fat. That's 44 to 59 grams if you're following a 1,600-calorie-per-day diet. Aim to get most from unsaturated sources and only about 12 grams per day in sat fat. And, obviously, the less trans fat, the better.

- Make a trade. Swap out sources of saturated for unsaturated fat when possible. Cook with olive or canola oil instead of butter, margarine, or shortening. Opt for lean red meat (check out page 166 for smart steak choices) and white meat, skinless turkey and chicken instead of dark meat. Also substitute your meat meals with seafood at least twice a week.

- Snack smart. Stock your home and office with plenty of fruits, veggies, peanuts, almond butter, and popcorn so that when you get hungry, you're less tempted to go for pastries, cookies, and potato chips.

- Be a small fry. You don't need to give up your favorite fried foods, but save them for special occasions, order smaller sizes, and share with friends. If you love fast food, check out the tips in chapter 14 and make it a goal to stop at sandwich shops more often than burger or fried chicken joints. Also keep dried fruit, veggies, nuts, or popcorn in your car at all times; when a snack attack strikes, you'll be prepared and zoom right by the drive-through.

almond butter nutrition

by the numbers

98

calories per tablespoon of almond butter

12

percent of your daily value of magnesium

2

grams of fiber

9

grams of fat (8 unsaturated, 1 saturated)

3

grams of protein

OLIVE OIL

The Slimming Story

Want to make peace with the scale once and for all? Extend the olive branch by swapping saturated fat sources such as butter for mono-unsaturated fat–rich olive oil. Olive oil increases satiety, helping tame your appetite so you eat less, and increases the release of the appetite-regulating hormone CCK in your gut. Plus, pairing the oil with carbohydrates works to keep blood glucose and insulin levels low, discouraging your body from storing fat.

More than keeping fat off your thighs, however, olive oil may actually increase your body's fat-burning power. Research shows that compared with a meal high in saturated fat, a meal prepared with olive oil boosts fat oxidation after eating. Experts aren't exactly certain of the reason, but they speculate that monounsaturated fatty acids may switch on genes related to fat burning and fat storage.

Olive oil's overall health-promoting qualities might help you shed excess weight as well. Extra-virgin olive oil (EVOO) is loaded with antioxidant polyphenols and may reduce inflammation. Inflammation is

FOIL SPOIL

Olive oil is delicate, and if not stored properly, it will lose some of its health-promoting antioxidants and could quickly become rancid, too. How to keep it fresh:

- Buy in small batches. Those economy-size bottles may seem like a money saver, but you're better off playing it safe by thinking small. Olive oil usually stays fresh for about six months.
- Keep it under wraps. Stash your bottle in a cupboard away from the heat of the stove and out of direct sunlight, both of which cause it to degrade faster.
- Use the sniff test. If it smells a bit off or rancid, toss it. The oil will leave an equally bad taste in your mouth.

your system's natural response to infection or injury, but it can become chronic over time and contribute to disease, including metabolic syndrome. Research shows that trading up to monounsaturated fats from saturated fats may also help you feel more energetic.

→ **Trim-Down Tip:** Olive oil is so versatile it's one of the only superfoods for weight loss you could eat every day without getting bored. Go ahead, try it! Aim to include olive oil in your meals at least once a day in place of saturated fat sources like butter, mayo, cream-based salad dressings, and vegetable oil. Try sautéing veggies in a few teaspoons, drizzle it over salad or on whole-grain bread, or toss it with pasta, cooked whole grains, or lentils.

The Amazing Proof

- Olive oil is one of the most important components of the Mediterranean diet, which is also rich in fruits and vegetables, whole grains, legumes, and fish. Studies show that eating like a Greek helps people lose weight and may stymie weight gain over time.
- Subjects who ate a diet in which the majority of their fat came from monounsaturated sources—olive oil, avocados, and nuts—actually lost weight and body fat over four weeks without making any other changes, according to a study in the *British Journal of Nutrition*. The control group, whose diet included mostly saturated fat, saw small increases in body weight and fat.
- Dieters who followed a low-cal meal plan that emphasized monounsaturated fat, protein, and complex carbohydrates lost almost

→ WANT TO EAT MORE OLIVE OIL
STARTING TODAY?

Replace premade, bottled salad dressings with a simple, fat-fighting homemade vinaigrette. Mix equal parts EVOO and vinegar (try balsamic or red wine), and add 1 teaspoon each of fresh chopped herbs, chopped garlic, lemon juice, or Dijon mustard, depending on your tastes.

> ## DON'T LIKE OLIVE OIL?
>
> Look for the word *light* on the label—it refers to the color and mild flavor, not the calorie count. Light olive oil is made using a fine filtration process, which bestows a more neutral flavor. Use this type when sautéing instead of butter or vegetable oil.

double the weight as a group who consumed the same number of calories but less total fat, less protein, and more carbs, a study in the *Archives of Internal Medicine* reports.

Trim-Down Tip: Even though olive oil is a slick health pick, it's still high in calories—119 per tablespoon—and going overboard may cause you to add pounds instead of dropping them. If you're counting calories, pour your oil into a stainless-steel spray bottle. The fine mist will coat salads, pans, and veggies lightly and evenly, helping you minimize your intake. (Two pumps nets about 40 calories, or less than a teaspoon.)

One More Major Reason to Eat Olive Oil

You'll likely live longer, and be healthier and happier.

Skipping saturated fat sources in favor of the monounsaturated fat, antioxidants, and other phytonutrients in olive oil is one of the best things you can do for your health. High blood pressure, elevated cholesterol, diabetes, heart disease, cancer, Alzheimer's disease, arthritis, and depression are only a few of the ailments that olive oil may help improve or keep at bay, research suggests. No wonder the flavorful oil has been referred to as liquid gold.

Like a Virgin?

If you're not sure what type of olive oil to toss in your basket, check this guide to what you'll find in stores:

- Extra-virgin: The cream of the crop, EVOO is worth its higher price tag when you're using the oil in a fresh salad or over veggies—anything that showcases its flavor. Made from the freshest, best olives, it touts the highest levels of healthy antioxidants and tastes incredibly rich and flavorful.
- Virgin olive oil (VOO): Although produced in the same way as extra-virgin olive oil, VOO is a slight step down from extra-virgin. For example, the olives used to make it may not have been pressed as quickly after harvest. (For California oils, if olives aren't pressed within twenty-four hours of harvest, they can't make the EVOO grade.) It may also be more acidic, which you may or may not notice. Regardless, it's still a tasty and healthy pick for your waistline, so if you're on a budget, this type could help you save a buck.
- Pure or light olive oil: If you're cooking, opt for this standard, inexpensive olive oil. It's more processed and may contain fewer antioxidants, but it withstands heat better than the extra-virgin and virgin varieties. And because its flavor is likely to be masked by whatever you're making, you needn't spend the money on EVOO.

....

→ **Trim-Down Tip:** Going out to eat? Skip the butter and ask your waitress to bring a small plate and some olive oil for dipping. Restaurant diners who received olive oil with their bread consumed 23 percent less bread than those spreading butter, a study in the *International Journal of Obesity* reveals. So even though those in the oil group took in more total grams of fat from their topping, they ended up consuming about 17 percent fewer calories overall.

....

olive oil nutrition

by the numbers

119

calories per tablespoon of olive oil

14

grams of total fat

10

grams of monounsaturated fat

2

grams of saturated fat

PEANUTS

The Slimming Story

Nibble on this: Despite their calorie and fat content (166 grams and 14 grams per ounce, respectively), peanuts may help lighten your personal load. Yep, the tasty nuts—technically legumes but closer to tree nuts—boast a barrel of nutrients and other qualities that make them a slimming calorie investment. Per ounce, you'll take in 7 grams of protein, more than you get from any other variety of nut (this is why they beat out almonds as our superfood nut), plus 2 grams of fiber and plenty of healthy unsaturated fat. The trimming trinity of hunger taming, these three nutrients work together to keep your stomach full and cravings suppressed. Protein and fiber also steady your body's blood glucose and insulin levels, an essential for staving off excess belly fat.

Like any good team, however, each nutrient brings its own slenderizing strengths to the table. Fiber reduces the number of calories you absorb from meals, and protein ups your calorie burn after eating. What's more, eating peanuts could boost your metabolism by as much as 11 percent. Experts aren't exactly sure why, but they know that your body fires through unsaturated fat more readily than the saturated kind.

What About the Butter?

If you love peanut butter and wonder why it didn't make our final list, check out the box on page 132 and give almond butter a chance. Whole peanuts, on the other hand, are perfect for snacking—they're portable, inexpensive, and easy to find just about anywhere. They also pair exceptionally well with salads, oatmeal, and other items. And with more protein than other nuts and a host of healthy unsaturated fat and fiber, peanuts had to be included among the superfoods—it was a no-brainer! But if the nuts aren't your bag, and you'd rather have the spreadable version, go ahead and make the swap; you'll still slim down.

But here's the thing: You won't actually absorb the full fat load from a serving of peanuts. (Don't worry: You *do* get all of the benefits of fiber described above.) Just as we suggested buying chunky almond butter in that superfood's section, we like peanuts because portions of the nut's lipid-containing cells remain intact even after chewing. The cells and their fatty acid passengers then travel through your digestive tract and out of your body without your hips, tummy, or other trouble spots being any the wiser. In a nutshell, peanuts are more than a tasty ballpark staple; they're a home run for diet success.

The Amazing Proof

- In a study of almost nine thousand people, those who ate nuts at least twice a week were 29 percent less likely to gain a significant amount of weight over twenty-eight months, even after researchers adjusted for weight-related variables, according to a study in *Obesity.*
- Eating a quick-digesting (read: glucose- and insulin-raising) meal with peanuts reduced the glycemic response by a full 55 percent, researchers from Arizona State University in Mesa found. What's more, the peanut group consumed 200 to 275 fewer calories over the course of the day compared with the control group.
- People following a diet rich in monounsaturated fat (totaling 15 to 20 percent of calories) that included peanuts or peanut butter daily lost 40 percent more weight after eighteen months than those who consumed less of the healthy fats, according to a study in the *International Journal of Obesity.* (Weight loss was similar between the two groups after a year, but the lower-fat group began gaining back pounds within the last six months, whereas the peanut group stayed steady.)

Three More Reasons to Eat Peanuts

1. *They're a super snack for warding off disease.* Peanuts' healthy fats could help lower cholesterol, plus they contain other healthy phytonutrients, including resveratrol (red wine's claim to fame),

WANT TO EAT MORE PEANUTS STARTING TODAY?

Sprinkle them on any salad. Peanuts lend a satiating texture to greens. Toss them in whole, chop them into small pieces, or even crush and mix them into salad dressing.

DON'T LIKE PEANUTS?

Grind peanuts in a food processor, then add to chili or spaghetti sauce. You'll never know they're there, but your body will thank you!

that may reduce your risk for heart disease, type 2 diabetes, and cancer. For example, women with risk factors for heart disease who ate only 1 ounce of unsalted peanuts (or 1 tablespoon of peanut butter) five times a week were 44 percent less likely to develop the condition than those who ate less, research from the Harvard School of Public Health reveals.

2. *They can keep you young inside and out.* The resveratrol you take in by eating peanuts may help sharpen your brain, and research suggests that nuts' niacin and vitamin E may lower your risk for Alzheimer's disease and may slow age-related cognitive decline. In your skin, those same two nutrients help buffer the effects of wrinkle-causing sun damage.

3. *Peanuts make a great good-night snack.* Pop a handful of the nuts to get a dose of tryptophan, the amino acid infamous for putting you to sleep after Thanksgiving dinner. It works by triggering your body to produce sleep-inducing melatonin. You also need tryptophan to make serotonin, which acts as a natural mood stabilizer.

Nuts for Peanuts!

Whether picking or partaking, you can get the most out of this crunchy superfood with these five tricks.

- Take a crack at whole peanuts. When snacking, shelling your own peanuts slows you down, which may help quell overeating.
- Buy in bulk. You could get a bargain. To make sure the bin is fresh, pick up a few whole peanuts and shake 'em. If you hear the nuts rattle inside their shells, it's a sign they may be dried out.
- Go naked. To avoid a dose of bloat-causing sodium, go for un-salted, dry-roasted, or raw nuts. Also skip boiled nuts, which have scads of sodium. And save those peanuts coated in honey, sugar, chocolate, or yogurt for a special treat, not an everyday snack.
- Be cool. Nuts can go rancid quickly, but they last longer if you store them in a cool, dry, dark place (that is, a cupboard away from the stove) or keep them in the fridge.
- Branch out. Not just for snacking, peanuts add a satisfying, protein-packed crunch to sweet and savory dishes alike: Use them whole, or place an ounce in a sandwich bag and use a meat tender-izer or the bottom of a mug to break into smaller pieces. Toss them into a stir-fry, noodles, or veggies; add to sauces, soups, and dips; or sprinkle chopped peanuts on yogurt, ice cream, and fruit par-faits.

peanut nutrition by the numbers

166
calories per ounce of peanuts

2
grams of fiber

14
grams of total fat

7
grams of monounsaturated fat

7
grams of protein

PUMPKIN SEEDS

The Slimming Story

Don't think of these crunchy bits as an autumn-only snack. Sprinkling them into your diet year-round can plant the seed for a more slender, healthy, energized you. Pumpkin seeds, sometimes called pepitas when shelled, abound with waist-whittling nutrients, including protein. One ounce of the kernels packs 8 grams, nearly as much as a cup of low-fat yogurt. Remember, you burn more calories digesting protein than you do fat and carbohydrates. Protein and fiber also provide the building blocks for metabolism-revving muscle, fill you up to curb overeating,

WANT TO EAT MORE PUMPKIN SEEDS STARTING TODAY?

Season your seeds for everyday snacking! Heat oven to 350 degrees. Spread raw seeds evenly on a baking sheet and coat with olive oil cooking spray and one of the following flavor combos (just enough to lightly dust the seeds). Cook until seeds are crisp, stirring frequently, about 20 minutes.

Spicy: Cayenne, smoked paprika, ground coriander, and salt

Sweet: Sugar, cinnamon, and nutmeg

Savory: Ground cumin, garlic powder, paprika, and black pepper

DON'T LIKE PUMPKIN SEEDS?

Mill pumpkin seed kernels in a food processor, and in less than thirty seconds your options for hiding them are endless: Mix them into mole or other sauces for rich flavor and texture, or use as a protein-packed thickener for soup, stew, and chili. They also add belly-trimming texture to hamburger, turkey burgers, and meatballs.

and steady your blood sugar and insulin levels, helping prevent the storage of excess fat.

Pumpkin seeds' fiber (about 2 grams per ounce) and healthy unsaturated fats work in similar ways to blunt cravings: They fill you up and keep blood glucose and insulin in check. And you'll take in both mono- and polyunsaturated fatty acids, which could give you a fat-burning boost postmeal.

Diet-friendly macronutrients aren't the only reason to start snacking on pumpkin seeds, however. Ounce for ounce, pepitas supply more natural magnesium than most other foods. You need the mineral so insulin can carry glucose out of blood and into cells that use it for energy; getting enough may help keep your system sizzling, protecting against diabetes and metabolic syndrome, both of which are related to obesity and excess ab fat. Unfortunately, most women in the United States don't get enough of the recommended 320 milligrams per day from their diet. Luckily, meeting your magnesium needs is as simple as munching about 2 ounces of pumpkin seeds. Two ounces also deliver about half your day's iron, which helps bring energizing oxygen to cells and may help fight fatigue—and maybe even that urge to skip your workout!

The Amazing Proof

- Snacking on pumpkin seeds instead of, say, chips increases your intake of protein, which could help you shed weight: Women who ate a diet consisting of 30 percent protein for four days showed an increase in satiety, fat burning, and metabolic rate compared with those who ate a similar diet with only 10 percent protein, report researchers from Maastricht University.
- As a woman's intake of magnesium goes up, her risk for metabolic syndrome (a condition characterized by belly fat) goes down, according to a study in the journal *Obesity*. For people with the highest intake of the nutrient—337 milligrams or more per day for women, or just over the amount in 2 ounces of shelled pumpkin seeds—the odds were 44 percent lower.

Four More Reasons to Eat Pumpkin Seeds

1. *Your heart goes pitter-patter for pepitas.* Along with cholesterol-lowering unsaturated fats and heart-healthy vitamin E, pumpkin seeds are rich in phytosterols, cancer-fighting compounds that may prevent the body's absorption of cholesterol from food and may also lower LDL levels. Meanwhile, magnesium promotes normal blood pressure.

Got Guts? Roast Your Own Seeds!

When Halloween rolls around, don't toss your jack-o'-lantern's seeds along with its stringy innards; instead, make your own body-trimming snack. Besides saving money, keeping a bowl or bag around to nibble on helps you resist the urge to binge on all those fun-size candy bars. Here's what to do:

1. De-slime the seeds. Pick out the white seeds from the stringy insides of your pumpkin. (Better yet, get your kids to do it.) Place in a bowl of water to further separate them from the pumpkin's pulp and strain out any residual pumpkin, then pour the seeds into a colander to drain.
2. Lay them out to dry. Line a baking sheet with a clean, absorbent towel and spread the seeds evenly. Let them sit overnight, allowing all the moisture to evaporate.
3. Toss and roast. Once the seeds are completely dry, heat oven to 275 degrees. Pour seeds into a bowl and toss with olive oil and sea salt. (Use about $1/2$ to 1 tablespoon oil and a sprinkling of salt per cup of seeds. Salt is okay here because you control the amount you use.) Set towel aside, spread seeds evenly on baking sheet, and cook until they're crisp, about 20 minutes, stirring frequently. You can eat pumpkin seeds whole, but they're probably larger than what you buy at stores, so chew them carefully and crunch only a few at a time rather than by the handful to avoid choking.

---

2. *The seeds may ease headaches.* Roughly half of people who suffer from headaches may be magnesium-deficient. Munching the seeds increases your intake of the nutrient, which relaxes blood vessels in the brain, potentially preventing or alleviating pain.

3. *They could reduce your risk for diabetes.* The higher one's intake of magnesium, the lower one's chance of developing the disease. People getting the most (about 300 milligrams or so for women) were 47 percent less likely to develop diabetes over twenty years compared with the low-intake group, according to researchers at the University of North Carolina in Chapel Hill.

4. *You'll stress less and sleep better.* Need to mellow out? Pumpkin seeds are rich in tryptophan, the calming amino acid your body uses to produce mood-stabilizing serotonin and melatonin, which may help you catch zzz's.

The Read on Seeds

Check out these tips for buying and storing the waist-shrinking super-food:

- Choose hulled pepitas. Cracking the shells between your teeth is a pleasant way to while away a lazy afternoon, but when you're short on time—you know, the other 364½ days a year!—opt for dry-roasted, shelled seeds. They make it a cinch to add hunger-curbing, calorie-burning protein to any meal or snack. For example, toss a tablespoon or two into trail mix, oatmeal, any kind of salad, pasta, quinoa, or rice pilaf.

- Skip the salt. Americans are seriously overdosing on salt—and it's not because of what comes out of your home saltshaker, but rather what manufacturers add to packaged food. Always opt for un-salted seeds (and nuts) when shopping.

- Keep them cool. Store your seeds in an airtight container in the refrigerator and they'll stay fresh up to six months. They also won't get lost way back in the pantry; seeing the seeds each time you open the fridge reminds you of their slimming powers—and how easy they are to add to meals.

pumpkin seed nutrition

by the numbers

146

calories per ounce of hulled pumpkin seeds

14

grams of total fat (10 grams unsaturated)

8

grams of protein

2

grams of fiber

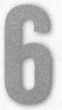

6 Super Fish and Meat

SARDINES

The Slimming Story

We know what you might be thinking: Sardines? *No thanks!* But before flipping to the next section, at least (a) find out what these mighty flab fighters can do for you (it's major); and (b) consider that they can be surprisingly tasty, depending on how you prepare them. (We swear! Check out the tips in this section.) Obviously, sardines are a tough sell, so they wouldn't have made the Drop 10 cut without a truly kick-butt combination of fat-burning nutrients plus other bonus benefits: You will reel in omega-3 fatty acids, protein, calcium, and vitamin D, all of which can help you shed weight; and the tiny fish are relatively inexpensive, environmentally sustainable, and lower in contaminants than those higher up on the marine-life food chain.

You probably already know that omega-3 fatty acids home in on helping your heart. They also target the area directly south—that is, your belly and other spots fat takes up residence. Research suggests that omega-3s switch on enzymes that tell your body to burn fat, while turning off those that encourage fat production and storage. Exercise seems to enhance the results and may trigger fat loss, but even without it, the fatty acids could prevent fat gain; a higher level of omega-3s in the body from dietary sources, for example, is associated with a lower level of body fat. Omega-3s also improve insulin sensitivity, potentially decreasing belly flab, and may increase levels of adiponectin, a hormone fat cells produce that speeds up metabolism and fat burning and may suppress appetite. As if that's not enough, omega-3s also help you maintain calorie-torching lean muscle mass.

There's more: The high-quality protein found in sardines provides the material needed to build lean muscle; plus, you'll fire through double the calories digesting it, compared with fats and carbs. Protein is extremely satiating, too, which keeps hunger at bay. Sardines' calcium, meanwhile, reduces enzymes related to fat production and may improve the breakdown of fat. Adequate levels of the mineral may also curb cortisol, a stress hormone linked to ab fat. As for vitamin D, research suggests having low levels of the nutrient at the start of a diet may hinder weight loss. Bottom line: Sardines' fat-melting benefits are packed in like a can of, well, you know. At least give 'em a try!

The Amazing Proof

- Among a group of overweight diabetics, those consuming omega-3-rich fish oil daily (the amount in about 6 ounces of sardines) saw a reduction in fat mass and had smaller fat cells after two months, compared with subjects taking a placebo, a study in *The American Journal of Clinical Nutrition* reports.

- As a woman's intake of calcium from food went up, the leaner she was likely to be, according to a study in *The American Journal of Clinical Nutrition*. Women who took in the most calcium (1,000 milligrams or more per day) weighed significantly less and had lower percentages of body fat and trimmer waists than those getting less of the mineral. But even those in the 600- to 1,000-milligram range were slimmer than those consuming less than 600 milligrams.

- Dieters who ate 25 percent of their calories from protein lost 59 percent more weight (more than 20 pounds) after six months compared with those who consumed a diet of only 12 percent protein, according to researchers at the Royal Veterinary and Agricultural University, Department of Human Nutrition, Centre for Advanced Food Studies, in Frederiksberg, Denmark. After a year, the high-protein group also had 10 percent less belly fat.

Four More Reasons to Eat Sardines

1. *They capture hearts and minds.* It's well-known that oily fish such as sardines keep your ticker healthy. That's why the American Heart Association recommends digging in to fat-rich fish twice a week. Their omega-3s are the stars: They give elasticity to arteries, lower triglycerides, raise levels of good cholesterol, and help beat disease-causing inflammation. Omega-3s may also reduce anxiety and improve brain function.

2. *Sardines are the perfect see-food.* Omega-3s' anti-inflammatory powers may protect against vision loss as you get older. And DHA, one specific fatty acid, plays a structural role in the retina. Women who consumed one or more servings of fish per week were 42 percent less likely to develop age-related macular degeneration, according to researchers at Harvard University.

3. *You'll build your bones and protect your joints.* The calcium in the fish works to strengthen bones, and omega-3s tamp down in-

---

SURPRISE! SARDINES ARE A SUPER GREEN SUPERFOOD

As if sardines' incredible fat-fighting and health-promoting powers weren't impressive enough, sardines are one of the least contaminated seafood options available. And those caught in the Pacific and Indian Oceans are among the most eco-friendly. Because they mature quickly, breed several times per year, have a relatively short life span, and eat a plankton diet (that is, marine organisms, not other fish), sardines aren't exposed to as much mercury and pollutants (like PCBs) as big swimmers such as tuna and swordfish.

Clean Sardines in Three Steps

Your fishmonger can do this for you, but if you want to try it your-self, here's how:

1. Remove the scales. Place the fish in a bowl of cold water and gently rub off the scales with your fingers.
2. Clean inside. Slice the fish lengthwise along the belly, then pull out and discard the innards with your fingers. Rinse well under cold water. The bones are edible—and a major source of the fish's calcium—so you don't need to remove them.
3. Prep for cooking. Because the fish are small and delicate, re-moving the head and attempting to fillet can be messy and leave you with a mangled piece, so cook sardines intact. (Skin and heads are edible, remember!) Brush with olive oil, season with salt and pepper, then grill, broil, bake, or pan-fry.

flammation associated with arthritis, helping to alleviate joint pain, tenderness, and morning stiffness. The calcium comes from the bones in sardines, which are tiny and soft. (Even canned brands touted as "boneless" offer a big calcium hit because they still have teeny, barely perceptible bones in them.)

4. *Your skin may get softer and smoother.* Omega-3s work to hydrate lipid-starved skin from the inside by helping to seal in moisture and soothe inflammation that can result from dryness. Plus, their anti-inflammatory action may fight wrinkle-causing free radicals.

Get Keen on Sardines

Both canned and fresh sardines will help you shed weight. Don't miss out! Forget what you think you know about sardines—that they're too fishy, salty, or slimy—and read on.

Why You Should Try Canned Sardines

- You can tone down their flavor. Yes, canned sardines may taste and smell a bit more like, well, fish than other seafood you're used to, but they're not as fishy as you might think. Peel open a can of sardines packed in water (their fishiness is less pronounced), and sniff for yourself! If the taste or smell is a turnoff, however, soak them in milk for an hour; the fishiness will disappear.

- They're a tummy-trimming alternative to tuna. Precooked and ready to eat, canned sardines aren't that different from other canned fish. Rinse them under cool water (to get rid of excess salt), mix them with chopped onion and bell peppers, then eat them on whole-grain crackers or spoon them over whole-grain bread. Or add a slice of Cheddar and broil for a tasty sandwich melt. You can also mix them into marinara. Their taste is surprisingly similar to that of tuna.

- You can't beat the price. Considering their diet prowess, nutrient value, and eco-friendliness, at around $2 per 3.75-ounce can, these babies may be one of the best health bargains in the supermarket.

- Or the convenience. They have a long shelf life, so if you keep a few cans in the cupboard, you'll always have a protein-packed, fat-torching meal option at the ready.

Buying tip: Opt for canned sardines packed in water rather than oil (to keep your calorie intake low), and look for those with the least amount of sodium. (You should still rinse before using.)

Why You'll Like Fresh Sardines

- There's nothing "fishy" about them. The freshest fish, including sardines, don't actually smell like the docks after a hot day; rather, they should smell only slightly briny. That said, if your "fresh" fish stinks, skip it. And even though sardines, which are about 8 inches long when sold fresh, do have a stronger seafood flavor than many other types of fish, they taste a lot milder than you might think.

- You'll get a bargain. Although not as cheap as canned, compared with some other options at the fish counter, sardines are a value. Don't be put off by the fact that they're sold whole; ask your fishmonger to clean and prepare them for you or check out the steps above.

WANT TO EAT MORE SARDINES STARTING TODAY?

Use canned sardines in recipes that call for anchovies, such as Caesar dressing. Or swap sardines for tuna when making a sandwich. Try this quick sammy recipe: Mix 1 can drained sardines with 1 tablespoon each chopped celery, chopped carrots, and low-fat mayo; 2 teaspoons chopped fresh parsley; and 1 teaspoon Dijon mustard. Serve between 2 slices whole-grain bread.

DON'T LIKE SARDINES?

Finely chopped, the fish hide well among the other bold fish flavors in a Manhattan clam chowder or seafood stew or a strong-tasting tomato-based pasta sauce such as puttanesca or arrabbiata.

- Sardines cook quickly. Once gutted, brush the whole fish with olive oil, season with salt and pepper, and throw them on the grill, under the broiler, or in the oven. Eat them whole or toss the meat with cherry tomatoes, chopped onion, olives, parsley, and a little olive oil. Sardines can also power up a simple whole-wheat pasta dish: Toss with garlic and olive oil and your favorite veggies.

→ **Buying Tip:** Look your sardines in the eyes. If their peepers are cloudy, dull, and sunken, the fish is probably bad. Eyes should be bright, the skin translucent, and the body firm.

sardine nutrition by

the numbers

140
calories per 3.75-ounce can of sardines in water

20
percent of your daily value of calcium (about 200 milligrams)

23
grams of protein

8
grams of total fat (5.5 grams unsaturated)

1
gram of omega-3 fatty acids

PROTEIN: THE METABOLISM-STOKING,
APPETITE-TAMING SUPERNUTRIENT

The phrase *high-protein diet* might bring to mind muscle-bound bodybuilders or that time you tried to go without carbs (shudder). A more accurate picture: You, only lighter and more toned, and a plate full of food such as eggs, fish, lean meat, and legumes, along with whole-grain pasta, brown rice, and veggies. In the real world, "high-protein" means getting 20 to 30 percent of your total daily calories from the nutrient (or 80 to 120 grams per day if you're following a 1,600-calorie diet), an amount research shows can jump-start weight loss and help you drop serious fat. The secret lies in protein's incredible pound-peeling properties. Here's what it can do for you:

- Sizzle an extra 100 calories per day. In order to break down the amino acids in protein-rich food, your body burns about double the calories it uses to digest fats and carbs. One study from Arizona State University in Mesa, for example, found that women who ate a diet consisting of 30 percent protein torched about 22 calories per hour after eating, compared with the 10 to 15 calories women on a low-protein diet burned (as measured 2½ hours after eating). That may not seem like a lot, but over the course of your day's eating, it could add up to an additional 100 or so calories—or about a pound in a month.

- Maintain metabolism-revving muscle. When you shed weight, you're not losing only fat. (We wish!) About 40 percent of those pounds can be traced to lean tissue, including lost muscle. Muscle, however, is what keeps your metabolism humming—it burns more calories while you're at rest than fat does. Feeding your body ample protein while dieting helps ensure your calorie-torching furnace burns hot. If you add in a strength-training workout or two each week, you'll stoke it even more. (Check out the moves in chapter 13 for ideas.)

- Flip off your hunger switch. Compared with carbs and fat, protein takes the top hunger-stifling spot. It may enhance the effect of leptin, a hormone that helps your body register fullness. Start incorporating protein into every meal and snack, and you're more likely to sail through the day without a growl from your stomach.
- Prevent the storage of excess belly fat. When you eat fast-digesting carbs, you get a spike in glucose and insulin, which can promote fat deposits, especially around your midsection. Eating protein along with those carbs helps temper this response, keeping blood sugar and insulin levels steady and you steadily burning.

How to Power Up Your Diet with Protein

- Pack it into every bite. Whether you're snacking on the go or sitting down to a proper meal, always include at least one protein-rich food. If you're not having a piece of fish or lean beef, for example, add hard-boiled egg whites, legumes, or edamame to salad or soup. If you're snacking on veggies and fruit, add a few nuts, a low-fat string cheese, or some yogurt, or whip up a protein-packed dip by mixing almond butter with yogurt.
- But don't go overboard. Only about the first 30 grams of protein you eat at each meal become muscle—any more than that could end up as fat. So when loading your plate, make sure you're also getting plenty of fiber from fruits, vegetables, and complex carbs, plus some unsaturated fat. Use this chart to help you keep track:

Superfood	Serving size	Grams of protein
Sardines	3.75-ounce can	23
Greek yogurt (nonfat)	1 cup	23
Flank steak	3½ ounces uncooked	21
Wild salmon	3 ounces uncooked	18

Lentils	1 cup cooked	18
Edamame	1 cup	17
Parmesan	1 ounce	10
Plain yogurt (nonfat)	1 cup	10
Pumpkin seeds	1 ounce (hulled)	9
Quinoa	1 cup cooked	8
Almond butter	2 tablespoons	7
Peanuts	1 ounce	7
Whole-wheat pasta	1 cup cooked	7

- Trim the fat. When choosing your main sources of protein, think lean to get lean—seafood, steak (check out page 166 for ideas), skinless white-meat chicken and turkey breast, eggs and egg whites, beans and lentils, edamame and tofu, and low-fat dairy (cottage cheese, yogurt, and milk).
- Stock your kitchen. Keep your cupboards and fridge full of different sources of protein that you can easily add to meals. Fish, poultry, and steak freeze well, and you'll typically find edamame only in the freezer section. Eggs can stay fresh in the fridge for at least three weeks. Canned wild salmon, canned beans, and quinoa are all good options, too. Some stores also sell vacuum-sealed bags of precooked lentils to make adding protein to anything extra easy!

STEAK

The Slimming Story

Meat lovers, rejoice! Not only won't beefing up your diet with lean cuts of red meat cause you to pile on pounds, but you also might shed more than if you avoided beef altogether. We're not advocating a steak dinner every night, but dining on a modest portion two or three times per week is one of the best ways to take in quality protein and iron, two nutrients that can make a big difference in determining your weight loss success.

Studies routinely find that when people are dieting, consuming 20 to 30 percent of their calorie allotment from protein leads to greater weight loss or fat loss than lower intakes do. It's no wonder: Protein is incredibly filling, helping you feel satiated on fewer calories and controlling hunger later, too. It also works to keep blood sugar and insulin from spiking, which over time can lead to excess fat, particularly around the middle. You'll rev up your metabolism as well; your body burns through about 25 calories to digest 100 calories of protein versus only 10 to 15 calories for the same amount of carbs and fat. What's more, protein is a must for maintaining muscle mass while dieting. And the more lean muscle you've got, the more calories you burn simply sitting still.

Thanks to the iron in steak, you may even be more jazzed to hit the gym, where you'll build more metabolism-stoking muscle. Red blood cells use the mineral to carry oxygen to the body's various organs, helping to give you energy. Between 9 and 16 percent of women are anemic, but many more may be iron-deficient, a milder condition that nonetheless can leave you dragging. You take in iron from plants, too, but your body absorbs it more readily from animal sources such as steak. So even though a 4-ounce serving provides only about 2 milligrams of your daily 18-milligram needs, it's substantial.

The Amazing Proof

- Women on a diet that included red meat lost more weight than those eating equal calories but little beef, reports a study published in *The American Journal of Clinical Nutrition*.
- Overweight people who regularly consumed meals consisting of about 30 percent protein improved their ability to burn fat, a study in the journal *Nutrition & Dietetics* shows.
- Researchers from the University of Illinois at Urbana-Champaign find that women on a low-calorie, 30 percent protein diet who walked for thirty minutes five times a week and logged two strength-training sessions weekly dropped more than 21 pounds after four months and lost fat mass, while a group that got the same amount of exercise but ate less protein shed only 14 pounds and less fat.

Three More Reasons to Eat Steak

1. *You'll snag all the benefits of B vitamins.* Eating steak delivers hefty doses of niacin and vitamins B_6 and B_{12}, as well as good amounts of the other B vitamins, all of which are critical for energy production and for healthy skin, hair, and eyes.
2. *You could strengthen your immune system.* Lean beef is one of your best sources of zinc, a mineral as important to your immune system as sleep and vitamin C! A mild to moderate deficiency could inhibit your body's normal defenses, whereas adequate levels ensure your immune cells can actively attack troublesome bugs.
3. *Steak may encourage clear, healthy skin.* The zinc in steak could also help regulate skin's oil production and your body's inflammatory response to acne, and its hefty niacin content (20 percent of your day's quota!) encourages smooth skin. The B vitamin niacin also helps defend against wrinkle-causing UV rays and environmental stress.

Steak Your Claim to Weight Loss

Beef's protein works to peel off pounds as long as you choose the leanest, healthiest types. Indulging too often in fatty cuts or greasy burgers, how-

ever, could tip the scale in the wrong direction. Use this advice to trim
the fat in more ways than one.

- Consider the cut. There are lots of different lean cuts of beef
  (meaning those with less than 10 grams of total fat and 4½ grams
  saturated fat per 3½-ounce serving), but in general, round and sir-
  loin steaks are lowest. Tenderloin (aka filet mignon) and flank
  steak are also good choices. If you need help choosing the best lean
  cut for what you're cooking, ask your butcher.
- Make the grade. When shopping, you'll encounter three different
  grades of beef, which indicate the amount of marbling (fat) the cut
  contains. Prime has the most, choice has less, and select has the
  least, so pick select cuts if possible; they have fewer calories and
  fat, and they won't lighten your wallet as much as the others—a
  win-win!
- Go for grass-fed. Beef labeled "grass-fed" comes from cows that
  graze in a pasture (their natural diet) versus those that eat
  grain-based feed. Their green diet results in meat with less saturated fat and more slimming, unsaturated fats; so if this pricier
  option fits in your budget, it's worth it to your waistline. Grass-fed
  (and local organic) beef is also better for the environment.
- Lose the lard. Before cooking your cut of steak, use kitchen scis-
  sors or a sharp knife to trim off visible fat along the edges. Or ask
  the butcher to do it for you.
- Pick a sound ground. If you're making meat sauce, chili, meat
  loaf, or burgers, choose ground beef with labels touting "92 percent lean" (or as high a percentage as you can find). Although "80
  percent lean" might sound like a diet-friendly choice, it means
  you're taking in 20 percent fat. Concerned that your meat loaf
  may be dry or crumbly? Beef with 8 to 10 percent fat (along with
  the eggs and whatever else your recipe calls for) should still be
  enough to keep it moist, especially if you add ground pork, as
  some recipes call for. (Give our loaf recipe on page 282 a try. It
  sneaks in extra veggies that also add moisture.)
- Hit the deli to slim your belly. Don't feel like firing up the grill or
  stove? Roast beef cold cuts typically come from top rounds, mak-

ing them a diet-friendly option for sandwiches. Ask at the deli counter for the leanest, freshest variety that's also lowest in sodium.

Ready to Start Cooking? You've Got Options!

1. *Grilling.* This method makes for a delicious, quick meal; it's best for more tender cuts of steak like flank and filet mignon. Avoid charring your meat, and keep flare-ups in check; both may be linked to a higher cancer risk. If you can, cook your meat a little to the side on your grill rather than directly over the flame.

WHERE'S THE BEEF?

A standard portion of steak, according to the USDA, is 3 ounces—about the size of a deck of cards when uncooked. That's not much, and cooking shrinks it down even more. If the thought of downsizing your dinner that much is disappointing, feel free to serve up a larger 5-ounce portion, which runs about 196 calories, and limit your intake to no more than twice a week. If even that amount seems slight, try these tips for a meatier-seeming meal:

- Chart it out. Think of your plate as a pie chart. Let your serving of steak make up about 25 percent, then fill up 50 percent with veggies and fruits and 25 percent with a fiber-rich side dish (try a whole-grain salad like quinoa or lentils) to get a full—and filling—plate for both your stomach and your senses.
- Slice to slim. Rather than serving up one small piece of steak and a side or two, cut your portion into strips or bite-size pieces and incorporate it into a veggie-loaded dish like steak fajitas or steak salad. Add beans for extra protein and fiber.
- Stack the deck. Grill up steak kebabs! But instead of having only one or two that have mostly meat and just a few veggies, load four or five skewers with mostly veggies and only two cubes of steak each. Serve with greens and lentils, quinoa, or brown rice.

2. *Broiling.* This method is similar to grilling, so consider broiling on cold days you don't want to go outside to the grill. Season with salt and pepper before placing your meat under the heat.

3. *Pan-frying or stir-frying.* Flank steak cooks in a flash in a pan or wok. And although "frying" is a dirty word in the diet world, you won't up the fat content of your meal as long as you use vegetable oil cooking spray instead of a large amount of oil or butter.

4. *Roasting.* Choose this technique for larger roasts and less tender cuts such as top round. Set your beef on a rack in a roasting pan, which allows the fat to drip off. Cook at 450 degrees for 10 to 15 minutes to seal in flavor, then turn your oven down to 350 degrees and roast until done.

5. *Slow cooking.* Don't want to babysit your beef? Tougher cuts (which are often leanest) and large roasts turn extra tender after a day in a slow cooker.

WANT TO EAT MORE STEAK STARTING TODAY?

Power up your salad with steak: Top 2 cups arugula with 3 ounces cooked, sliced flank steak, 2 medium steamed beets (cut into wedges), 1/4 cup reduced-fat feta cheese, and 1 tablespoon chopped walnuts. For dressing, mix 1 tablespoon orange juice, 1 teaspoon Dijon mustard, 1 teaspoon olive oil, and 1 teaspoon white wine vinegar. Drizzle over salad.

DON'T LIKE STEAK?

Use equal amounts of ground beef and ground turkey when preparing burgers, meatballs, and meat loaf. Or slip lean ground beef into casseroles, chili, or stew.

steak nutrition by the numbers

137

calories per 3½ ounces (uncooked) of lean flank steak

21

grams of protein

5

grams of total fat

2

grams of saturated fat

. . . .
WILD SALMON
. . . .

The Slimming Story

If you're not already hooked on this star of the sea, it's sure to lure you in after you read this! Although best known for its ability to keep your heart healthy and brain sharp, salmon (including lox) is awash in body-trimming benefits that will have you swimming in a two-piece suit before you know it. Yep, even though it's a so-called fatty fish, salmon, with its omega-3 fatty acids, could help your body burn flab more effectively. The fats alter the expression of certain genes, shifting your body to burn fat rather than store it. Plus, the micronutrients may increase levels of the hormone adiponectin, a key regulator of metabolism, fat oxidation (aka fat burning), and appetite. Omega-3s may also make you more sensitive to insulin, the hormone responsible for moving sugar from your blood and into cells, which burn it for energy, possibly helping to reduce belly fat.

Salmon's healthy fats work with its protein load—you take in 18 grams per 3 ounces—to keep you feeling full, so you can cut calories sans hunger. Omega-3s and protein also help you maintain muscle, which, because muscle burns more calories than fat, keeps your metabolism humming. Protein itself encourages extra calorie burning in a different way, too; you sizzle through more while simply digesting it than you do other nutrients.

Vitamin D is another key weight loss helper you'll net from salmon. Having higher levels of the nutrient may help you lose weight more efficiently. Although experts aren't entirely sure why, they speculate that the vitamin sets up a roadblock for hormones that would otherwise encourage your body to produce and hang on to fat rather than burn it.

The Amazing Proof

- In a study analyzing the diets of thirty-five thousand women published in *Public Health Nutrition*, those who ate oily fish such as salmon two to four times per week had the lowest basal metabolic indexes, a common measure of body fat.

- Overweight subjects who consumed fish oil supplements daily (containing the equivalent amount of omega-3s in a 5-ounce fillet of wild salmon) and walked three days a week for forty-five minutes shed about 3½ pounds of fat over twelve weeks, whereas those taking a placebo lost very little, a study from the University of South Australia reports.
- Researchers at the University of Minnesota in Minneapolis find that the higher a person's levels of vitamin D at the start of a reduced-calorie diet program, the more weight and abdominal fat she lost after eleven weeks.

One More Major Reason to Eat Salmon

It keeps you healthy head to toe, inside and out.

Only 36 percent of people eat fish regularly, yet adding fish to your plate two or three times per week is one of the smartest decisions you can make. Oceans of studies link its high content of omega-3 fatty acids and other nutrients with a lower risk for heart disease, heart attack, stroke, cancer, and vision problems. Omega-3s may also help alleviate depression, anxiety, arthritis, dry skin, and more.

Go Wild for Salmon!

When shopping for fresh salmon, your best bet by far is wild Alaskan (sometimes called Pacific), which is low in contaminants and hailed as one of the world's best-managed fish from an environmental perspective. Atlantic salmon, on the other hand, is endangered in the wild, so you will find only the farmed variety at supermarkets. Raised from eggs in pens set up in the ocean, farmed salmon sounds like a good solution to overfishing in theory, but in practice it's a different story.

At aquafarms, pens can crowd in up to a million fish, and the close quarters may lead to outbreaks of bacteria and sea lice. As a result, some farms use large doses of antibiotics, which may contribute to antibiotic resistance. The salmon are also typically fed food pellets made of fish further up the food chain, and they may contain high levels of pollutants linked to cancer, such as PCBs and dioxins. In fact, farmed salmon could contain as much as five times the chemical load of a wild Alaskan fillet. And because they don't eat the krill that give wild salmon its pinky-orange hue, farm-raised fish are actually off-white. They get their coloring from chemicals.

Salmon farmers stand by the safety of their practices and the healthfulness of their fish, but unless you know where your fish comes from and the operations of the farm—U.S. products are typically better than imports—there's no way to know what, besides omega-3s and other nutrients, your fish contains. Unfortunately, fresh wild salmon can be expensive. If the cost is out of your budget, you have two options. First, try wild salmon in a can or pouch, both of which you'll find for a fraction of the price of fresh fish. Like tuna, it's precooked and ready to eat, making it a good choice for salads, salmon burgers, and pasta dishes. Or, if you'll eat only the fresh stuff, many experts say you're better off eating the domestically farmed fish than none at all; salmon is so good for you (and your waistline) that the benefits outweigh the risks.

Feel Like a Fish Out of Water When It Comes to Seafood?

Before you dive into cooking salmon, follow these tips for choosing and storing your catch of the day.

At the Fish Counter

- Get fresh. Some markets get salmon deliveries daily, others only once or twice per week. Ask your fishmonger what days a new batch arrives and try to shop then.
- Be cool. Make sure the fish is splayed out on a thick bed of fresh, not half-melted, ice.
- Check the hue. Look for fillets that are bright, glistening, and firm to the touch. If one is dull or brown around the edges, move on.
- Sniff out what's good. The freshest picks are nearly odorless save for a slight briny aroma. If you detect a strong smell, something's fishy. Skip it.

In Your Kitchen

- Cook it quickly. Kept in the fridge, fresh fish will last only a day or two. If you aren't making your salmon right away, it freezes well.
- Freeze out freezer burn. If you spy a sale, buy one or a few large fillets, slice them into 3- to 5-ounce portions, and freeze them. To thwart ice crystals, wrap fillets in plastic wrap first, then place in a plastic freezer bag. If you cook for one, wrap fillets individually; otherwise, wrap your family's portions together.
- Don't stress if you don't want to eat the skin (it may harbor traces of PCBs and mercury). If you buy salmon with the skin still on, cook it that way. Removing it from raw fish can be tough, and you may end up wasting a lot of the meat. After it's cooked, however, salmon skin peels off easily.

Banish Salmon Boredom

A broiled or grilled piece of salmon is simple to make and simply delicious, but it's easy to get stuck in a rut. Don't be afraid to get creative or use the fish in place of other types of protein in your favorite recipes—it's as versatile as chicken.

WANT TO EAT MORE SALMON STARTING TODAY?

Join the salmon club! Pan-fry a 3-ounce piece of fish in 1 teaspoon olive oil. Stack with 1 slice cooked turkey bacon, 2 slices tomato, 2 teaspoons light mayonnaise, and romaine between 1 whole-grain bun.

DON'T LIKE SALMON?

Consider buying smoked salmon; its flavor disguises some of the fishiness. Slip it into a cooked dish with bold flavors, such as an omelet with veggies and feta cheese, and you're less likely to notice you're eating seafood!

Here are a few ideas to get you thinking beyond the fillet:

- Go crazy for kebabs. Buy a center-cut piece of salmon, which is the thickest part, and cut it into cubes. Marinate for an hour in olive oil infused with citrus juice or herbs (dill is delish), then load up skewers with the fish and your favorite veggies. Grill 4 minutes on each side.
- Have a bowl. Salmon makes a tasty, tummy-trimming addition to vegetable chowders and bisques. Add cubed, raw salmon to simmering soup 5 minutes before serving; it will cook in the liquid.
- Be a burger queen. Chop raw salmon and mix with soy sauce and diced onion in a bowl. Stir in egg whites and whole-wheat bread crumbs until you get a texture you can mold into patties. Grill 3 minutes on each side.
- Create a slimming slice. Salmon can perk up homemade pizza. Cover a whole-wheat pizza crust with marinara sauce and part-skim mozzarella. Cook as directed on the crust's package, adding small pieces of canned salmon a few minutes before it's done.
- Use your noodle. Combine diced raw salmon with a small amount of olive oil, lemon juice, and salt and pepper, then toss with just-drained whole-grain pasta. The heat of the noodles flash-cooks the fish in seconds.
- Pick a lox. Use finely sliced smoked salmon (also known as lox) as you would lunch meat in sandwiches. Spread a little low-fat cream cheese on whole-grain bread, stack with lox, red onion, tomato, and lettuce.

wild salmon nutrition

by the numbers

124
calories per 3-ounce fillet (uncooked)

18
grams of protein

5
grams of total fat

3.5
grams of unsaturated fat

1.3
grams of omega-3 fatty acids

7 Super Eggs and Dairy

The Slimming Story

Take a crack at eating more eggs. Yep, no longer the fat- and cholesterol-raising bad-health bombs people once thought they were, these little guys—yolks and all—are powerful partners in your quest to get lean. Their most important function: helping you conquer hunger. Eggs' high-quality protein (one egg packs 6 grams) makes them incredibly filling for a mere 72 calories each. In fact, eat eggs in the a.m. and not only will they curb your appetite until your next meal, but they'll also fill you up enough so you take in fewer calories the rest of the day, research shows.

Even better, eggs also trigger your body to burn more calories, because protein requires more fuel to digest than carbs or fat do. Protein is also vital for building and maintaining lean muscle, which revs up your metabolism. And eggs help prevent the spikes in blood sugar and insulin that promote fat storage.

We didn't have to scramble to find a few more reasons to recommend eggs. They are loaded with choline, a compound that blocks fat absorption and breaks down fatty deposits, and is one of the few natural sources of vitamin D, adequate levels of which may help you drop weight more easily. Plus, you'll get more of the hunger-taming unsaturated fat than the heart-harming saturated kind. To top it off, they're easy to prepare, versatile, and *cheap-cheap-cheap*!

→ **Trim-down tip:** Both yolks and whites contain protein, but the yolks are higher in calories. If you're trying to cut back, use one whole egg and two egg whites when making an omelet or an egg sandwich. (An egg white has a mere 17 calories.)

The Amazing Proof

- After eight weeks, dieters who ate two scrambled eggs, toast, and jelly for breakfast five days a week lost 65 percent more weight and 16 percent more body fat and had a waist that was 34 percent trimmer than those who had a bagel breakfast with the same number of calories but no eggs, according to a study in the *International Journal of Obesity*.

Hatch a Plan to Fit Eggs into Your Diet

Eating eggs in the a.m. is the most obvious way to dine on the fat fighters, but there are dozens of ways to sneak more egg protein onto your plate. Check out these fresh ideas.

- Snack: Hard-boiled eggs are a perfect on-the-run snack. In their shell, they'll stay fresh in the fridge for up to a week.
- Lunch: Slip slices of hard-boiled egg into any sandwich, or make a fried egg the main event. Fry using vegetable oil cooking spray, then stack your egg between two slices of whole-wheat toast along with your favorite veggies and a slice of cheese.
- Dinner: Toss a poached egg with whole-wheat pasta, olive oil, and veggies, or serve one sunny-side up over salad.

WANT TO EAT MORE EGGS STARTING TODAY?

Eggs tame your appetite no matter when you crack 'em. But because people tend to skimp on protein when they're in a rush in the morning—which can lead to more intense snack attacks later in the day—it's a good idea to make a batch of hard-boiled on Sunday and grab one to go every day on your way out the door.

DON'T LIKE EGGS?

Eggs don't have to take center stage on your plate for you to harness their slimming superpowers. Sneak them into your diet by eating egg-containing recipes such as whole-grain crepes, pancakes, waffles, and muffins (check out the recipes on pages 262–263), plus meat loaf (recipe on page 282) and burgers (see page 283).

- Overweight women who ate two eggs in the morning consumed 163 fewer calories at lunch and fewer calories over the next thirty-six hours than they did when they ate a breakfast consisting of the same number of calories but no eggs, a study in the *Journal of the American College of Nutrition* reports.

Four More Reasons to Eat Eggs

1. *They won't harm your heart.* Yes, eggs are high in dietary cholesterol, but research suggests that eating eggs may not necessarily raise cholesterol levels in your blood, nor is egg consumption linked with an increased risk for heart disease, except among people with diabetes. So unless your doctor tells you otherwise, feel free to have a whole egg a day. Want more? Add all the egg whites you want!

2. *Eggs are a beauty superfood, too.* Add eggs to your plate and you'll net multiple nutrients that feed your skin, hair, and nails, including ample amounts of complexion-smoothing vitamin A and the

B vitamin biotin, which keeps skin moisturized and calm and promotes healthy hair and nails. You also get a dose of hydrating vitamin E.

3. *Your future eyes will look bright.* Egg yolks contain lutein and zeaxanthin, two carotenoids that act as antioxidants to promote eye health and guard against age-related vision loss.

4. *They help with hangovers.* Having a hard time seeing the sunny side of anything after a night out? Beat a path to the egg carton: Eggs are rich in the amino acid cysteine, a substance that breaks down acetaldehyde, a toxin in alcohol that can lead to hangovers. Bring on brunch!

Find a Good Egg

It won't matter to your waistline what type you buy—getting the hunger-squashing protein and nutrients is what matters—but there are other factors to consider. Use this guide to decide what's best for you.

If you're on a tight budget: By all means, go for an inexpensive dozen. And pick white or brown, whichever you prefer; the shell color signals only a different breed of hen, not better quality, nutrition, taste, or anything else.

If you have grocery bill wiggle room: Consider eggs enriched with omega-3 fatty acids. To produce them, farmers feed hens omega-3-rich flaxseed and/or other sources of the fatty acids. Although fortified eggs don't pack as much of the fat-fighting nutrients as fish—you'll find eggs with up to about 350 milligrams each, which is less than you get from an ounce of salmon—even a little extra may help you stay healthy.

If you're concerned about additives: Go organic. To qualify for that label, farmers feed hens a hormone-free, vegetarian diet and nothing else.

If animal welfare is a priority: Choose eggs from a small, local farm, or research the practices of companies that sell organic eggs. You might be tempted to look for the labels *cage-free* or *free-range,* but the definition of those terms isn't stringent when it comes to eggs, and the hens may not actually, as you might imagine, spend all day happily clucking outdoors.

egg nutrition by the numbers

72
calories per 1 large whole egg

17
calories per egg white

6
grams of protein per 1 large egg

5
grams of total fat
(3 grams unsaturated)

PARMESAN

The Slimming Story

Say cheese! You'll certainly want to take before and after pics of yourself if you add a little of this dairy dynamo to your diet. Parmesan has one of the highest amounts of calcium among cheeses: A 1-ounce serving delivers 336 milligrams—more than a cup of skim milk! That's enough to put you about one-third of the way toward optimal fat burning and seeing better results on the scale. Most women don't get the recommended 1,000 milligrams of calcium per day, and that insufficiency can trigger a rise in two hormones that not only impede fat burning, but actually tell your cells to store fat. An adequate level of calcium, on the other hand, especially if it comes from dairy, suppresses the double-trouble hormones, encouraging cells to release fat that your body then uses as fuel. Calcium also binds to a small portion of the fat in your gastrointestinal tract, saving you from absorbing some calories. The research is convincing: If you're low in calcium, upping your dairy intake will help you lose more weight if you're dieting or help you trade fat for lean muscle if you're not.

Parmesan is a big cheese in the diet world for a few other reasons, too. A 1-ounce serving packs 10 grams of protein—more than the same amount of chicken breast. As we've already noted, protein is the most satiating of all nutrients and burns more calories during digestion than either carbs or fat. But limit yourself to about an ounce of Parm a day—it does contain 111 calories and 7 grams of fat, after all. Don't be put off by that fat content, though: It helps you feel physically and emotionally full—you get to indulge in a food that's often a diet no-no. And it's a lot easier to be satisfied with smaller amounts of Parm than with blander cheeses, thanks to its strong and satisfying flavor.

→ **Trim-Down Tip:** Sensitive to lactose? You may still be able to eat Parmesan, because hard cheeses tend to have less. To test it out, sample a small amount and wait twenty minutes to see how you react.

The Amazing Proof

- Compared with those who ate less than a serving of dairy per day, overweight adults who consumed three servings daily (with about 1,200 milligrams of calcium total) dropped 4.8 pounds of body fat after twelve weeks without making any other changes to their diet, according to a study in *Obesity Research*.
- Women who ate an ounce of full-fat cheese a day gained significantly less weight over a nine-year period than those who didn't, a study in *The American Journal of Clinical Nutrition* finds.

Three More Reasons to Eat Parmesan

1. *It helps beef up bones.* Dietary calcium is your skeleton's best friend: Without it, your system starts stealing from the stockpile in your bones to maintain its tightly regulated blood levels. Take in at least 1,000 milligrams each day and you'll have enough to go around.
2. *Cheese keeps you smiling.* Calcium helps maintain the integrity of your teeth's enamel. Research shows people who get enough of the mineral are less likely to have severe gum disease.

The Grate Debate

Regardless of the brand or form you choose, Parmesan is rich in fat-trimming calcium, so buy whatever appeals to your taste buds and/or budget most. That said, if the cheese sprinkles from the pasta aisle are all you know, consider sampling the hunks of Parm in the dairy case or gourmet cheese section of the market. (If you do stick with sprinkles, check the ingredients list to be sure what you're buying is all cheese and not a lot of fillers.) Flavor varies widely, and a block of the fresh stuff or a container of the freshly shredded cheese will likely give you a richer, more satisfying taste for your calories. If you go with the block, you may still want to grate, shave, or shred it once you get home to make your 1-ounce portion appear more plentiful.

3. *You'll absorb more vitamins.* Several of your body's most important nutrients, including the antioxidant beta-carotene, are fat-soluble. Tossing an ounce of Parm into your spinach salad or sprinkling it over a baked sweet potato, for example, improves your uptake of the veggies' nutrients.

Become a Cheese Whiz in the Kitchen

Pasta isn't the only thing Parmesan pairs well with. Try these eating ideas:

- Melt in sandwiches. Parm is a slimming upgrade from the neon orange, rubbery varieties you may have been using.
- Make a fat-fighting fondue. Nuke 1 ounce shredded Parm, ½ cup low-fat (1 percent or 2 percent) milk, and 1 tablespoon Dijon mustard. Dip in broccoli, sliced bell peppers, or other favorite veggies.

WANT TO EAT MORE PARMESAN STARTING TODAY?

Dress up a salad with two superfoods: Mix 1 tablespoon grated Parmesan with 2 tablespoons nonfat plain yogurt, 1 tablespoon lemon juice, and fresh dill to taste; drizzle over greens.

DON'T LIKE PARMESAN?

Swap Parm for other cheese in sandwiches, wraps, quiches, and omelets—anywhere stronger flavors tend to prevail, such as this roast beef on rye sammy: Mix 1 tablespoon light mayo with 1 teaspoon horseradish; spread on 2 slices rye bread; place 3 ounces lean roast beef, 2 slices tomato, 1 ounce thinly sliced Parmesan, and ¼ cup greens between bread.

- Swap for salt. With all its nutrients, this cheese is a perfect partner for cooked veggies. Pass the Parm!
- Stir into soup. You'll love the creamy, sharp flavor Parmesan adds to a bowl of minestrone, French onion, tomato, or lentil soup.
- Supercharge your snack. Eat thin slices or shavings with an apple or pear to complement the sweetness.

Parmesan nutrition
by the numbers

336
milligrams of calcium per ounce of Parmesan

111
calories

10
grams of protein

7
grams of fat

YOGURT

The Slimming Story

You're gonna have a cow when you hear about everything this nutritionists' dream food can do for you! Shall we start with helping you sizzle serious fat? An 8-ounce serving of plain, low-fat, and nonfat yogurt packs 400 to 500 milligrams of calcium—almost half of your day's quota of the mineral, which makes yogurt a gold mine when you consider that most of us don't get enough calcium to meet our body's needs. When your calcium intake is low, your body assumes you're undernourished and releases a pair of hormones to regulate levels of the mineral. Unfortunately, these hormones also encourage your system to store fat while hampering your ability to burn it. When you do get enough (1,000 to 1,300 milligrams per day), however, those hormones halt their diet sabotage and you burn fat efficiently.

Calcium also hooks up with dietary fat in your gut, preventing the absorption of a small portion of the calories you eat. Plus, the mineral slows down fat cells' production of cortisol, a hormone that encourages flab buildup in the belly.

If you're tempted to pop a calcium supplement, consider this: Dairy sources like yogurt produce better results. Why? By eating yogurt, you also take in tons of body-trimming whey protein. Like any protein-rich food, yogurt is incredibly filling; gives you a calorie-burning boost after eating; helps to steady insulin levels, thwarting fat storage; and provides the building blocks for metabolism-enhancing muscle. But yogurt's whey has a special edge: It delivers more of the amino acid leucine than other commonly eaten protein sources, sending fat cells a signal to release their lipids (aka fat), which your muscles then use for fuel.

→ **Trim-Down Tip:** Check nutrition labels and opt for yogurt fortified with vitamin D. Higher levels of D may enhance weight loss by encouraging your body to let go of fat stores so you can burn them for energy. Plus, vitamin D helps your body absorb calcium.

The Amazing Proof

- People on a low-calorie diet that included yogurt lost 61 percent more fat overall and 81 percent more belly fat than those on a similar eating plan but without yogurt, according to a study from the University of Tennessee in Knoxville.

→ **Trim-Down Tip:** Don't dump the watery layer that settles on the top of a carton of yogurt—that's the fat-fighting whey protein! Stir it in instead.

- Subjects who ate a breakfast rich in calcium (543 milligrams, or slightly more than the amount in a cup of low-fat plain yogurt) and vitamin D (8.7 micrograms, or about 58 percent of your daily quota; check yogurt labels to see how much yours contains) increased postmeal fat burning by 75 percent, compared with those who dined on a meal lower in the two nutrients, a study in the *European Journal of Clinical Nutrition* reports. The calcium group also consumed fewer calories later that same day and the following day.
- Women who increased their calcium intake to about 1,000 milligrams per day by eating dairy saw a greater increase in postmeal fat burning after one year than those who took in less than 800 milligrams, researchers at Purdue University find.

Four More Reasons to Eat Yogurt

1. *Its healthy bacteria help beat bad bugs.* Most manufacturers add probiotics to yogurt—microorganisms that join up with the good bacteria in your body and help strengthen your defenses against germs that can cause colds, flus, and diarrhea. They also keep your digestive system healthy overall and may lower your risk for gum disease and some cancers.
2. *You'll strengthen your bones.* Aside from serious fat frying, dairy's calcium fortifies bones, helping to prevent fractures and warding off osteoporosis. Milk gets all the attention, but yogurt actually has more calcium per serving.

3. *You could help control your blood pressure.* A review of studies by researchers at Monash University in Clayton, Australia, confirms that consuming two or more servings of low-fat dairy a day is linked to a reduced risk for high blood pressure. Dairy is rich in multiple nutrients that likely play a role, including calcium, magnesium, and potassium, as well as peptides (small, proteinlike compounds), in preventing the constriction of blood vessels.

4. *Yogurt may give you a preperiod lift.* The calcium and vitamin D in D-fortified yogurt could keep you smiling in the days before your period. PMS sufferers who took both nutrients daily had the same improvement in mood and lessening of anxiety as those taking a hormone used to treat the condition, a study in the *International Journal of Gynecology & Obstetrics* reports.

The Scoop on Yogurt

Believe it or not, many of the yogurt cups stacked in the dairy case are more akin nutrition-wise to dessert than to a superfood for weight loss. Here's how to choose one to help you lose:

- Think plain and slimming. If you're used to flavored yogurt, switch to plain and add your own enhancements. Fruit varieties

---

Lovin' Spoonfuls

Yogurt is so versatile, there are countless tasty ways to eat and use it. Check out these ideas and let them spark your own culinary creativity:

- Experiment with toppings. Fresh or dried fruit, nuts, seeds, honey—you've got options! Why not try something new every day for a week?
- Spoon on flavor. Yogurt itself makes a tasty topping. Add a dollop of plain to oatmeal, chili, soup, or a baked potato.
- Blend for your belly. Making a smoothie? Use nonfat yogurt instead of skim milk to take in more fat-blasting calcium.

often contain added sugar (and calories) and have less calcium, because the yogurt has to share carton space.

- Be on sugar patrol. Even plain varieties can contain added sugar. Yogurt naturally has about 12 grams per 6 ounces, so check ingredients lists to ensure you're not getting any extra.
- Face the fat. Whether you go for nonfat or low-fat is a matter of personal taste. Both can help you trim down, although you'll save an extra 10 to 20 calories by picking the former.
- Get the best of both worlds. Greek yogurt is thicker and tangier than regular and could contain about twice the filling protein, too. The catch: It has less calcium. Because both nutrients help you shed weight, try alternating between the two varieties.
- Love bugs. Probiotics are the health-promoting bacteria added to yogurt, but not all brands have high levels. Look on labels for the phrase *live and active cultures,* or seek out the National Yogurt Association's Live & Active Cultures seal.
- Know fro yo. Frozen yogurt is an ideal skinny treat, but it's not your best source for all the slimming nutrients described in this chapter. Enjoy it now and then, but don't think of it as a superfood.

WANT TO EAT MORE YOGURT STARTING TODAY?

Yogurt's taste and creamy texture make it the perfect pound-peeling swap for fatty sour cream and mayonnaise. Go half and half or make a direct trade with mayo in potato, chicken, egg, or tuna salads; and use yogurt for sour cream in Mexican dishes and dips. (Because Greek yogurt is thicker, it tends to work best.)

DON'T LIKE YOGURT?

Trim the fat from homemade baked goods and get more flab-fighting calcium by using yogurt instead of oil. Try the recipe for Whole-Wheat Blueberry Pancakes with Three-Berry Compote on page 262.

yogurt nutrition by the numbers

110
calories per cup of nonfat plain yogurt

40
percent of your daily value of calcium

25
percent of your daily value of vitamin D in fortified yogurt

10
grams of protein

Greek yogurt nutrition by the numbers

130
calories per cup of nonfat plain Greek yogurt

25
percent of your daily value of calcium

23
grams of protein

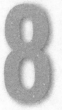

8 Super Tasty Extras

COFFEE

The Slimming Story

The perks of coffee extend well beyond shaking off a.m. grogginess; raising a mug of caffeinated joe could help lower your weight. The caffeine in a cup of coffee increases your resting metabolic rate, the calories your body burns throughout the day to keep its systems humming, by up to 15 percent. What's more, that boost seems to last a good three to four hours. For the average woman, that means about 25 calories a day off the books. Although that number might seem like small beans, it adds up to as many as 2½ pounds lost per year. From drinking coffee! Have two cups—one in the morning and another at least four hours later for two separate spikes in metabolism (more caffeine in a sitting may not mean a higher calorie burn)—and you could trim 5 pounds by next year without making any other changes to your eating routine.

Along with calories, you could burn more fat, too. The caffeine in coffee seems to activate metabolic pathways that trigger cells to let go of stored fat, allowing you to use it for fuel. Java's peppy partner seems to block signals of muscle fatigue and discomfort during exercise, which means both cardio and strength training feel easier. In other words, if you sip before your sweat session, you'll probably work out harder and longer—sizzling a good chunk of extra calories in the process. What's more, caffeine may also block the body's receptors for adenosine, a chemical that causes postexercise achiness. Should next-day muscle malaise cramp your style, coffee may ease it enough that you could at least get out for a walk. Brava, java!

→ **Trim-Down Tip:** If you know caffeinated coffee gives you the jitters or keeps you up at night, sip decaf. Although you may not see the metabolism or exercise benefits, the chlorogenic acid found in all types of coffee may help prevent insulin resistance, which is linked to obesity and diabetes.

The Amazing Proof

- Study subjects who consumed 50 milligrams of caffeine (the amount in half a cup of coffee) got a short-term boost in metabolism compared with those who took a placebo, according to researchers from the University of Copenhagen in Denmark.
- A study in *The American Journal of Clinical Nutrition* finds that women who increased their coffee consumption even by a little over the course of twelve years gained less weight than those who cut back on java.
- The day after stimulating their quadriceps (doing squats, for instance), women who consumed the amount of caffeine in two cups of joe felt 48 percent less leg pain within an hour, research from the University of Georgia reveals.

Four More Reasons to Drink Coffee

1. *It benefits your bean.* Coffee is a no-brainer for mental health. Caffeine helps you process information more quickly, potentially leading to fewer errors in your day-to-day life. It may also help ease headaches; it's associated with a lower risk for depression; and it may block inflammation linked to Alzheimer's disease.

Plus, the powerful antioxidants in coffee could reduce cell damage that may contribute to Parkinson's disease.

2. *The brew boosts heart health.* The antioxidants and acids in coffee may work together to soothe inflammation that damages your ticker, possibly leading to heart disease. But opt for drip coffee or espresso from a machine that uses paper pods: The filters catch cafestol, a lipid found in unfiltered coffee that might raise cholesterol.

3. *Coffee could help ward off cancer.* Phytoestrogens, antioxidant flavonoids, and other compounds in coffee may limit DNA damage and stifle the growth of cancer cells and tumors. Coffee has been linked to a lower risk for breast, oral, skin, brain, and pancreatic cancers.

4. *It could help you dodge diabetes.* Research suggests that people who down either regular or decaf coffee daily are less likely to develop type 2 diabetes. The chlorogenic acid in coffee might help prevent insulin resistance, a harbinger of the disease.

Harness Coffee's Power

Sipping is only a start! Here's how to achieve the biggest better-body bang from every cup:

- Go for basic black. It goes without saying that sugary syrups and whipped cream are enemies of your waistline, but you should also opt out of milk, especially the full-fat variety, and sugar. These additives may reverse the fat-torching benefits of your mug by causing insulin levels to rise. If you can't stomach your usual blend black, try a lighter roast, which is milder and may be easier to drink. Or add a splash of skim, and sip before hitting the gym—you'll still rev up your workout, if not calorie burning.

- Give espresso a shot. If you like espresso better than coffee, go ahead and sip it instead. (But do go for the filtered kind to protect your heart from cholesterol-raising compounds.) Espresso has about a third less caffeine than coffee does, however, so you may want to order a double shot to achieve coffee's full metabolism-boosting effect.

- Set your limit. Your body can build a tolerance to caffeine after only two or three cups, hindering its slimming benefits. Megajolts may also leave you jittery and unable to sleep and could increase levels of fat-promoting stress hormones. Aim to sip no more than a cup or two in a sitting and no more than about three cups a day. (And by cup, we mean 6 to 12 ounces, not the vase-size vessels coffee shops serve up.)

Coffee Talk

Whether you're a lifelong java fan or letting the idea of drinking more coffee percolate, these tips will help you brew a tasty pot:

- Know beans. The taste of coffee varies, depending on the bean's birthplace. Varieties grown in Africa, the Caribbean, Hawaii, and Mexico tend to give a lighter, less bitter flavor, whereas beans from

Labels to Look For

Coffee packages are sometimes stamped with logos that give you a hint about how the beans were grown and by whom. Here are three of the most common:

USDA organic. This emblem tags coffee grown using eco-friendly practices and without most conventional pesticides.

Fair Trade Certified. This black-and-white stamp indicates that coffee farmers received a competitive price for their goods and that a portion of the profits went on to fund projects such as schools in their communities.

Rainforest Alliance. The seal from this nonprofit organization means your beans grew on farms full of native trees rather than on a cleared plantation.

South and Central American countries produce a richer, fuller-bodied cup.

- Do the daily grind. Coffee gets its flavor from beans' delicate oils, which are released during grinding. They degrade quickly, though, so use freshly ground beans to make a tastier mug.

- Measure success. The standard ratio for drip coffee is 2 level tablespoons per 8 ounces of cold water, but experiment with more water or fewer grounds to find what works for you.

- Stay fresh. To avoid stale beans (and coffee that tastes like day-old dregs), keep your beans in an opaque, airtight container away from heat and light. They'll last up to three weeks.

Caffeine Caution

For all its benefits, when it comes to coffee, you can have too much of a good thing. Pay attention to a few warnings if you fall into any of the following categories:

If you're new to coffee: Buying your brew at a café can give you more caffeine than you bargained for. A cup of Starbucks joe, for example, can

WANT TO DRINK MORE COFFEE STARTING TODAY?

Double up daily. Start your morning with a cup, then pour another around lunchtime or in the early afternoon to get a second spike in metabolism, keeping your calorie burn high all day. If you're already drinking two cups a day, you probably don't need more but should space them out for maximum benefits.

DON'T LIKE COFFEE?

Sip green tea. You'll take in about a third of the caffeine per cup, but you'll get a dose of catechins, compounds that may give you an extra calorie-burning boost. They're in decaffeinated tea as well, so if you're sensitive to caffeine, it's a good option.

have double the kick you'd get from a home brew. That extra could leave newbies feeling more panicky than perky. If you're unsure of how you'll react, start with a half-caf.

If you have trouble sleeping: The caffeine in a cup of coffee is thought to lose its oomph after about five hours, but the more caffeine you take in, the longer it takes your body to flush it out. If you find yourself counting sheep rather than sawing logs, stick to caffeinated in the a.m. only, then go decaf after noon.

If you have type 2 diabetes: Although coffee could help lower your risk for the disease, once you've got it, limiting caffeine is a good idea. Talk to your doctor about what's safe for you.

*coffee nutrition by
the numbers*

330

milligrams of caffeine per 16-ounce serving of
Starbucks Pike Place Roast

95

milligrams of caffeine in an 8-ounce cup of home-brewed coffee

2

milligrams of caffeine in an 8-ounce cup of decaffeinated coffee;
there's a small amount even in decaf blends

2

calories per 8-ounce cup of black drip coffee

DARK CHOCOLATE

The Slimming Story

You can stop rubbing your eyes. That's no misprint: Chocolate can help you lose weight. Its pound-peeling power is actually taking effect as you read this, before you even take a bite. How so? If you start out on a diet plan knowing it regularly "allows" you to indulge a little in something as pleasurable as chocolate, you'll improve your odds of sticking with the program. You're also less likely to binge and more likely to make smarter choices for the long haul.

With dark chocolate, however, the waist-whittling power isn't all in your head, which is why it made our superfood list over other treats. With less sugar than the milk variety, dark chocolate delivers a super-rich, intense flavor that blows taste buds away and leaves you satisfied with a small amount. (A good thing—it does pack a calorie punch, after all.) And believe it or not, dark chocolate (at least 70 percent cocoa) supplies a full 3 grams of fiber per 1-ounce serving, versus milk chocolate's 1 gram. That, along with its fat, produces feelings of satiety, which could quiet your appetite and silence cravings. Plus, even though the treat is relatively high in saturated fat, it comes in the form of stearic acid, a portion of which the body converts to the more diet-friendly oleic acid, a monounsaturated fat. (Stearic acid also doesn't raise cholesterol.)

The candy aisle hero has some ab-flattening abilities, too. Loaded with antioxidants, dark chocolate may improve insulin sensitivity, which could help ward off belly-bulging metabolic syndrome. And for chronically harried people, eating dark chocolate daily seems to lower levels of the stress hormone cortisol. (Elevated levels of cortisol, and chronic stress in general, are associated with a wider waistline.) But even if you're not constantly anxious, chocolate could give you a mood lift by stimulating neurochemicals in the brain that produce a sense of happiness and relaxation. That may be exactly the boost you need to resist emotional eating and instead hit the gym or go for a walk, or at least stick to your diet.

➜ **Trim-Down Tip:** Limit your serving of dark chocolate to about 1 ounce per day. (Check labels to approximate how big a piece that gives you; it varies depending on the thickness of the particular bar.) Even though dark chocolate is a superfood for weight loss, at about 170 calories per ounce, its waist-trimming abilities max out if you overdo it, possibly causing you to pile on pounds instead of melting them off.

The Amazing Proof

- After snacking on about 3½ ounces of dark chocolate, study subjects felt more satisfied and less hungry and had reduced cravings for sweet, salty, and fatty foods than after gobbling the same amount of milk chocolate, researchers from the University of Copenhagen in Denmark report. Two and a half hours later, they also took in 15 percent fewer calories from a pizza buffet.

➜ **Trim-Down Tip:** Don't try to stifle your cravings! Instead, daydream a little about your treat's taste and texture before indulging. That may help you feel satisfied with a single portion.

- When women were deprived of chocolate for a week, they experienced more intense, chronic chocolate cravings and scarfed up approximately double the amount when it was eventually allowed than did a group that was allowed to eat chocolate, a study from the University of Toronto finds.
- People who treated themselves to chocolate every day weighed less, had a slimmer waist, and were less likely to have metabolic syndrome than those who didn't eat the sweet, according to a study in *Nutrition Research*.

Four More Reasons to Eat Dark Chocolate

1. *It's a special treat for your heart.* Antioxidant-loaded dark chocolate appears to reduce inflammation that may lead to hardened

arteries. Eating a small amount regularly could also help increase blood flow to the heart, prevent blood clots by making platelets less sticky, lower total and LDL cholesterol, and reduce your risk for hypertension.

2. *Dark chocolate cuts off cancer cells.* Indulge in the dark stuff and you'll take in a potent phytonutrient compound that fights fast-growing cancers such as colorectal cancer. It works with enzymes in your body, causing cancerous cells to die while leaving normal cells alone.

3. *Your brain benefits big-time.* Research suggests the antioxidants in dark chocolate may protect brain function as you age, but they might also provide more immediate benefits. The flavonols in dark chocolate trigger the production of nitric oxide, which increases blood flow and may improve both vision and certain cognitive functions, research from the University of Reading in England indicates.

4. *You'll be treating your skin, too.* The antioxidant flavonols and polyphenols in cocoa might also work with your sunscreen to help protect you from sunburn, according to research reported in *The Journal of Nutrition.* The flavonols help increase blood flow as well, which may improve hydration and bring glow-bestowing oxygen to your skin.

Choose the Best Chocolate

Feel like a kid in a candy store trying to pick among all the different bars? Follow these tips to make the most slimming selection:

- Go to the dark side. Opt for a bar with at least 70 percent cocoa (aka cacao solids). The higher the percentage, the better it is for your body. Some brands go up to 87 percent, but there's a trade-off: a slightly bitter taste. Typical dark chocolate contains only about 50 to 55 percent cocoa, so 70 percent is a good middle ground. The darker types may be a little pricier, but because you'll eat (and crave) less, the cost could be a wash.

WANT TO EAT MORE DARK CHOCOLATE
STARTING TODAY?

Drizzle it over anything! You'll melt when you sample tasty combos such as dark chocolate and pretzels, graham crackers, apples, or other fruit. Simply nuke in the microwave for a few seconds to soften, then pour.

DON'T LIKE DARK CHOCOLATE?

Ease your taste buds into very dark (70 percent cocoa) chocolate by starting with regular dark varieties (50 to 55 percent cocoa), then buying bars in the 60 percent range and so on. Mixing with other flavors (try the ideas below) can also help mellow the taste.

- Pick a perfect pairing. Dark chocolate mixed with caramel or toffee is delicious, but manufacturers add sugar and remove some of the healthy cocoa when making these combos. If you want to mellow the taste of pure dark chocolate, look for bars that mix in spices (mint and ginger are yummy), or eat it plain with fresh fruit or nuts, which give you a bonus hit of fiber.
- Be single-minded. Instead of a standard 3½-ounce bar, look for dark chocolate in smaller servings to help you control portions. If you can't find them, portion out your treat at home: After breaking off a 1-ounce piece, wrap up the rest and stash it in the cupboard before enjoying your treat.
- Savor the flavor. Slow down and take small bites, letting each melt on your tongue so you can fully experience the cocoa taste. It will help you feel more satisfied and resist the urge to have another piece.

Think Outside the Bar

Plain, dark chocolate by itself is a special luxury, but it's not the only way to enjoy this superfood for weight loss.

- Make a smoothie move. Chop up an ounce of dark chocolate (or use nibs—whole, shelled cacao beans) and blend with fruit and skim milk or yogurt.

- Ditch fake choco topping. Instead of drenching fro yo with sugary chocolate sauce, go with the real thing! Either melt an ounce of dark chocolate and pour, or sprinkle finely chopped bits on top.

- Sample a s'more. Who says you have to be camping? Top half of a whole-grain graham cracker with 2 teaspoons dark chocolate chips and 1 marshmallow. Microwave until the chocolate melts.

- Get into the mix. Combine 1 ounce dark chocolate chips with 1 tablespoon each raisins and nuts for a sweet grab-and-go snack.

- Make a toasty treat. Spread 1 slice whole-grain toast with 1 tablespoon melted dark chocolate chips. Top with 2 sliced strawberries.

- Drink it up. Blend 1 ounce melted dark chocolate with 6 ounces steaming skim milk.

dark chocolate nutrition
by the numbers

170

calories per ounce of dark chocolate with 70 to 85 percent cocoa

19

percent of your daily value of energizing iron

3

grams of fiber

drop *10* inspiration

"I learned to take care of myself."

NAME: Lisa Dailey
AGE: 33
OCCUPATION: Work-at-home mom
FAMILY STATUS: Married, three children
HEIGHT: 5 feet 7 inches
STARTING WEIGHT: 160
DROP 10 WEIGHT: 146
LOST: 14 pounds in fifteen weeks

My story: "I have done tons of diets and taken every diet pill on the market. Last summer, I tried them again and lost weight but put it all back on. I wanted to do something that wasn't a quick fix—and to teach my daughters that it's important to be healthy and active and that the size of your dress does not define you as a person."

Biggest challenge to losing weight: "My husband is deployed in Afghanistan, and we don't live near family, so I have an almost non-existent support network. When I started the plan, I had good weeks and bad weeks and eventually buckled down when it came to my eating."

Why Drop 10 clicked: "When I started feeling healthier, the desire to take care of myself kicked in. If I don't put myself first once in a while, nobody else will. I have found a happy place where I don't feel the desire to splurge on unhealthy treats, and my stress levels are lowering, so I'm not tempted by that second glass of wine after the kids go to bed."

How my body changed: "I lost 19$\frac{1}{2}$ inches off my waist, hips, and thighs! I've even noticed that my shadow no longer has love handles."

Success tip: "I use dry-erase markers to write motivational sayings on my bathroom mirror. I find it very helpful—I'll write things like 'Failing to plan = planning to fail' and 'I may not be perfect, but parts of me are fantastic.' Now, I'm more confident and ready to take on new challenges!"

THE
SUPER PLANS
2

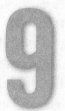

Thirty-one Days to Slim!
The No-Diet Superfood Weight Loss Plan

For all of you who would rather count anything besides calories, you're in the right place. If you've tried meal-plan diets only to find yourself dropping out more than dropping dress sizes, welcome! Or maybe you detest formal diets? Whatever your beef, this chapter is dedicated to you—anyone who is not able, not ready, or simply not interested in following a menu plan but who still wants to make a change for the better. One diet does not fit all, yet everyone deserves a chance to succeed at weight loss. This is yours.

This flexible program is full of effortless, simple tips for upgrading your existing diet to the superfoods system. It's meant to work gradually: You adopt new behaviors a little at a time, so you painlessly replace the fattening junk in your diet with slimming superfoods. This approach is an incredibly easy way to feel healthier and more energized. Even better, it will help you steadily shed inches. (Of course, if you'd rather follow a formal menu plan, we've got a great one in chapter 10!)

Think of this chapter and the tips you read here as an all-you-can-eat buffet of skinny habits and superfoods. Sample each one, but revisit only those you like. Because you pick and choose what works best for your life, schedule, and taste buds, you're more likely to be successful in the long run than you would be on standard diets.

What to do: Each day for a month, test-drive a new tip. If you skip a day, don't worry about it. If you want to jump ahead, go for it. The key is to keep following the tips and enjoying the foods you like and forget the ones you don't. The only thing you shouldn't do: Feel pressure to keep up with every tip. You're the boss, and you decide what's working and what's not. If you truly like them all, that's awesome! But even if you end up ditching multiple tips, by the end of the month, you'll still have picked up enough healthy habits and new ways of thinking about food to have a huge impact on the quality of your diet, your health, and what you see on the scale. That's right: no calorie counting, no meal plan to follow, no thinking—just shrinking. Your "thinner in thirty-one days" plan starts now!

Day 1: Rise and Dine on Eggs

Your mother was right: Breakfast is the most important meal of the day—eating first thing in the morning switches on your calorie-burning machinery. In fact, breakfast eaters are up to 50 percent less likely to be obese than those who routinely skip it, according to a study from Children's Hospital Boston. One of your best a.m. options? Protein-packed eggs: They kick your metabolism into high gear, and research shows that eggs have an all-day effect on suppressing appetite, so you feel less hungry and consume fewer calories for the next twenty-four hours.

➡ **Try It:** Bored by hard-boiled? Over over easy? Bake a veggie-filled frittata (try our recipe on page 255) on Sunday, and eat it all week. Nuke a slice each a.m. and enjoy with low-fat yogurt and whole-grain toast.

Day 2: Fight Fat with Fiber

Believe it: The more you fill your stomach with fiber, the better your chances of flattening your belly. Aside from warding off hunger and fat-promoting spikes in insulin, increasing your fiber intake to 34 grams daily can prevent the absorption of up to 120 calories per day from your meals. That's more than 12 pounds a year! The recommended daily intake is 34 grams, but most Americans eat only about half that amount of fiber. Closing the gap is as easy as munching a few fiber-rich superfoods throughout the day.

→ **Try It:** To close the gap between the number of fiber grams you're likely getting now and the optimum level, toss 1 cup of blueberries (4 grams) into yogurt at breakfast; add ¾ cup of lentils (12 grams) to a lunchtime salad or sandwich wrap; snack on almonds (3 grams per ounce); and whip up mashed sweet potatoes for dinner (a medium potato has 4 grams). Presto—you surpassed your daily goal!

Day 3: Power Up Your Workout

Exercise does more than sizzle calories and rev your metabolism; it can melt away the blues and bolster self-confidence, thwarting emotional eating and making it easier to stick with your healthy-eating goals. Check out chapter 13 for fitness ideas, then get moving! But be sure to fuel your workouts with energizing fare.

→ **Try It:** An hour or so before you exercise, sip a small cup of coffee, which may help you work out longer and harder without feeling the extra exertion. If it's been several hours since your last meal, nosh on a small snack such as a kiwifruit or some low-fat yogurt. Whatever you choose, don't fill up completely; a stuffed stomach can leave you sluggish.

→ H_2-OH, YEAH!

Don't forget to hydrate before and after your workout. If you're engaging in moderate exercise (versus, say, regularly running marathons), skip the sports drinks. They often have added sugar and calories. Water is free of both and hydrates just as well.

Day 4: Get a "Fast" Food Fix

Stock your cupboards and fridge with superfoods you can use to put together portable meals and snacks on the fly. Think canned wild salmon or almond butter for sandwiches, and goji berries, peanuts, and apples for between-meal bites. It's also an excellent idea to make a batch of quinoa and lentils each week, then stash them in storage containers in the fridge so they're ready to go when your stomach says, "Feed me now!"

→ **Try It:** Make a quick salmon-salad wrap to take with you and eat anywhere: Combine a can of wild salmon with low-fat mayo and onion; roll up with lettuce and tomato in a whole-wheat tortilla.

Day 5: Defat Your Favorites

Craving mac 'n' cheese, pizza, or other comfort food? Eat it! You don't need to deprive yourself; if you do, you're more vulnerable to binge attacks down the road. Instead, trim the fat by adding a few slimming superfoods: Toss plenty of low-calorie, high-fiber vegetables into a smaller portion of noodles, or pile veggies on a slice of cheese pizza. You'll still feast, but for fewer calories. Case in point: When people ate vegetables with a meal, they consumed a full 20 percent fewer calories than when eating a no-veggie meal, but they still felt satisfied afterward, a study in *The American Journal of Clinical Nutrition* reveals.

→ **Try It:** Stir a cup of frozen or lightly steamed broccoli, mushrooms, or artichoke hearts into mac 'n' cheese, or order them as toppers on your pizza. Also check out the veggie-packed comfort food recipes in chapter 11.

Day 6: Schedule Snack Time

Eating consistently throughout the day keeps your stomach full, your blood sugar levels steady, and you from wanting to devour everything in the office vending machine or in your kitchen late at night. Plan to have a meal or small snack every three or four hours. (If you usually don't remember to eat until your stomach starts growling angrily, set an alert on your computer or smartphone.) The best hunger-taming options run about 150 to 200 calories and contain a mix of protein, fiber, and healthy fats.

→ **Try It:** Stash superfood snacks in the places where you spend time. Keep Parmesan and apples in your office fridge, or air-popped popcorn, peanuts, dried cherries, or goji berries in your car or cupboards.

Day 7: Reserve a Table at Chez Moi

Love to eat out or order in? Consider showing your stove a little love and you'll save cash and calories. Research suggests that the more often you hit restaurants, the more likely you are to overeat and be overweight. Start by planning your week's menu and shopping ahead of time, getting everything you need so you're ready to prep a meal the moment you're hungry.

→ **Try It:** If you're not following the formal Drop 10 menu plan, flip to chapter 11 for easy superfood-stuffed recipes that even a cooking newbie can make.

Day 8: Play Up Protein

Chances are that this fat-shedding MVP (which boosts your calorie burn and helps you feel fuller longer) is sitting on the sidelines of your diet: Americans take in only about 15 percent of their day's calories from protein, according to the USDA. Aim to bump up your intake to 20 to 30 percent, or about 120 grams per day, by incorporating a protein powerhouse into every meal and snack. Potent picks include lean steak, wild salmon, lentils, edamame, yogurt, pumpkin seeds, peanuts, almond butter, and quinoa.

→ **Try It:** Double up on protein-packed superfoods to make double trouble for flab. Stir-fry your favorite frozen veggies with shelled edamame and serve over quinoa.

Day 9: Fill the Veggie Void

Produce is filling and naturally low in calories, so the more of it you eat, the less hungry you'll be for junky snack foods and the easier it will be to eliminate excess calories and fat from your, er, bottom line. In fact, women who increase their produce intake are 24 percent less likely to become obese, a study in the *International Journal of Obesity* reveals. Challenge yourself to work in at least 5 cups of veggies per day. It's a lot easier than you think!

→ **Try It:** Snack on broccoli, edamame, or other crudités at least once per day. Then, when preparing each of your meals, stop and think about what (and how much) produce you can add. Mushrooms, kale, artichokes, and sweet potatoes go with almost anything: scrambled eggs or an omelet, soup, sauces, pasta, stir-fry—you name it! Or start each lunch and dinner with a veggie-loaded salad.

WHAT COUNTS AS A SERVING?

Superfood	Serving
Artichoke	1 cup cooked artichoke hearts or 1 whole large artichoke
Broccoli	1 cup chopped florets
Edamame	1 cup shelled or 2¼ cups in the pod
Kale and other greens	1 cup cooked or 2 cups raw
Mushrooms	1 cup cooked or raw
Sweet potato	1 cup cooked or mashed (about 1 large potato)

Day 10: Focus on Real Food

If you're tempted to stock up on diet foods (processed goods remade with fewer calories or fat), think twice. The "light" impostors are rarely satisfying emotionally or physically and often lead people to think incorrectly they can eat with abandon as long as the product is labeled *low*-whatever. Ditch the fake stuff and stick with the real thing, channeling your efforts into serving up a sensible, scaled-back portion instead.

→ **Try It:** The next time you need a treat, savor an ounce of rich, dark chocolate with at least 70 percent cocoa or a cube of real Parmesan. For more ideas, check out page 298–301 for 24 superfood-packed, portion-specific indulgences.

Day 11: Celebrate Success

Don't be a slave to the number on the scale! Reward yourself for the healthy habits you've adopted and stuck with thus far, such as meeting your fiber quota (see Day 2) or eating 5 cups of veggies a day (Day 9). Behavior-based bonuses might help people lose more weight than prizes for pounds lost, a study in *Obesity Reviews* indicates. Besides, if you've been exercising, you may be replacing some fat with lean muscle, which weighs more but takes up much less space on you.

→ **Try It:** Today, treat yourself to a pedicure, new earrings, or other nonedible reward for the healthful goals you've already met. Do it again for any good-for-you habit you stick with for at least a week. Your goal can be as simple as switching your usual snacks for superfood nibbles such as popcorn, blueberries, edamame, or pumpkin seeds. Even a seemingly small change like this can have a big impact on your weight and health.

Day 12: Flip Your Fat Script

Eating fat helps you feel satiated, so you consume fewer calories overall. What type of fat you eat, however, is important. Unfortunately, the ratio of slimming unsaturated to saturated fat is off for most Americans. Shifting the balance so you take in more of the good mono- and polyunsaturated fats and less of the saturated stuff gives you a leg up on getting lean. The best sources of diet-friendly fats include almond butter, avocado, olive oil, peanuts, pumpkin seeds, salmon, and sardines.

→ **Try It:** Trade creamy salad dressings for olive oil and vinegar, and sauté in olive oil instead of butter. Leave Cheddar off sandwiches and replace it with slices of avocado, and grill salmon patties instead of hamburgers at your next barbecue. Also swap out a morning doughnut for low-fat yogurt mixed with almond butter, and ditch that bag of potato chips for a handful of peanuts.

Day 13: Enjoy Dessert

No fooling! If you've been following the tips so far, you're already incorporating more slimming superfoods into your diet. Good job! Allowing yourself a small splurge every day keeps you satisfied and motivates you to continue making healthy choices. The trick: Choose a treat that excites your sweet tooth without overloading you with calories and fat.

→ **Try It:** Spoon up about half your usual helping of ice cream (or, better yet, a true half serving, which is ¼ cup), then fill the other half of your bowl with sliced cherries, diced kiwifruit, or fresh pomegranate seeds. Or sprinkle an ounce of chopped dark chocolate over a bowl of fruit. For more sweet superfood ideas, flip to page 298.

Day 14: Join the Slow-Food Movement

Unless you're competing in the Coney Island hot-dog-eating contest, the only prize you get for wolfing down meals quickly is extra calories. It takes about twenty minutes for satiety signals to kick in, so the faster you munch, the more likely you are to add a paunch. Practice pacing yourself at every meal by chewing food longer, eating meals in separate courses, and choosing foods that require more time to consume. It's also helpful to portion out meals at the stove rather than putting serving dishes—and seconds—on the table within easy reach.

→ **Try It:** When making a noodle dish, use fusilli or penne whole-grain pasta, because you can spear one or two at a time. (Spaghetti could encourage you to twirl up bigger mouthfuls.) Or snack on a whole artichoke, taking the time to scrape out the flesh from each petal. When eating popcorn, pop only a kernel or two into your mouth at a time rather than a whole fistful.

Day 15: Fit a Salad into Every Sandwich

Whether you've got a hankering for ham or treasure your turkey, slip extra veggies, fruits, and other superfoods between your slices of whole-grain bread or in a whole-wheat wrap. You'll take in more filling fiber and fat-fighting vitamin C.

→ **Try It:** Kale, avocado, apple slices, mushrooms, and artichoke hearts all team up well with cold cuts. Lunching on tuna or chicken salad? Stir chopped broccoli, edamame, or diced apple into your mix, and top with a leaf or two of kale.

Day 16: Milk Your Diet

Wish there were a magic bullet for bikini season? Poof—granted! Most women don't get enough calcium, which can make your body's flab-burning equipment run about as well as an old, battered jalopy. But boosting your intake by eating low-fat dairy such as nonfat yogurt, skim milk, and cottage cheese, as well as Parmesan, throws metabolism into overdrive, helping you sizzle fat.

→ **Try It:** To reach your target 1,000 milligrams of calcium a day, spoon up nonfat yogurt (488 milligrams per cup) at breakfast or as a snack, add 1 ounce of shredded Parm (336 milligrams) to your lunchtime salad or sandwich, and sip a small smoothie made with nonfat yogurt and your favorite superfood fruits after dinner.

Day 17: Eat Breakfast for Lunch

If noon rolls around and you start thinking, "Salad, sandwich, soup, *again?*" bypass your usuals and throw your taste buds a curveball by making a traditional breakfast food for lunch. Omelets, oats, and yogurt parfaits prepared with whole-grain cereal all fit the bill. To keep you full, be sure whatever you make has a mix of protein, fat, fruits or veggies, and whole-grain carbs.

→ **Try It:** Turn a bowl of old-fashioned oatmeal (already one of the most satiating foods around) into a supersatisfying lunch by stirring in a tablespoon of almond butter or crushed peanuts, a dollop of creamy nonfat yogurt, and a helping of your favorite superfood fruit. Or turn eggs into a Mexican meal by scrambling a mixture of 2 egg whites, 1 whole egg, ¼ cup canned black beans (rinsed and drained), 2 tablespoons part-skim mozzarella, 1 tablespoon chopped onion, and a sprinkle of salt, pepper, and paprika. Top with ¼ cup store-bought salsa, and serve over 1 slice whole-wheat toast.

Day 18: Take a Coffee Break

Pour yourself a cup of coffee to perk up both you and your metabolism. If you're tempted to dump in fake sweeteners, don't—it may backfire. Artificial sugars could trigger cravings for high-calorie foods. In fact, people who used them saw their body mass index (a measure of body fat) increase 47 percent over eight years compared with those who refrained.

→ **Try It:** Skip the supersize mug and pour an 8-ounce cup, then sip your java black; cream and sugar could cancel out the calorie-burning benefits.

Day 19: Whet Your Appetite to Block Hunger

People who had an 80-calorie appetizer consisting of three key elements—fat, protein, and fiber—prior to eating went on to consume 43 percent fewer calories during their next sitting, according to a study in the journal *Obesity*. These calorie counts don't make room for, say, a giant plate of mozzarella sticks, but you've got plenty of nutritional options among the superfoods.

→ **Try It:** Top 1 multigrain crispbread with 1 tablespoon avocado and 1 tablespoon hummus. Or make a refreshing cucumber-yogurt salad: Combine 3 ounces nonfat plain yogurt, ¼ cup half-inch-thick cucumber slices, 2 teaspoons chopped peanuts, 1 teaspoon lemon juice, and 1 teaspoon chopped fresh dill.

Day 20: Pump Your Plate with Wholes

Carbs are like lovers: The best ones leave you feeling fulfilled and happy; the wrong ones, unsatisfied and hungry for more. Whole grains are chock-full of fiber that keeps blood sugar and insulin levels steady, warding off hunger. Refined carbs (white bread, cookies, and the like), on the other hand, can lead to the spikes that ramp up your appetite and encourage your body to store fat.

→ **Try It:** Weed out the whites in your diet by swapping white rice for quinoa, white noodles for whole-grain pasta, and white bread for whole wheat. Also trade refined-grain cereals such as cornflakes for whole-grain cereals or oatmeal, and potato chips for air-popped popcorn.

Day 21: Resize Servings

One of the easiest ways to trim down is to shift the balance of food on your plate. Instead of making a serving of meat or starchy carbs the main focus, take only about half as much of these as you normally would and bulk up your helpings of fruits, veggies, whole grains, and low-fat dairy. You'll still feel that you're getting your fill, but you'll end up taking in many fewer calories and much less fat.

→ **Try It:** Load your plate with at least two different kinds of fruits and vegetables. Lightly sauté artichoke hearts and kale in olive oil, for example. Or serve a baked sweet potato and a side of fresh kiwifruit and cherries.

Day 22: Play Healthy Hooky!

You're doing *great*! To celebrate, forget about losing weight today. When slimming habits start to become second nature and you're eating healthfully most of the time, it's okay to have a free day once in a while to really indulge, whether it's a birthday, a party, or any old Tuesday. Not being perfect all the time is healthy, especially for your psyche. That said, a free day isn't an excuse to binge until you waddle home clutching your gut. Whatever you eat, do it slowly so you can heed your body's satiety signals. Halfway through your plate, ask yourself, Would I keep eating if this were an apple? When the answer is no, you're done.

→ **Try It:** Even when you're not focused on losing, it's easy to sneak in superfoods. If you go out for dinner, for example, order steak (try a petite filet mignon) and leave room for a little apple pie or a rich piece of artisanal dark chocolate, then linger over coffee.

Day 23: Rethink Tube Food

If your appetite switches on along with the TV, prepare a slimming snack before you start clicking so you don't grab chips or cookies while you watch. Portion out a sensible serving in the kitchen, put the rest away, and bring only that portion to the couch with you. When you hit the bottom of the bowl, you're finished for the night. Try it and watch what happens after a few weeks—*you'll* be the biggest loser.

→ **Try It:** Upgrade your usual TV munchies to air-popped popcorn (check out page 118 for ways to spice it up), salted edamame, or an apple, fresh blueberries, or pomegranate seeds. For more smart snack ideas, turn to page 286.

Day 24: Give Fat the Slip

You'll be amazed how easy it is to trick your stomach into being satisfied with fewer calories and less fat. People who had a meal made with hidden pureed veggies automatically consumed up to 360 fewer calories the rest of the day, research from Pennsylvania State University in University Park discovers. Veggies add weight and fiber to dishes, but not many calories. Give it a whirl! All you need is a blender or food processor.

→ **Try It:** Lightly steam a serving of broccoli, kale, or sweet potatoes, puree, then mix into a bowl of soup or a helping of pasta sauce. Or trade half the ground beef in lasagna, meat loaf, or pasta sauce for chopped button mushrooms.

Day 25: Spoon Up Soup

Because of the amount of water in broth-based soups, they fill you up on fewer calories than other foods. Whether you choose to have your bowl as a starter or the main event, it will go a long way toward helping you beat hunger and slim down. Soups are a snap to make at home, but for a fast fix, look for canned or boxed varieties low in sodium and fat and rich in vegetables and fiber. (Boxed soups come in containers that resemble large juice boxes, and they may taste fresher.)

→ **Try It:** Slurp up veggie-based soups such as minestrone, and add ½ cup of lentils for an extra serving of filling fiber.

Day 26: Friend a Farmer

Instead of heading to your usual grocery store, take a walk through a farmers' market or stroll around a large health food supermarket. Both spots stock the freshest fruits, veggies, eggs, and other slimming goodies and display them in a way that's a feast for your eyes. The presentation is inspiring—there's no way *not* to be tempted by the yummy-looking, good-for-you fare!

BORN IN THE CSA

Community-supported agriculture, better known as CSA, is essentially a subscription service for farm-fresh goodies. You buy a share of a farm's harvest by paying up front, then you pick up your box at a designated spot (often a farmers' market) weekly or biweekly during the harvest season. Fruits and vegetables are the items usually on offer in CSAs, but you can also find CSAs specializing in meat, eggs, and dairy. CSAs ensure that your fridge stays stocked with fresh produce, and you support nearby farms while getting to sample all sorts of foods you won't find in many supermarkets. For more info, check out www.localharvest.org/csa.

→ **Try It:** Along with taking in the healthy-foods eye candy, chat up the farmers or shop clerks. Ask for hints on how to eat less familiar superfoods such as kale, pomegranate, quinoa, or sardines. If you're getting bored with a superfood you eat often (such as apples, broccoli, whole-grain pasta, or salmon), quiz them for fresh prep ideas.

Day 27: Go Fish

Fatty fish such as wild salmon and sardines are rich in flab-fighting omega-3 fatty acids and vitamin D, which may speed up your weight loss results. Make it a goal to have either of these seafood picks at least once a week instead of your usual dinner standby.

→ **Try It:** Salmon and fresh sardines cook quickly, which means they're an ideal choice for your weeknight menu. Marinate in a mixture of lime juice, garlic, and cumin, then grill or broil (about 10 minutes per inch of thickness), flipping once.

Day 28: Spice Up Your Weight Loss

Trying to lose weight by eating plain fish and veggies (or naked anything, for that matter) night after night is like riding a bike with no seat—you won't get very far before you get tired and give up. So keep an arsenal of spices and seasonings on hand to excite your taste buds. Think of cayenne, turmeric, rosemary, sage, cinnamon, curry, and any other underused spices in your cabinet as your secret stick-with-it weapons.

→ **Try It:** Experiment with different spices to find the ones you like best, then keep a few in shakers on the table or on the counter so you can give salmon, veggies, or anything else a kick.

Day 29: Fix a Slimming Side Dish

If you find yourself reaching for, say, frozen Tater Tots or french fries to round out your dinner plate, ask yourself if the rubbery, freezer-burned bits are actually worth the calories. In the time it takes for these same-old carbs to bake, you can upgrade to a side dish that tastes better and will help you shed fat, not pack it on.

→ **Try It:** Lentils and quinoa complement nearly any entrée and cook in about fifteen minutes. Prep a batch of either, and toss with olive oil, your favorite herbs, and spices, plus edamame and fresh or frozen veggies. Can't surrender fries? Try this easy recipe: Peel 3 medium sweet potatoes (about 1 pound), and cut into 2-inch-long wedges; brush with 1 tablespoon canola oil, and lay out on a cookie sheet. (Cover sheet with foil for easy cleanup.) Season potatoes with a dash of salt. Bake at 425 degrees until slightly browned and tender, 15 to 30 minutes. Serve warm.

Day 30: DIY with Convenience Foods

We understand the appeal of processed foods such as frozen dinners and boxed mixes: They're fast and easy. The problem is that they're also great hiding places for calories, extra fat, and belly-bloating sodium, and they short you on slimming nutrients such as vitamin C, calcium, and fiber. If you plan ahead, however, putting real food on the table is every bit as quick and simple.

→ **Try It:** Once a week, instead of vegging out in front of the tube, veg out for real in the kitchen with your favorite superfood-containing recipes. Cook up a big batch of homemade soup, throw together a large casserole or anything else you like, and stash it in the freezer. Most of the superfood recipes in chapter 11 freeze well, but the Vegetable Meat Loaf (page 282), Lentil Burgers (page 283), and Kale and White Bean Potato Soup (page 270) are particularly good choices.

Day 31: Freeze Out Fat and Calories

Nothing beats fresh fruits and vegetables for snacking and in salads, but filling your freezer with a few bags of the frozen stuff will save you cash and help you eat healthfully because you'll always have fiber-rich, filling produce on hand to add to meals. The same goes for lean steak and wild salmon. When you see a bargain, buy extra, then separate them into portions and freeze. Transfer to the fridge for thawing the morning before you plan to prepare them.

→ **Try It:** The next time you hit the grocery, grab a bag each of frozen broccoli, artichoke hearts, edamame, and blueberries. When prepping dinner, make it a goal to add a few cups of at least one to your pasta, casserole, side dish, or whatever else you're whipping up.

Keep Going!

What a difference a month makes! Review all the tips to see which ones have become part of your regular routine and which you passed up. Revisit at least one you didn't try or one you did but that didn't stick, and give it another go. Happy eating!

drop 10 inspiration

"I finally lost those last stubborn pounds!"

NAME: Alyssa Pentis

AGE: 22

OCCUPATION: Graduate student

FAMILY STATUS: Single

HEIGHT: 5 feet 5 inches

STARTING WEIGHT: 166

DROP 10 WEIGHT: 154

LOST: 12 pounds in five weeks

My story: "I lost a lot of weight during college, but I couldn't shed the last 5 to 10 pounds no matter what I tried."

Biggest challenge to losing weight: "Portion control. I am a pretty healthy eater, but I was cooking recipes that were intended for two. And I would get bored exercising and stop."

Why Drop 10 clicked: "The meals were so easy to prep and cook—in 10 or 15 minutes. Plus, the plan helped me with my portion control because everything was measured out. And I really used those indulge-and-snack calories! You have to be happy—you can't deprive yourself, especially of dark chocolate. The workout was easy. I could do the sets anywhere when I traveled."

How my body changed: "I lost inches off my belly and dropped a pants size. Like most people, I'd always had the hardest time shrinking my lower half, but I just bought shorts and jeans in a smaller size—that's the best payoff I could ask for!"

Success tip: "I learned the importance of shocking your body. One week, I plateaued and lost no weight. The following week, I changed my workout and tried some new meals on the plan and lost 2 more pounds."

The Drop 10 Menu:
Five Weeks of Satisfying, Fat-Melting, Superfood-Packed Breakfasts, Lunches, Snacks, and Dinners

Whether you want to shed 10, 20, 30 pounds, or more, the Drop 10 diet can transform your body fast and forever by harnessing the slimming powers of the superfoods you've read about so far. This diet won't leave you listening to a growling stomach all day. Instead, you listen to your taste buds, choosing among 140 delicious, hearty meals and recipes packed with foods scientifically proven to help burn fat, rev up your metabolism, and tame even the most ravenous of appetites. You also pay attention to your cravings: Snacking and indulging in your favorite goodies are encouraged. Drop 10 is so easy, so flexible, and so yummy, you'll start thinking of it as a way of life rather than a weight loss program.

You'll remember it's a diet, though, when you step on the scale after only one week and already see the pounds starting to drop away. Combined with the fun, fat-blasting, body-toning workouts in chapter 13, the Drop 10 meals are designed to help you erase a total of 10 pounds over the course of five short weeks. If your goal is to zap more, hit repeat and keep going another five weeks or as long as you like. There's so much variety among the superfoods, meals, and treats, you'll never get bored—but you will adopt new eating habits and find new superfoods and fat-fighting dishes that will help keep you slim and healthy for life. And now, without further ado, let the thinning begin!

How to Use the Drop 10 Diet Plan

- Fill up on satisfying, fat-melting meals. Starting on page 225, you'll find five weeks' worth of quick meals and easy recipes, designed by our nutrition expert, Heather K. Jones, RD. Choose one superfood-packed dish from each meal category (breakfast, lunch, dinner, and snacks) every day to build the 1,400-calorie base of your 1,600-calorie menu. (Don't worry, the math will work out! Keep reading.)

- Customize the menu to your tastes. Flexibility is a dieter's best ally, and you get plenty of it here, starting with how you can tailor the plan to meet your needs. You can eat a brand-new dish at every meal, plus snacks, or stick to a rotating group of your favorites. Each meal has similar calorie counts (around 350 calories for breakfast, 450 calories for lunch or dinner, and 150 calories for a snack), so you can mix and match however you like. Any way you go, you'll enjoy delicious meals that will keep you satiated and steadily shedding pounds and inches.

- Hit all the superfoods at least once. You'll lose no matter which meals and snacks you choose to eat—that's the beauty of the Drop 10 plan. But for truly wow results, eat a range of meals that fill your diet with as many of the superfoods as possible, and aim to try each superfood at least once. (Yep, that includes sardines. If you haven't already, turn to page 154 to read about them; you do not want to miss out on their incredible benefits.) The science is convincing, and if you try them, the scale will convince you, too.

- Add your favorite foods. In addition to the filling 1,400 daily calories the basic meal plan delivers, you get to spend another 200 "happy" calories per day by eating or drinking anything you want: chips, candy, french fries, wine, whatever! Check out chapter 12 to get some ideas, and refer to it often during the five weeks. If you don't see your must-haves, it's easy to look up calorie counts at NutritionData.Self.com.

- Feel free to splurge. Birthday parties (with cake and ice cream), girls night out (two rounds, please!), Sunday fun days (mmm, barbecue)—life would be pretty boring if you couldn't indulge when the occasion calls for it. That's why Drop 10 lets you roll over up to four days' worth of happy calories (800 total) to blow all at once if you'd like. You'll quickly see that achieving diet success has little to do with what you might think of as diet food.

- Feed the whole family with superfoods! When you've got a hungry crowd to handle, turn to chapter 11 for forty delicious meals that each make four or more servings. Or, if you find a recipe (or more!) that you especially love, make it and freeze extra portions to enjoy at later meals.

- Eat out the Drop 10 way. For date nights and lunches with co-workers, or on those days when you barely have time to breathe, much less pack or prepare a meal, you can skip the menu ideas here and get your superfoods from a restaurant or fast-food place instead. The same goes for, say, a friend's dinner party or brunch at your parents'. (For the best fat-sizzling results, however, try to eat from the menu plan as often as possible.) Either way, the key is to stay within your calorie limits for the day and fill your plate with superfoods. Check out chapter 14 for eating-out picks that contain superfoods and for related calorie information from a supersized list of restaurants. Likewise, chapter 14 lists calories for various splurge-worthy meals you might encounter while out to eat or at someone else's home. For example, you can order a lunch that adds up to roughly 450 calories or choose to use your lunch and happy calories together for a bigger meal that's 650 calories. Balance your calories like your checkbook—never spending more than you've got—and you'll be in good shape. Literally!

The Drop 10 Menu

Now that your appetite has been whetted by learning how easy and flexible the Drop 10 plan is, it's time to eat. Each scrumptious meal and snack—organized here by type, including grab-and-go store-bought options—delivers the perfect balance of metabolism-stoking protein, skinny carbs, and healthy fats that will help you say goodbye to a grumbling stomach, sugar crashes, and wild cravings and hello to a slimmer, more energized, and healthier you. We hope you're hungry!

Belly-Shrinking Breakfasts

(Choose One Daily; Each Option Totals About 350 Calories)

Don't be tempted to skip this important meal; eating breakfast wakes up your metabolism, priming it for a day of calorie burning. Plus, because you won't be so ravenous come lunch, you might end up eating less throughout the day. In fact, studies show that people who regularly eat in the a.m. are thinner than those who don't. If you're usually not hungry first thing, you don't need to force spoonfuls of yogurt down your throat as soon as your eyes pop open. Wait a little while, and eat either after you've dressed or when you get to work. The key is that you have something, especially the mix of protein, fruits, vegetables, healthy fats, and whole grains you'll find in these tasty meals.

EGGCELLENT A.M. OPTIONS

1. **Veggie Scramble**

   Cook 10 cherry tomatoes and 1 cup sliced mushrooms in a nonstick pan until soft. Add 1 whole egg and 1 egg white; scramble until cooked. Serve with 1 slice whole-grain toast topped with 1 tablespoon almond butter and 2 teaspoons honey.

2. **Filling Frittata**

   Cook ½ cup each of chopped red onion and chopped kale in an ovenproof 6-inch skillet coated with cooking spray for 3 minutes. Add 2 ounces low-sodium deli turkey breast, chopped; cook until heated through, about 2 minutes. Remove from heat. Stir in 1 whole egg and 1 egg white, beaten; ½ cup part-skim ricotta; and 2 teaspoons chopped fresh basil. Heat under broiler until frittata puffs, 2 to 3 minutes.

3. **Salmon Scramble**

   Cook 10 cherry tomatoes and ¼ cup chopped onion in a nonstick pan until soft. Add 1 whole egg, 1 egg white, and 2 ounces chopped nitrate-free smoked wild salmon; scramble until cooked. Serve with 1 cup fresh blueberries and ½ cup low-fat plain Greek yogurt.

4. Egg Muffin

Scramble 1 egg in a nonstick pan. Serve on a whole-wheat English muffin with 1 slice (1 ounce) Cheddar. Enjoy with ½ an apple.

5. Baked Eggs

Sauté 1 cup sliced mushrooms and 2 cups chopped kale in an ovenproof skillet coated with cooking spray until mushrooms are tender and kale wilts, about 7 minutes. Remove from heat. Stir in 1 whole egg and 1 egg white, beaten; 2 tablespoons grated Parmesan cheese; and 2 teaspoons chopped fresh basil. Heat under broiler until egg mixture puffs, 2 to 3 minutes. Serve with 1 slice whole-wheat bread topped with 1 tablespoon almond butter.

SLIMMING SMOOTHIES

6. Berry Smoothie

Blend 1½ scoops whey protein powder with ½ cup fresh blueberries, ¼ cup rolled oats, and 1 cup almond milk. Add water to thin or ice to thicken.

7. Blueberry-Almond Smoothie

Blend 1 cup fresh or frozen blueberries, 1 tablespoon almond butter, 6 ounces low-fat plain Greek yogurt, and ½ cup skim milk until smooth. Thin with water if necessary.

HOT AND COLD CEREAL

8. Hot Quinoa

Top 1 cup cooked quinoa with ½ cup skim milk, ¼ cup diced apple, 1 tablespoon raisins, 1 tablespoon slivered or chopped almonds, and a dash of cinnamon.

9. Make-Ahead Muesli

Mix ½ cup rolled oats (not instant) with 2 tablespoons chopped walnuts, 2 teaspoons raw honey, and a dash of cinnamon in a bowl. Add 1 cup water, cover with plastic wrap, and refrigerate overnight. Serve cold topped with 1 apple, chopped.

10. Crunchy Cereal

Top 1 cup Kashi GoLean cereal and 1 cup skim milk with ½ cup fresh blueberries and 1 tablespoon pumpkin seeds.

11. Peanutty Oatmeal

Cook ½ cup rolled oats in 1 cup skim milk as directed on package. Top with ¼ cup fresh blueberries and 2 tablespoons unsalted peanuts.

FRUIT, VEGGIES, AND YOGURT

12. Loaded Yogurt

Top 6 ounces low-fat plain Greek yogurt with ¼ cup fresh blueberries, 2 tablespoons chopped almonds, and 2 tablespoons pomegranate seeds. Serve with ½ an oat bran bagel spread with 1 tablespoon trans-fat-free margarine.

13. Yogurt Parfait

Layer 9 ounces low-fat plain Greek yogurt with 1 cup fresh blueberries and 2 tablespoons unsalted peanuts in a bowl.

14. Lärabar Parfait

Crumble 1 Peanut Butter Cookie Lärabar (made with peanuts and dates) on top of 6 ounces low-fat plain Greek yogurt.

15. Sweet Sweet Potato

Bake or microwave a medium sweet potato until soft. Cut open; sprinkle with cinnamon and 2 tablespoons chopped walnuts; drizzle with 2 teaspoons honey. Serve with 6 ounces low-fat plain Greek yogurt.

16. Broiled Grapefruit

Drizzle 1 teaspoon honey over 2 grapefruit halves. Heat under broiler until honey starts to bubble and brown, about 5 minutes.

Serve with 1 slice whole-wheat toast topped with 1½ tablespoons almond butter.

17. Baked Apple

Core an apple and place it in a small ovenproof dish. Fill hole in apple with 2 tablespoons chopped walnuts, and drizzle with 2 teaspoons honey. Pour a small amount of water into baking dish. Bake at 350 degrees for about 25 minutes. Serve with 6 ounces low-fat plain Greek yogurt.

18. Artichoke-Parmesan Crispbreads

Top 2 high-fiber crispbreads with 1 cup chopped canned (rinsed and drained) artichoke hearts. Top each with ½ tablespoon grated Parmesan. Microwave until cheese melts, 30 to 60 seconds. Serve with 6 ounces low-fat plain Greek yogurt drizzled with 1 tablespoon honey.

WHOLE-GRAIN BITES

19. Honeyed Waffles

Spread 2 teaspoons almond butter and 2 teaspoons honey on 2 toasted whole-grain waffles. (Look for whole-wheat flour as the first ingredient.) Top with ½ small banana, sliced.

20. Almond Muffin

Spread 1½ tablespoons almond butter on a whole-wheat English muffin. Serve with 1 kiwifruit.

21. Salmon-Stuffed Pita

Fill a 6½-inch whole-wheat pita with 2 ounces nitrate-free smoked wild salmon, 3 slices red onion, and 1 wedge Laughing Cow Light Creamy Swiss cheese.

BREAKFAST QUICKIES

22. Eat and Run

1 hard-boiled egg, 1 cup fresh cherries, 3 tablespoons unsalted peanuts.

23. Hit the Trail

Combine ¼ cup unsalted peanuts with ¼ cup multigrain pretzels, 2 tablespoons dried cherries, and 2 tablespoons pumpkin seeds.

24. Wake-up Call

1 Almond & Coconut Kind Fruit & Nut bar and a 16-ounce coffee skim latte

25. Coffee Shop Special

Starbucks Perfect Oatmeal with Nut Medley Topping and a tall (12-ounce) nonfat Caffè Latte.

Munchie-Taming Lunches
(Choose One Daily; Each Option Totals About 450 Calories)

More than an excuse to take a break from work, lunch is a time to recharge with filling, fat-fighting fare. These scrumptious dishes are packed with veggies and other superfoods that allow you to enjoy a large, satisfying portion without the giant calorie load. That helps stave off cravings and keeps your metabolism humming, which keeps you losing inches. If you begin to miss old trips to the drive-through or deli, take a walk before or after eating your Drop 10 lunch to get that change of scenery minus the unwanted calories. On the other hand, don't let busy days bump lunch to the bottom of your to-do list; doing so sets you up for an out-of-control foraging session later. Eating before you get to the point of wanting to gobble up anything and everything in sight—even if it means taking bites between phone calls and email—keeps your appetite steady and you ready to power through the rest of the day.

TEN WAYS TO SET YOURSELF UP FOR SUCCESS

Think of the superfood meals in this chapter as your weight loss weapons and the tips below as specialized training. Follow them while you are on the Drop 10 plan to get the most pound-peeling power out of everything you put in your mouth.

1. *Slow down!* Speeding through meals could be a ticket to stronger cravings and extra helpings. Women who took twenty-nine minutes to eat not only consumed fewer calories but also felt more satisfied than when they ate in only nine minutes, a study from the University of Rhode Island in Kingston notes. To hit the brakes, rest your fork or sip water between bites.

2. *Relax, already.* Feeling harried? Log some couch time, or set aside a few moments to breathe deeply—whatever helps you chill out. Some relaxing every day can lower stress hormones that may spur overeating, a study from Harvard Medical School finds.

3. *RIP, MSG.* On this plan, you'll eat plenty of fresh, whole foods, but sometimes you need to reach for premade eats, for whatever reason. When you do, limit those with monosodium glutamate (MSG). The flavor enhancer may interfere with your body's ability to regulate appetite. Watch out for *monosodium glutamate* on labels, or *hydrolyzed soy protein* or *autolyzed yeast*, both of which contain MSG.

4. *Weigh your success.* If you're on the Drop 10 diet, you probably have a scale. Use it! Dieters who weighed themselves at least weekly lost more weight than those who didn't, according to research from the Minneapolis Heart Institute Foundation. (Whether you step on the scale once a week or more frequently, weigh yourself in the buff and at the same time of day on the same scale for consistency.) Seeing the numbers plummet can be a great motivator, but it shouldn't be your only one. Because the scale doesn't account for lost inches and gains in lean muscle, also pay attention to how your clothes fit, how you look in the mirror, and how energized you feel.

5. *Drink to a slimmer you.* Don't forget that liquid calories count toward your bottom line. Americans guzzle an incredible 458 calories a day from drinks such as juice and soda, according to a report in the journal *Obesity*. Those liquid calories can lead to weight gain, because people don't necessarily compensate by eating less. Craving a soda? Sip a glass of seltzer or club soda (zero calories!) with a squeeze of lemon instead, or save up those happy calories. (Diet sodas aren't the answer: the artificial sweeteners may signal to your brain that you've consumed sugar, which could cause a chain reaction of excess insulin, a blood sugar crash, and, eventually, a ramped-up appetite.)

6. *Sleep off the munchies.* Eating snacks is a must on this plan, but if you find yourself extra hungry, you may need to log more zzz's than bites. Getting fewer than seven or eight hours of sleep could cause spikes in ghrelin, an appetite-stimulating hormone, and dips in leptin, which suppresses hunger. Can't get into the habit of tucking in at a reasonable hour? Hit the sack fifteen minutes earlier each night for a week, then thirty minutes, and so on until you're logging enough horizontal hours.

7. *Tune in to your food.* If you regularly chew and view, switch off the TV during mealtimes and move from the coffee table to the kitchen or dining table instead. When you're distracted, you may have a hard time recalling later how much you ate, so you might snack without realizing how many calories you've already taken in. Your brain is also more likely to register plated eats on a table as bona fide meals, which means you're less prone to excess grazing between meals.

8. *Grow your veggie love.* Not crazy about all the superfood vegetables? To win yourself over, employ the powers of two superfoods you probably do like: grated Parmesan and olive oil. Adding a favorite topping to veggies only three times can train you to enjoy the produce more later, even when you serve them without the extras, according to a study in *Appetite*.

9. *Close your kitchen at night.* Regularly munching after eight p.m. is linked to weight gain, according to researchers at the University of Kansas in Lawrence. After packing up any leftovers from dinner and doing the dishes, switch off the kitchen lights and mentally lock up the cupboards and fridge until morning. If you tend to sit in the kitchen reading the paper or paying bills, find another spot in the house to avoid temptation. Out of sight, out of mind!

10. *Cut yourself some slack.* Everybody messes up at some point. It is not grounds for throwing in the towel; one overindulgence (or several!) does not a busted diet make. If you didn't budget enough happy calories for, say, those extra ribs you ate at the picnic, simply get back on track at your next meal. Just remember that every bite is an opportunity to start fresh. You can do this!

SAMMIES AND WRAPS

1. Chicken-Avocado Wrap

Top a 10-inch whole-wheat tortilla with a 4-ounce boneless, skinless chicken breast, cooked; ¼ avocado, sliced; and 1 medium tomato, sliced. Wrap. Serve with 1 cup fresh blueberries.

2. Sardine Salad Sandwich

Mix 3 ounces chopped canned sardines (packed in water, drained) with 1 small chopped carrot, 2 tablespoons chopped fresh parsley, 1 tablespoon lemon juice, and 1 teaspoon olive oil. Serve with 2 slices whole-wheat bread and 1 apple.

3. BALT

Layer 3 pieces center-cut bacon, 4 slices avocado, lettuce, 2 thick slices tomato, and 1 tablespoon olive oil mayo between 2 slices whole-wheat bread. Serve with 1½ cups sliced fresh strawberries drizzled with 1 tablespoon balsamic vinegar.

4. Open-faced Turkey-Brie Melt

Top 1 slice whole-wheat bread with 2 ounces thinly sliced low-sodium turkey, 1 ounce Brie, 2 thin slices avocado, and 1 teaspoon low-sugar raspberry preserves; broil until cheese melts. Serve with 6 ounces nonfat raspberry yogurt.

5. Mushroom Sandwich

Place 1 portobello mushroom (brushed with ½ teaspoon olive oil and grilled or broiled), 1 slice Havarti (1 ounce), and ¼ cup sliced roasted red pepper on 2 slices whole-grain toast spread with 1 tablespoon olive oil mayonnaise mixed with ⅛ teaspoon ground cumin. Serve with ½ cup fresh cherries.

6. Spicy Sardine Sammy

Mix 3 ounces canned chopped sardines (packed in water, drained) with 2 tablespoons each chopped celery and chopped water chestnuts. Add 2 teaspoons olive oil mayonnaise, 2 teaspoons chopped cilantro, and a squeeze of Sriracha sauce. Serve in a 6½-inch whole-wheat pita, and enjoy with 1 kiwifruit.

7. Egg Salad Pita

Mix 2 chopped hard-boiled eggs with 1 small chopped carrot, 1 small stalk chopped celery, 2 tablespoons chopped parsley, and 2 teaspoons olive oil mayonnaise. Serve in a 6½-inch whole-wheat pita, and enjoy with 1 apple.

SOUP 'N' SALAD

8. Loaded Lentil Soup

Prepare 2 cups canned low-sodium lentil soup, and mix in ¼ cup fresh chopped kale, ¼ cup diced carrot, ¼ cup canned black beans (rinsed and drained). Serve with 1 whole-grain cracker and 1 ounce Cheddar on the side.

9. **Two-Bean Chili**

Sauté ½ cup chopped onion in 1 teaspoon olive oil until soft. Stir in 1 cup chopped tomatoes, ¾ cup canned kidney beans (rinsed and drained), ½ cup canned black beans (rinsed and drained), ½ cup water, 1 teaspoon chili powder, and ½ teaspoon cumin. Simmer, stirring occasionally, until chili has reduced slightly, about 15 minutes. Top with ⅓ cup avocado cubes and 2 teaspoons chopped fresh cilantro.

10. **Steakhouse Salad**

Coat 2 cups mushrooms with olive oil cooking spray. Roast at 450 degrees until mushrooms are tender, about 30 minutes, stirring once or twice. Place over 3 cups arugula. Top with 1 cup canned (rinsed and drained) artichoke hearts, 1 cup sliced cherry tomatoes, 3 ounces sliced grilled skirt steak, 1 tablespoon grated Parmesan, 2 teaspoons lemon juice, and 1 teaspoon olive oil. Enjoy with ½ cup fresh blueberries.

11. **Artichoke-Pasta Salad**

Mix 1 cup chopped canned (rinsed and drained) artichoke hearts into 1 cup cooked whole-grain pasta. Add 1 cup halved cherry tomatoes, 2 tablespoons chopped fresh basil, 1 tablespoon olive oil, and 1 tablespoon balsamic vinegar. Sprinkle with 1 tablespoon pine nuts.

12. **Sweet Potato and Quinoa Salad**

Mix ½ cup cooked quinoa with 1 cup cooked, cubed sweet potato and ½ cup chopped red bell pepper. Dress with 2 tablespoons chopped fresh cilantro, 1 tablespoon olive oil, 1 tablespoon lemon juice, and a pinch of ground cumin.

13. **Smoked Salmon Salad**

Toss 3 cups mixed greens with 1 cup cucumber slices, 1 chopped carrot, 1 chopped tomato, 2 teaspoons olive oil, and 2 teaspoons lemon juice. Top with 3 ounces nitrate-free smoked salmon.

Enjoy with 1 slice whole-wheat toast spread with 1 tablespoon almond butter and 1 teaspoon honey.

14. Poached-Egg Salad

Place 1 poached egg over 2 cups arugula tossed with 1 baked sweet potato (cut into wedges), ¼ cup black olives, ¼ cup chopped cucumber, 2 tablespoons chopped Cheddar, 2 tablespoons chopped onion, 1 tablespoon balsamic vinegar, and 2 teaspoons olive oil.

15. Power Protein Salad

Combine a 4-ounce can of sardines (packed in water, drained) with 2 cups steamed broccoli, ½ cup cooked quinoa, and 2 cups mixed salad greens. Dress with 2 teaspoons olive oil and 2 teaspoons lemon juice; top with 2 teaspoons chopped fresh parsley.

16. Chicken-Cherry Salad

Combine ¾ cup cooked quinoa with ½ cup pitted fresh cherries and 4 ounces cooked boneless, skinless chicken breast. Serve on top of 3 cups mixed salad greens; dress with 2 teaspoons olive oil and 2 teaspoons lemon juice.

17. Crispy Kale and Quinoa Salad

Toss 3 cups kale with 2 teaspoons olive oil and 1 teaspoon reduced-sodium soy sauce. Spread kale on a baking sheet and bake at 350 degrees until kale is golden brown and crispy, about 15 minutes, tossing once. Mix baked kale with 1 cup cooked quinoa, and top with 2 teaspoons chopped fresh cilantro and 2 teaspoons lime juice. Serve with 1 kiwifruit.

HOT AND HEARTY

18. Curry-Yogurt Salmon

Mix 2 ounces low-fat plain Greek yogurt with ¼ teaspoon curry powder and freshly ground black pepper. Coat a 6-ounce wild salmon fillet (with or without skin) with yogurt mixture; broil on a baking sheet coated with vegetable oil cooking spray until fish is cooked through, about 12 minutes. Remove skin, if necessary. Drizzle with lime juice. Serve with 2 cups steamed broccoli and ½ cup cooked brown rice.

19. Breakfast for Lunch

Prepare 2 whole-grain pancakes (made from a mix) topped with ¼ cup fresh blueberries and 2 tablespoons light syrup. Enjoy with 1 slice Canadian bacon, 1 scrambled egg, and 1 orange cut into sections and sprinkled with 2 tablespoons pomegranate seeds and 1 tablespoon shredded coconut.

20. Pork Stir-fry

Sauté 4 ounces pork tenderloin (cut into strips) with 1 cup broccoli florets, ⅓ cup frozen shelled edamame, and ¼ cup sliced onion in 2 teaspoons olive oil mixed with 1 teaspoon sesame oil and ¼ teaspoon reduced-sodium soy sauce. Serve over ½ cup cooked quinoa.

21. Asian Peanut Pasta

Cook 2 ounces soba noodles as directed on package. Toss with 1 teaspoon sesame oil and 1 teaspoon lime juice. Mix with 2 cups broccoli, ½ cup edamame, 1 carrot sliced into thin rounds, and 1 tablespoon chopped peanuts. Top with 1 teaspoon chopped fresh cilantro and a squeeze of Sriracha sauce (if desired).

22. Tomato-Poached Eggs

Sauté 1 cup chopped mushrooms and 1 chopped garlic clove in 1 teaspoon olive oil. Stir in 2 cups spinach; add 2 cups low-sodium tomato sauce. When sauce heats through and bubbles slightly, add 2 eggs and cover. Poach eggs in sauce until cooked, about 5 minutes. Top with 1 tablespoon grated Parmesan. Serve with 1 slice whole-wheat bread.

23. Veggie Stir-fry

Heat 1 teaspoon sesame oil over high heat. Stir-fry 2 cups broccoli, 1 cup sliced red bell pepper, ½ cup shelled edamame, and

4 ounces cubed tofu. Top with 2 teaspoons chopped fresh cilantro, 1 teaspoon lime juice, and a squeeze of Sriracha sauce (if desired). Serve with ½ cup cooked brown rice.

24. Steak and Potatoes

Microwave 1 medium sweet potato until tender, about 8 minutes. Serve with 2 cups steamed broccoli, 3 ounces grilled skirt steak, and 1 slice whole-wheat bread topped with 1 tablespoon almond butter.

25. Chili Sweet Potato

Top 1 large baked sweet potato with 1 cup canned vegetarian chili with beans, 1 tablespoon low-fat plain yogurt, and 1 teaspoon chopped fresh chives (optional). Serve with 2 kiwifruit.

Fat-Sizzling Snacks
(Choose One Daily; Each Option Totals About 150 Calories)

Think about the last time you planned to eat healthfully but ended up devouring an entire pizza or gorging on whatever the vending machine popped out. You were probably starving right before your first bite, right? In the battle of wills between good diet judgment and a stomach that's been empty for hours, a growling belly usually prevails. That's why it's crucial to plan for and eat these slimming snacks: Doing so keeps your energy up and hunger down, so you won't make choices that stymie your weight loss success. Whether you eat these yummy options between breakfast and lunch, or between lunch and dinner (or split them up, munching half in the morning and half in the afternoon), depends on your schedule and hunger level. The important thing is that you eat every three to four hours during the day. So, for example, if you eat breakfast around nine a.m. and have lunch at twelve-thirty or one but won't eat again until seven p.m., then snack midafternoon. With so many delicious, grab-and-go, filling choices, you won't need the vending machine.

EASY MUNCHIES

1. Italian Popcorn

Pop a 100-calorie bag of microwave popcorn. Sprinkle with 2 tablespoons shredded Parmesan, ½ teaspoon dried oregano, and a few shakes of red pepper flakes.

2. Hot Popcorn

Toss 1 tablespoon unsalted peanuts with ½ teaspoon chili powder, ⅛ teaspoon red pepper flakes, and a 100-calorie snack bag of popcorn.

3. Soy in Shell

Toss 1 cup cooked edamame in pods with ¼ teaspoon salt.

4. Sweet and Spicy Seeds

Toss 1 cup pumpkin seeds with 1 tablespoon olive oil, 1 tablespoon sugar, 1 teaspoon cinnamon, and a shake of cayenne pepper. Spread seeds in an even layer on a foil-covered baking sheet. Bake at 350 degrees until seeds are golden brown, 30 minutes, stirring every 10 minutes. Makes six 2½-tablespoon servings.

5. Kale Chips

Lightly coat 3 cups kale leaves (center ribs removed) with 1 tablespoon olive oil. Sprinkle with ¼ teaspoon salt. Bake at 350 degrees until kale is brown and crispy, 10 to 15 minutes.

6. Fruit and Fiber

Top 1 slice Pepperidge Farm 100% Whole Wheat Cinnamon Swirl Bread with Raisins with 1 tablespoon almond butter and serve with ¼ cup sliced pear.

7. Mini-Pizza

Split a 100-calorie English muffin; top with 2 tablespoons marinara sauce and 1 tablespoon grated Parmesan. Broil until warm.

8. Nutty Banana

Spread 1 medium banana with 2 teaspoons almond butter.

9. Hot Apple Pie

Top a thinly sliced apple with 1 tablespoon chopped walnuts, 1 teaspoon honey, and a sprinkle of cinnamon. Microwave until warm, 30 seconds.

FAST GRABS

10. Pomegranate Spritzer

Mix ½ cup pomegranate juice with 8 ounces seltzer. Add a squeeze of lime juice. Enjoy with ⅓ cup peanuts (measured in shells).

11. Apple and Cheese

Serve ½ small apple with 1 ounce Parmesan.

12. Apple and Cheese 2

Enjoy 1 mozzarella string cheese and 1 apple.

13. Cocoa Berries

Mix ½ ounce dark-chocolate-covered blueberries with 3 tablespoons goji berries.

14. Goji Trail Mix

Combine 2 tablespoons goji berries with ¼ cup whole-grain cereal and 2 tablespoons unsalted peanuts.

PARFAITS AND PUDDING

15. Greek Treat

Top 4 ounces low-fat plain Greek yogurt with 1 tablespoon granola cereal and 1 teaspoon honey.

16. Berry-Oat Parfait

In a glass, spoon 1 layer each: 6 ounces nonfat vanilla yogurt, ¼ cup fresh blueberries, 1 tablespoon toasted oats.

17. Pomegranate-Chocolate Pudding

Enjoy 1 snack-size reduced-fat chocolate pudding topped with ¼ cup pomegranate seeds.

18. Blueberry-Cocoa Parfait

Top ½ cup fresh blueberries with ⅓ cup ricotta cheese and ½ teaspoon cocoa powder.

QUICK DIPS

19. Warm Artichoke Dip

Drain 1 can (14 ounces) artichoke hearts. Chop artichokes and mix with 6 ounces low-fat plain Greek yogurt, ¾ cup grated Parmesan, 2 chopped garlic cloves, and 2 tablespoons chopped fresh parsley. Microwave until warm, about 4 minutes, stirring every 2 minutes. Makes six ¼-cup servings. Serve with 15 baby carrots for dipping.

20. Salty South of the Border Bites

Serve 10 baked tortilla chips and 1 cup red bell pepper strips with 2 tablespoons guacamole for dipping.

21. Peanut-Yogurt Dip

Dip 1 cup cucumber slices in 2 teaspoons peanut butter mixed with a few drops reduced-sodium soy sauce and ⅓ cup plain nonfat Greek yogurt.

22. Almond-Chocolate Apple

Melt ½ ounce dark chocolate; mix with 1 teaspoon almond butter. Use as a dip for ½ an apple, sliced.

23. Edamame-Yogurt Dip

Mash ¼ cup shelled edamame; stir into 3 ounces low-fat plain Greek yogurt. Stir in 1 teaspoon lemon juice, 1 teaspoon chopped fresh parsley, and a pinch of cayenne pepper (optional). Serve with 2 crispbread crackers for dipping.

24. Hummus Dippers

Enjoy ¼ cup hummus with 10 baby carrots and 1 cup broccoli florets.

25. Indian Yogurt Dip

Stir ⅛ teaspoon curry powder, 1 teaspoon chopped fresh cilantro, and a pinch of cayenne pepper (optional) into 3 ounces low-fat plain Greek yogurt. Serve with 15 baby carrots and 1 cup red bell pepper slices for dipping.

Thinner Dinners
(Choose One Daily; Each Option Totals About 450 Calories)

If dinner tends to be your downfall, your taste buds are going to love what's coming. These mouthwatering, nutrient-dense options serve up hearty portions that leave you feeling full and satiated—not overly stuffed the way you might be used to—but still steadily shrinking. The trick is in their balance of lean protein (including meat-free options such as lentils and beans), slow-digesting whole grains and produce, and healthy, satisfying fats. After enjoying these powerhouses, you'll no longer need to raid the fridge for leftovers or snacks during prime time. Instead, you'll hit the sack at night feeling satisfied, slimmer by the day, and proud of your diet accomplishments.

PERFECT PASTAS

1. Veggie Pasta

Sauté ½ cup chopped red onion, 1 chopped garlic clove, and a pinch of red pepper flakes (optional) in 2 teaspoons olive oil until onion is soft, about 5 minutes. Add 2 cups chopped tomato and ½ cup frozen artichoke hearts, thawed and drained; cook 5 minutes. Pour sauce over 2 ounces whole-grain pasta (cooked as directed on package); top with 2 teaspoons chopped fresh basil and 1 teaspoon chopped fresh parsley. Serve with ½ cup steamed sugar snap peas.

2. Tuna and Artichoke Pasta

Sauté 1 cup frozen artichoke hearts (thawed and drained), 1 tablespoon chopped pitted olives, and 1 teaspoon chopped garlic in 1 teaspoon olive oil for 5 minutes. Add 1 cup halved grape tomatoes and 2 tablespoons white wine; simmer until wine reduces slightly, about 5 minutes. Toss artichoke mixture with 2 ounces whole-grain linguine, cooked; 3 ounces canned-in-water chunk light tuna, drained; 1 teaspoon lemon juice; 1 teaspoon dried rosemary; and salt and pepper to taste.

3. Broccoli-Peanut Noodles

Combine 1 tablespoon peanut butter with 1 teaspoon lime juice and a pinch of red pepper flakes (optional). Toss with 1 cup cooked whole-grain pasta. Top pasta with 2 cups steamed broccoli, 4 ounces grilled boneless, skinless chicken breast, 1 teaspoon chopped fresh cilantro, and ½ tablespoon chopped peanuts.

4. Pesto Pasta

Mix 1 cup cooked whole-grain pasta with 1 tablespoon prepared pesto and 1 tablespoon grated Parmesan. Serve with 2 cups steamed broccoli and 3 ounces grilled skirt steak.

5. Garlicky Broccoli Pasta

Boil 3 cups broccoli florets. After 10 minutes, add 3 ounces whole-grain pasta and cook as directed on package. Drain pasta and broccoli (save 1 cup pasta cooking water). In 1 teaspoon olive oil, sauté 2 chopped garlic cloves with a pinch of red pepper flakes (optional). Toss broccoli-pasta mixture with garlic and oil.

Sprinkle with 1 tablespoon grated Parmesan. Add a bit of pasta water to thin the sauce, if desired.

FILLING SALADS

6. Grilled Steak Salad

Toss 2 cup greens with ¾ cup corn kernels, ¼ cup each sliced carrot and red onion, ½ cup halved grape tomatoes, 3 ounces grilled flank steak, ½ ounce blue cheese, and 2 tablespoons store-bought olive oil vinaigrette.

7. Greek Lentil Salad

Mix 1 cup cooked lentils with 2 cups spinach, 1 cup halved cherry tomatoes, and 4 ounces cooked and chopped boneless, skinless chicken breast. Top with a dressing of 1 tablespoon crumbled feta, 1 teaspoon olive oil, 1 teaspoon lemon juice, and a few shakes of dried oregano.

8. Broccoli-Shrimp Salad

Whisk 1 teaspoon olive oil with 1 teaspoon lemon juice and a pinch of curry powder. Toss dressing with 2 cups steamed broccoli, 1 cup cooked lentils, and 4 ounces cooked shrimp. Top with 2 teaspoons chopped fresh cilantro.

9. Steak and Pumpkin Seed Salad

Grill 3 ounces skirt steak. Serve with a salad made of 3 cups spinach, 1 cup chopped broccoli, ¼ cup avocado cubes, 1 tablespoon roasted pumpkin seeds, and 1 tablespoon chopped fresh cilantro. Dress with 2 teaspoons lemon juice and 1 teaspoon olive oil. Enjoy with a 4-inch whole-wheat pita.

10. Citrusy Quinoa Salad

Combine 2 cups mixed greens with ¾ cup cooked quinoa and 1 orange (segmented, rind and white pith removed). Top with 4 ounces cooked boneless, skinless chicken breast, 2 tablespoons grated Parmesan, and 1 teaspoon olive oil.

SEAFOOD

11. Mediterranean Baked Salmon

Rub 4 ounces wild salmon with 1 teaspoon olive oil. In a baking dish coated with 1 teaspoon olive oil cooking spray, place salmon, 1 sliced red bell pepper, ½ sliced fennel bulb, and 10 small black pitted olives. Sprinkle with 2 teaspoons chopped fresh oregano and season with freshly ground black pepper. Bake at 375 degrees for 10 minutes; stir the veggies; bake until cooked through, 15 to 20 minutes more. Drizzle with lemon juice. Serve with ½ cup cooked quinoa.

12. Salmon with Pumpkin Seed Pesto

In a food processor, combine ½ cup roasted pumpkin seeds, 1 tablespoon grated Parmesan, and 2 garlic cloves; pulse until seeds are almost ground. Add ¾ cup fresh basil, ¾ cup fresh parsley, 2 tablespoons lemon juice, and 2 tablespoons olive oil. Pulse until combined; you may want to add a tablespoon or so of water to thin the sauce. (Makes 6 servings, about 1 cup total; refrigerate the extra for up to a week.) Serve on top of a 4-ounce cooked wild salmon fillet. Enjoy with 1 cup steamed green beans and ¾ cup cooked brown rice.

13. Beach Treat

Prepare a frozen crab cake with a side sauce of 1 tablespoon olive oil mayonaise mixed with ¼ teaspoon chili powder and a splash of lime juice. Toss 1 sweet potato, sliced into wedges, with 2 teaspoons olive oil and 1 teaspoon Old Bay seasoning (optional); roast until tender. Serve with 20 steamed asparagus stalks.

14. Italian Fish Stew

Sauté 1 cup chopped red onion and 1 chopped garlic clove in 1 teaspoon olive oil. When onion softens, add 2 cups chopped fresh tomatoes. When tomatoes break down and sauce simmers, add 4 ounces halibut and ½ teaspoon dried oregano. Simmer until fish is cooked, about 10 minutes. Top with 1 tablespoon grated Parmesan and 1 teaspoon chopped fresh parsley. Serve with 1 slice whole-wheat bread and a salad made of 3 cups mixed greens, ½ cup sliced mushrooms, and 10 small black olives. Dress salad with 1 teaspoon olive oil mixed with 1 teaspoon lemon juice.

15. Indian-Spiced Broccoli with Shrimp

Toss 3 cups broccoli with 1 teaspoon olive oil, ½ teaspoon ground cumin, ½ teaspoon ground coriander, and ¼ teaspoon cayenne pepper (optional). Spread broccoli on a baking sheet; roast for 10 minutes at 425 degrees. Toss 4 ounces shrimp with 1 teaspoon olive oil. Add to sheet with broccoli; roast until shrimp are cooked, about 10 minutes more, stirring once. Top with 2 teaspoons lemon juice mixed with 2 teaspoons chopped cilantro. Serve with ¾ cup cooked brown rice.

STEAK, POULTRY, AND PORK

16. Steak and Squash

Sauté ½ cup chopped red onion and 1 chopped garlic clove in 1 teaspoon olive oil until soft, about 5 minutes. Add 2 cups chopped tomato; cook until a sauce forms. Pour sauce over 3 cups cooked spaghetti squash (cut in half, scrape out seeds and pulp, and bake rind side up for about 40 minutes at 375 degrees; when cooked, separate strands by running a fork down the squash from stem to bottom). Top squash with 2 tablespoons chopped fresh basil. Broil 4 ounces flank steak about 7 minutes, turning once. Serve steak with squash.

17. Garlicky Kale and Bean Sauté

Sauté 2 cups chopped kale with 1 chopped garlic clove in 1 teaspoon olive oil until kale is tender. Stir in ¾ cup canned white beans (rinsed and drained); heat until beans are warmed. Top with 1 tablespoon grated Parmesan, and serve with 3 ounces grilled skirt steak.

18. Cheesy Baked Quinoa

Mix 1 cup cooked quinoa with 2 cups steamed kale, 2 tablespoons grated Parmesan, 1 teaspoon chopped fresh parsley, and ½ teaspoon chopped fresh sage. Bake at 350 degrees until cheese melts, 5 minutes. Serve with 3 ounces grilled skirt or flank steak.

19. Asian Slaw and Steak

Toss 3 cups chopped napa cabbage with 1 cup sliced red bell pepper, 1 teaspoon each chopped fresh mint and cilantro; top with 1 tablespoon chopped peanuts, 1 teaspoon sesame oil, and 1 teaspoon lime juice. Serve with 3 ounces grilled skirt steak and ¾ cup cooked brown rice.

20. Chicken with Mushrooms and Peppers

Sauté a 5-ounce boneless, skinless chicken breast in a nonstick pan coated with cooking spray until cooked through, about 10 minutes; remove from pan and keep warm. In same pan, sauté 1 cup chopped red bell pepper, 1 cup chopped mushrooms, and ½ cup chopped red onion in 2 teaspoons olive oil until vegetables are tender, about 5 minutes. Add 1 cup chopped tomatoes and 2 teaspoons chopped fresh oregano; cook until tomatoes break down into a sauce, about 8 minutes. Place vegetable mixture on a plate; top with chicken, 2 tablespoons grated Parmesan, and 2 teaspoons chopped fresh basil. Serve with 1 slice whole-wheat bread.

21. Summer Barbecue

Grill a 3-ounce turkey burger; place on a whole-wheat English muffin bottom; top with ¼ avocado, sliced; 1 small tomato, sliced; ½ ounce Cheddar; and muffin top. Serve with 2 cups cubed watermelon.

22. Cherry Pork Tenderloin

Cook 4 ounces pork tenderloin. Top with a cherry salsa made with ½ cup pitted fresh cherries, 1 teaspoon chopped fresh cilantro, 1 teaspoon lime juice, and 1 chopped scallion. Serve with 1 cup cooked brown rice tossed with chopped fresh cilantro and lime juice to taste.

VEG OUT!

23. Sweet Potato and Lentils

Combine 1 cup cooked lentils with 1 cooked medium sweet potato, cubed; 2 cups spinach; 2 teaspoons olive oil; and a pinch of cayenne pepper (optional). Top with 1 teaspoon chopped fresh cilantro and a squeeze of lime juice. Eat with 1 kiwifruit.

24. Quinoa and Pepper Sauté

Sauté 1 cup chopped red bell pepper, ½ cup chopped red onion, and ¼ teaspoon smoked paprika in 1 teaspoon olive oil until vegetables are soft, about 5 minutes. Add 2 cups kale; sauté until kale wilts. Serve vegetable mixture over 1 cup cooked quinoa. Sprinkle with 2 tablespoons grated Parmesan and 2 teaspoons chopped fresh parsley. Serve with a tangerine.

25. Stuffed Chiles

Stuff a mild Anaheim chile (or other mild pepper) with a mixture of 1 cup cooked quinoa, ½ cup tomato sauce, ½ cup frozen corn kernels, and 2 tablespoons diced onion; bake 20 minutes. Top with 2 tablespoons grated Parmesan.

You've Reached Your Weight Loss Goal—Now What?

Congratulations! Your first order of business: Celebrate! Bask in your success by going shopping, treating yourself to a spa day, or blowing off chores and spending the afternoon with your family. Whatever you decide, you deserve it. You've earned it.

Next up, make a pledge to keep the weight off and maintain your trim, healthy new figure. The best part is, you already know how to do it. On the Drop 10 diet, you've lost more than extra pounds; you've also ditched the poor eating habits that caused you to put them on in the first place. And what you've gained, aside from a sexy, svelte body, are a slew of new behaviors and a wealth of knowledge about the foods and meals that help fill you up on fewer calories, stave off cravings, burn and resist fat, rev your metabolism, and keep your energy level high. As we mentioned in chapter 1, the Drop 10 diet and the superfoods approach aren't fads you pick up and drop the way you might other diets; rather, they're a collection of healthy foods, habits, tips, ideas, recipes, and ways of thinking that slowly become a part of your everyday life.

You will need to transition, however, from the weight loss stage of the plan to the maintenance stage. Here's how:

- Adjust your calorie intake. Continue to eat your favorite superfoods and the Drop 10 meals and snacks, but add about 200 calories to your daily 1,600-calorie intake. These aren't bonus happy calories for splurges; they're calories you spend on superfoods and other healthful, whole foods, and that you spread evenly over all your day's meals and snacks. To do it, slightly increase the serving sizes of dishes and foods you're already eating. For example, instead of a 3-ounce fillet of wild salmon, have 4 ounces. After one week, weigh yourself. If you have lost any more weight but would rather maintain the optimum weight you've worked so hard to achieve, add another 200 calories. If you've gained, drop your intake by about 100 calories. Keep tweaking your meals until your weight stabilizes, giving you an idea of how many calories per day you need to stay right where you are. Also keep weighing in regularly to stay on top of your stats so you know if and when you need to make additional changes.
- Broaden your meal horizons. Keep planning your menu each week, incorporating the superfoods and as many meals and snacks from this book as you like. But don't be afraid to branch out, too. Search for recipes online or in cookbooks, or swap them with friends. Aim to make the thirty superfoods the centerpiece of your diet, but also remember that it's important to take in a range of other fruits, vegetables, whole grains, lean protein, low-fat dairy, and foods rich in healthy unsaturated fats. Also check out the tips on the following page to help you stay on track as you

begin eating superfood-packed meals and making recipes not included in the menu plan.

- Keep moving. Hands down, exercise is one of the most useful tools to keep fat from coming back. Research suggests that working out not only might help reduce your biological drive to eat following weight loss (aka a ramped-up appetite), it also encourages fat burning versus fat storage. All this is in addition to the calories you sizzle during exercise itself. Need more convincing? Consider data from more than six thousand participants in the National Weight Control Registry: Regular exercise sessions (think at least three hours of moderate-intensity physical activity per week) helped these participants keep off an average of 74 pounds for more than five years. Whether you keep following the Drop 10 superworkouts in chapter 13 or explore others (we know firsthand that *SELF* magazine and Self.com are chock-full of good ones each month), vow to make fitness a part of your regular routine and your new slimmed-down self will be here to stay.

Ten Stay-Slim Tips For Life

We hope you stash this book in your kitchen and use it for planning menus and making slimming, healthy meals. After all, the healthy habits that got you to your trim new self will help you stay that way for life! So keep logging your meals and calories in your food journal (remember, you can find data for almost anything at NutritionData.Self.com) and, of course, go on indulging (in moderation) in your favorite treats. But it helps to have a few extra tricks up your sleeve as you begin to focus on maintaining your amazing success.

1. *Be on portion patrol.* It's human nature to clean your plate—and the more you're served (or serve yourself), the more you're likely to eat. For example, when researchers at Pennsylvania State University in University Park gave people standard-size meals for eleven days, then supersized them by 50 percent, diners took in 423 more calories per day. If you need help sticking to sensible

portions when eating meals off the Drop 10 plan, downsize your dishes: Smaller plates hold less. Also, if you have trouble eyeballing servings, whip out measuring spoons and cups. It's worth taking a little extra time now so you won't see pounds appear later.

2. *Come up with coping strategies.* Emotional eaters are thirteen times more likely to be overweight or obese, according to researchers at the University of Alabama in Tuscaloosa. If you tend to eat to soothe stress, it's crucial to separate food from your mood, especially now that you will probably be making more food choices away from the plan. Search online for meditation and breathing exercises, have a go-to pal you can call to let off steam, go for a walk—whatever! Just be sure you've got a plan in place before the urge to overeat takes hold.

3. *Keep the kitchen fires burning.* It's okay to eat out once in a while, but by maintaining more control over what goes in your mouth, you can better maintain those low numbers on the scale. Also brown-bag your lunch as often as possible. You can prep tomorrow's lunch today: Before cleaning up the kitchen after dinner, make your meal while leftovers, condiments, and other items are already out.

4. *Plan menus, make grocery lists, and shop in advance.* This goes double for those weeks when you're extra busy and may be tempted to wing it. The better prepared you are to eat healthfully, the more apt you are to follow through. Our brain is more rational when we are making decisions about the future, according to a study from Harvard University. Researchers found that online shoppers who ordered groceries at least five days in advance selected healthier fare than those who shopped for next-day delivery. Make lists, and decide on your meals a week ahead of time to stay on track—and stay off the phone with the pizza delivery guy.

5. *Adopt a see-food approach.* If you tend to forget about fruits and veggies when they're in the produce and crisper drawers, move 'em on up! Place them front and center in your fridge. Also stock nuts and other superfood snacks in cupboards you open often. You're more likely to eat what's directly in your line of vision.

6. *Give away your "fat" clothes.* Got enough different sizes in your closet to stock an entire store? Pare down to what fits you right now. Hanging on to stuff that's too big "just in case" is setting yourself up for failure. Don't doubt your new habits, abilities, or resolve! Believe you can keep the weight off, then make it happen.

7. *Catch weight creep before it starts.* Although it can seem like 5 or 10 (or more) pounds suddenly appear overnight, they actually add up one at a time. And the more in tune you stay with your body, the better equipped you are to waylay fat so it doesn't sneak back on you. You were probably weighing yourself regularly during the weight loss phase of the Drop 10 diet, so keep it up. At least once a week at the same time of day, hop on the scale wearing nothing but your birthday suit. You'll keep tabs on your weight this way, as well as reaffirm your success and stay motivated to eat healthfully. It really works! Women who had dropped pounds and then weighed themselves daily for the following eighteen months had the lowest recurrence of regain, according to a study in *The New England Journal of Medicine.* One thing to remember: Your weight may fluctuate from 1 to 3 pounds from one week to the next; what counts is the overall trend. Is your weight mostly steady week after week, or is it steadily adding up? If it's the latter, revisit the tips and tools in this book to get back on track.

8. *Perform the jeans test.* Weighing yourself regularly is important, but the number on the scale shouldn't be your only measure of success. Zip up your favorite pair of skinny pants once a week, especially if you're keen on wearing flowy tops, unstructured dresses, and boyfriend jeans. Those clothes can make it easy to miss a little extra fat, but a sleek pair of denims doesn't hide much.

9. *Be realistic about calories in and calories out.* People are notoriously bad at eyeballing servings and guessing calorie loads. Likewise, we tend to overestimate the number of calories we burn during a workout and thus how justified we are in splurging afterward. In fact, women ate about 120 more calories following

252 • THE DROP 10 DIET

a bout of intense exercise than they did after a lighter workout that burned the same number of calories, according to a study from the University of Ottawa. The fix: Don't simply estimate your calorie intake; look it up! Check NutritionData.Self.com, or, when you go out to eat, pick up nutrition brochures or research menus and nutrition info online beforehand. Also think of an especially tough workout as a bonus or a way to balance overestimations and miscalculations, not an excuse to have a second piece of cake.

10. *Train your brain.* Saying sayonara to bad fat for good is as much about how you think about food as what you actually eat—the two are intimately connected. Remember that you have power over what goes in your mouth. Keep these quick tips in mind to keep you on track:

- Press pause. Before mindlessly or rashly gobbling up a bag of cookies or grabbing stale doughnuts from the conference room, take a few deep breaths to contemplate what you're doing and why. Are you truly hungry? Is whatever you're eating really going to make you happier? Is the taste or binge (and its aftereffects) worth the extra sugar, fat, and calories? Sometimes a brief check-in with yourself drums up the extra willpower you need to move on.

- Take your mind off food. Be creative in finding ways to distract yourself from cravings, urges to eat treats, or extra helpings. Thinking about something else entirely can work to replace those mental images of food. How about playing a quick game on your phone? Games such as solitaire actually increase activity in the same areas of your brain that light up when you think about food.

Now go on and eat, drink, and be slim! You've got the tools you need to sustain your new figure and newfound energy for life.

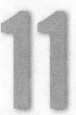

The Drop 10 Recipes:
Simple, Fat-Fighting, Superfood-Loaded Meals and Snacks for the Whole Family

The quick, single-serving meals in the preceding chapter gave you a taste of just how delicious "diet" food is on the Drop 10 plan. Ready for more? Want to spread the tummy (and tummy-shrinking) love to your family and friends? Whether you're cooking for just you, a pair of picky teenagers, or your entire book club, these easy recipes—for pancakes, tacos, pasta, chocolate treats, and more—are as scrumptious and satisfying as they are slimming. Research shows that cooking at home helps you painlessly trim calories, fat, and body weight—which is reason enough to toss those take-out menus and skip store-bought junk. These amazingly easy, crowd-pleasing dishes offer forty more delicious options.

Quickie Breakfasts

If you're wondering how you'll fit a homemade meal into your wake-then-no-break a.m. schedule, you're not alone: A lack of time is one of the most common barriers to eating healthfully, research suggests. But that's not an issue here. These recipes take little time to prep or can be made ahead. Plus, you'll net so much extra energy from eating the nutrient-packed dishes, you'll sail through your morning to-do list with time to spare.

Apple-Yogurt Cups

SERVES 4

2 apples, diced
2 cups nonfat plain Greek yogurt
$1/3$ cup ground flaxseed
$1/4$ cup agave nectar or honey
$1/2$ cup golden raisins

Set out 4 large wine or parfait glasses. In each, layer $1/4$ apple, $1/4$ cup yogurt, 2 teaspoons flaxseed, 1 teaspoon agave nectar, and 1 tablespoon raisins. Repeat layer in each glass.

THE DISH 263 calories, 4 g fat (0 g saturated), 46 g carbs, 6 g fiber, 13 g protein

Kale, Potato, and Onion Frittata

SERVES 4

Vegetable oil cooking spray

1 yellow or white onion, sliced

1 pound kale, trimmed, blanched 3 minutes in boiling water, drained, squeezed, and coarsely chopped

2 cloves garlic, chopped

2 cups boiled diced potatoes

2 whole eggs

2 egg whites

$1/2$ teaspoon paprika (preferably smoked)

Heat oven to 400 degrees. In a medium cast-iron skillet coated with cooking spray, cook onion over medium heat, stirring, for 5 minutes. Add kale and garlic; stir 5 minutes. Add potatoes. In a bowl, whisk eggs, egg whites, 2 tablespoons water, and paprika; stir into vegetable mixture. Cook over medium-low heat 1 minute. Transfer skillet to oven; bake until eggs are set and center is slightly runny, 6 to 8 minutes. Turn oven to broil and broil until top is golden, 1 minute.

THE DISH 153 calories per serving, 3 g fat (1 g saturated), 24 g carbs, 4 g fiber, 9 g protein

Banana-Coffee-Crunch Smoothie

SERVES 2

3 cups sliced banana

2 cups diced pear

2 cups cooled coffee

1 cup nonfat plain Greek yogurt

2 tablespoons honey

1/2 tablespoon chopped walnuts

1/2 teaspoon rum extract

Puree all ingredients in a blender. Pour into 2 glasses.

THE DISH 306 calories per serving, 10 g fat (1 g saturated), 51 g carbs, 1 g fiber, 9 g protein

Tucson Breakfast Burrito

SERVES 6

$1^1/_2$ tablespoons vegetable oil

1 red or green bell pepper, chopped

$^1/_2$ medium onion, chopped

$1^1/_2$ pounds thickly sliced lean deli roast beef, julienned

$^3/_4$ cup low-fat, low-sodium chicken, beef, or vegetable broth

2 cups store-bought tomato salsa, divided

1 cinnamon stick

Salt to taste

1 large whole egg plus 1 large egg white, whisked lightly

6 flour tortillas, warmed

Heat oil in a skillet over medium heat. Sauté pepper and onion for 3 minutes. Stir in meat; continue sautéing until meat is browned and crispy but not burned. (Scrape meat from the bottom occasionally.) Stir in broth and $^1/_2$ cup salsa, and add cinnamon stick. Bring mixture to a boil. Reduce heat to medium; cook until most of the liquid evaporates but meat remains moist. Salt to taste. Remove cinnamon stick. Mix eggs into meat mixture; cook until eggs are just firm, 1 or 2 minutes. Spoon $^1/_6$ of mixture onto each tortilla and roll up. Place on a plate and spoon $^1/_4$ cup salsa over each burrito.

THE DISH 265 calories per serving, 9 g fat (3 g saturated), 25 g carbs, 7 g fiber, 25 g protein

Sweet Potato Biscuits

SERVES 8

    1 medium sweet potato (about 5 ounces)
    2 tablespoons chilled unsalted butter, cubed
    1¼ cups whole-wheat biscuit mix
    ½ cup low-fat buttermilk
    ¼ teaspoon ground allspice

Wrap sweet potato in a paper towel. Microwave on high until soft, 4 minutes. Scoop flesh into a bowl and mash; set aside. Heat oven to 400 degrees. In a bowl, rub butter into biscuit mix with fingertips until large pea-size crumbs form. Add sweet potato, buttermilk, and allspice; mix until just combined. Transfer dough onto a cookie sheet; form into a 12 x 4-inch rectangle. Cut into 8 rectangles with a serrated knife and separate slightly. Bake until biscuits are firm to the touch, 8 to 10 minutes. Transfer to a wire rack to cool. Once cool, store in an airtight container for up to three days.

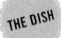 THE DISH

124 calories per biscuit, 5 g fat (3 g saturated), 15 g carbs, 2 g fiber, 3 g protein

Pumpkin Muesli

SERVES 1

1/4 cup pumpkin puree
1/4 cup quick-cooking oats
1/2 cup nonfat plain yogurt
2 tablespoons honey
1 teaspoon grated lemon zest
2 tablespoons slivered or chopped almonds
1 hulled sliced fresh strawberry

In a bowl, combine pumpkin and oats. Cover with plastic wrap and microwave 20 seconds; set aside 10 minutes (so oats absorb puree). In another bowl, mix yogurt, honey, and zest. Swirl in pumpkin mixture, and top with almonds and berry slices.

THE DISH 377 calories per serving, 9 g fat (1 g saturated), 67 g carbs, 6 g fiber, 12 g protein

Berry-Cinnamon Breakfast Quinoa

SERVES 4

1 cup 1 percent milk
1 cup quinoa, rinsed and drained
2 cups fresh raspberries or blueberries
$\frac{1}{2}$ teaspoon cinnamon
$\frac{1}{3}$ cup chopped walnuts
4 teaspoons honey or molasses
$\frac{1}{2}$ cup low-fat plain yogurt

In a medium saucepan, bring milk, 1 cup water, and quinoa to a boil over high heat. Reduce heat to low; cover and simmer until quinoa absorbs most of the liquid, 15 minutes. Turn off heat; let stand covered 5 minutes. Stir in berries and cinnamon; transfer to 4 bowls; top with walnuts. Top each bowl with 1 teaspoon honey and 2 tablespoons yogurt before serving.

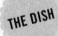

THE DISH

341 calories per serving, 11 g fat (2 g saturated), 53 g carbs, 8 g fiber, 12 g protein

Granola with Cranberries and Almonds

SERVES 4

$1/2$ cup roasted shelled pumpkin seeds
Vegetable oil cooking spray
$1/2$ cup unsweetened cranberry juice or apple juice
$1/3$ cup maple syrup
$1/3$ cup brown sugar
$1^1/2$ teaspoons cinnamon
2 cups old-fashioned oats
$1/2$ cup chopped roasted almonds
$1/4$ teaspoon salt
1 cup dried cranberries

Heat oven to 350 degrees. Spread pumpkin seeds on a baking sheet. Bake until lightly toasted, 8 to 10 minutes. Set aside to cool. Reduce oven temperature to 325 degrees. Spray another baking sheet with cooking spray; set aside. In a small saucepan, cook juice, syrup, sugar, and cinnamon over medium heat, stirring constantly, until sugar dissolves. In a bowl, mix pumpkin seeds with oats, almonds, and salt. Pour maple mixture over oat mixture; stir until combined. Spread mixture onto prepared sheet. Bake 20 minutes. Remove sheet from oven. Stir in cranberries, then bake until granola browns, 10 to 15 minutes more. Cool completely before serving.

THE DISH 377 calories per serving, 15 g fat (2 g saturated), 58 g carbs, 6 g fiber, 10 g protein

Whole-Wheat Blueberry Pancakes with Three-Berry Compote

SERVES 6

Pancakes

1 cup whole-wheat flour

$1/2$ cup all-purpose flour

1 tablespoon baking powder

$1/2$ teaspoon salt

$1^1/_4$ cups skim milk

3 tablespoons vegetable oil

1 egg, beaten

1 tablespoon maple syrup or honey

1 cup fresh or frozen blueberries (thawed if frozen)

Compote

Vegetable oil cooking spray

$1/3$ cup sugar

1 tablespoon lemon juice

$1/2$ cup fresh hulled and sliced strawberries

1 cup fresh blackberries

$1^1/_2$ cups fresh blueberries

6 tablespoons nonfat plain Greek yogurt

In a bowl, combine flours with baking powder and salt. Mix in milk, oil, egg, and syrup until smooth. Fold in 1 cup fresh or frozen blueberries. Heat a griddle or frying pan coated with cooking spray over medium-high heat. Using a $\frac{1}{4}$-cup measure, pour batter onto griddle. Cook until browned, 1 to 2 minutes; flip over and cook until golden. Remove from pan; keep warm. Compote: In a small saucepan, combine sugar, juice, strawberries, blackberries, and remaining $1\frac{1}{2}$ cups fresh blueberries, with 3 tablespoons water; bring to a simmer over medium heat, and cook until blueberry skins pop, 5 minutes. Let cool for 5 minutes before serving. To serve, spoon compote over pancakes and top each with 1 tablespoon yogurt.

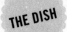

THE DISH   318 calories per serving, 9 g fat (1 g saturated), 51 g carbs, 6 g fiber, 11 g protein

Warm Portobello Caprese English Muffins

SERVES 2

Vegetable oil cooking spray

4 portobello mushroom caps

1/4 teaspoon each salt and freshly ground black pepper

2 whole-grain or multigrain English muffins, halved and toasted

8 slices tomato

2 tablespoons balsamic vinegar

4 large fresh basil leaves

3/4 cup shredded part-skim mozzarella

Heat broiler. Heat a medium skillet coated with cooking spray over medium-high heat. Place mushroom caps in skillet, sprinkle with salt and pepper, and cook until just tender and juicy, 3 to 4 minutes per side. Transfer to a baking sheet. Top each muffin half with a mushroom cap, 2 slices tomato, 1/2 tablespoon vinegar, 1 basil leaf, and 3 tablespoons mozzarella. Broil until cheese melts and bubbles, 2 to 3 minutes.

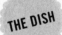

330 calories per serving, 10 g fat (5 g saturated), 41 g carbs, 5 g fiber, 21 g protein

Energizing Lunches

The drive-through can be a tempting midday stop, but consider this: The more you eat out, the more likely you are to be overweight. Fast food is often loaded with saturated fat, sugar, and calories, while it skimps on the fiber-rich veggies and whole grains that keep you full and focused on things other than a growling stomach. Give these easy-to-make lunches a spin and you'll see that healthy food can be as convenient and craveworthy as your favorite combo meal.

Artichoke-and-Beef Lettuce Wraps

SERVES 4

1 can (13 ounces) artichoke hearts, rinsed, drained, and thinly sliced

1/2 pound lean deli roast beef, sliced into thin strips

1 small zucchini, thinly sliced

1 cup canned chickpeas, rinsed and drained

1/4 cup grated reduced-fat Parmesan

1/4 cup packed fresh basil

2 tablespoons capers, chopped

1/4 cup lemon juice

1 teaspoon olive oil

1/2 teaspoon salt

1/4 teaspoon freshly ground black pepper

16 lettuce leaves (such as butter or romaine)

In a bowl, place artichokes, beef, zucchini, chickpeas, Parmesan, basil, capers, juice, and oil; add salt and pepper. Toss to coat. Wrap 1/4 cup filling in each lettuce leaf; serve.

THE DISH 280 calories per 4 wraps, 10 g fat (3 g saturated), 26 g carbs, 5 g fiber, 23 g protein

Bean and 'Bello Burger
SERVES 4

4 tablespoons canola oil, divided

2 medium portobello mushrooms, diced

1/2 red onion, diced

1/2 green bell pepper, diced

1 can (15 ounces) black beans, rinsed and drained

1/4 teaspoon paprika

1/4 teaspoon garlic powder

1/8 teaspoon freshly ground black pepper

2 egg whites

6 tablespoons bread crumbs

1 tablespoon honey mustard

1 tablespoon Worcestershire sauce

4 whole-wheat buns

1/2 cup barbecue sauce

4 lettuce leaves

4 tomato slices

Heat 2 tablespoons oil in a large skillet over medium heat. Cook mushrooms, onion, and bell pepper, stirring occasionally, until pepper softens, 4 to 5 minutes. Add beans, paprika, garlic powder, and black pepper. Cook, smashing beans with the back of a spoon, 1 to 2 minutes more. Transfer mixture to a bowl; mix in egg whites, bread crumbs, mustard, and Worcestershire. Form into 4 patties. Wipe out skillet; heat remaining 2 tablespoons oil over medium heat and cook burgers until browned and firm, 6 to 7 minutes per side. Place on bun bottoms; top each with 2 tablespoons barbecue sauce, a tomato slice, a lettuce leaf, and a bun top.

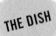

THE DISH 475 calories per burger, 18 g fat (2 g saturated), 61 g carbs, 11 g fiber, 18 g protein

Spiced Lentil Tacos

SERVES 4

1 tablespoon olive oil

1 cup finely chopped onion

1 clove garlic, chopped

$1/2$ teaspoon salt

1 cup dried brown lentils, rinsed

1 package ($2^1/4$ ounces) taco seasoning

$2^1/2$ cups vegetable broth

$1/2$ cup fat-free sour cream

1 chipotle chile in adobo sauce, finely chopped
   (or half for less heat)

2 teaspoons adobo sauce

8 taco shells

$1^1/4$ cups shredded lettuce

1 cup chopped fresh tomato

$1/2$ cup shredded reduced-fat Cheddar

Heat oil in a large skillet over medium-high heat. Cook onion and garlic with salt until onion softens, 3 to 4 minutes. Add lentils and taco seasoning. Cook until spices are fragrant and lentils are dry, 1 minute. Add broth; bring to a boil. Reduce heat, cover, and simmer until lentils are tender, 25 to 30 minutes. In a bowl, mix sour cream with chile and adobo sauce. Uncover lentils; cook until mixture thickens, 6 to 8 minutes. Mash with a rubber spatula. Spoon $1/4$ cup lentil mixture into each taco shell. Top with 2 heaping teaspoons sour cream mixture, lettuce, tomato, and cheese.

THE DISH 249 calories per 2 tacos, 7 g fat (2 g saturated), 37 g carbs, 10 g fiber, 12 g protein

Sweet Potato Soup

SERVES 1

1 tablespoon reduced-fat sour cream

1 teaspoon orange juice concentrate

1 small (4-inch) whole-wheat pita

1/2 clove garlic

Vegetable oil cooking spray

1 teaspoon extra-light olive oil

1 small carrot, peeled and grated

1/4 cup chopped onion

1/4 teaspoon cinnamon

1/4 teaspoon salt

1 cup low-sodium nonfat chicken broth

1 small sweet potato, cooked, peeled, and quartered

In a bowl, mix sour cream with concentrate; refrigerate. Rub pita with garlic; coat with cooking spray and toast in toaster oven; cut into 6 wedges. Heat oil in a medium saucepan over medium heat. Cook carrot and onion with cinnamon and salt until onion softens, 3 to 4 minutes. Add broth and sweet potato. Bring to a boil. Simmer on low, stirring occasionally, until mixture thickens, 4 to 5 minutes. Transfer to a blender and puree until smooth. Top with sour cream mixture and serve with pita.

THE DISH 394 calories per serving, 9 g fat (2 g saturated), 71 g carbs, 11 g fiber, 12 g protein

Chopped Salad with Crispy Sardines

SERVES 4

¼ cup lemon juice

2 tablespoons olive oil, divided

2 cloves garlic, finely chopped

1½ teaspoons dried oregano

1 teaspoon chopped fresh mint

½ teaspoon freshly ground black pepper

3 medium tomatoes, chopped

1 large cucumber, seeded and chopped

1 yellow bell pepper, chopped

1 can (15 ounces) chickpeas, rinsed and drained

¼ cup crumbled feta cheese

¼ cup thinly sliced red onion

2 tablespoons chopped, pitted kalamata olives

2 cans (4 ounces each) sardines with bones,
   packed in olive oil or water, drained well

⅓ cup all-purpose flour

In a bowl, whisk juice, 1 tablespoon oil, garlic, oregano, mint, and black pepper until well combined; set aside. In another bowl, combine tomatoes with cucumber, bell pepper, chickpeas, feta, onion, and olives. Drizzle with vinaigrette; toss to coat. Heat remaining 1 tablespoon oil in a large skillet over medium heat. Toss sardines in flour, shake off excess, and cook until crisp and browned, 2 minutes on each side. Remove from pan. Divide salad mixture among 4 plates; top with sardines before serving.

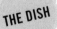

THE DISH 411 calories per serving, 18 g fat (4 g saturated), 42 g carbs, 9 g fiber, 23 g protein

Kale, White Bean, and Potato Soup

SERVES 6

1 tablespoon olive oil

1 large onion, diced

5 cloves garlic, chopped

4 cups chicken or vegetable broth

4 medium potatoes, diced

1 large turnip or rutabaga

2 cans (15 ounces each) cannellini beans,
    rinsed and drained

3 cups kale

6 tablespoons grated Parmesan

Heat oil in a large pot over medium heat; sauté onion and garlic 2 minutes. Stir in broth, 2 cups water, potatoes, and turnip; cover and bring to a boil. Reduce heat; simmer 25 to 30 minutes. Add beans and kale; cook until kale is soft, 5 to 10 minutes more. Divide soup among 6 bowls. Top with cheese before serving.

THE DISH

429 calories per serving, 6 g fat (2 g saturated), 78 g carbs, 15 g fiber, 21 g protein

Edamame Noodle Salad with Lemon Dressing

SERVES 2

4 medium carrots, peeled and grated (or 1½ cups
    julienned carrots)
1½ cups cooked shelled edamame
1 cup cooked whole-wheat spaghetti or lo mein noodles
1 cup corn
1 cup chopped tomato
½ cup chopped yellow bell pepper
⅓ cup thinly sliced shallots
2 tablespoons chopped fresh cilantro
3 tablespoons lemon juice
3 tablespoons rice vinegar
1 tablespoon olive oil
2 cloves garlic, chopped
1 teaspoon finely chopped ginger
½ teaspoon kosher salt
¼ teaspoon freshly ground black pepper

In a bowl, combine carrots, edamame, spaghetti, corn, tomato, bell pepper, shallots, and cilantro. In another bowl, whisk juice, vinegar, oil, garlic, ginger, salt, and black pepper; pour over salad and toss to coat. Cover and chill at least 1 hour before serving.

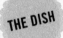 **THE DISH** 427 calories per serving, 13 g fat (1 g saturated), 67 g carbs, 15 g fiber, 19 g protein

Grilled Chicken Pitas with Kiwifruit Raita

SERVES 4

1 pound boneless, skinless chicken breasts

1 tablespoon olive oil

1 clove garlic, chopped

1/2 teaspoon freshly ground black pepper

1 1/2 cups nonfat plain Greek yogurt

3/4 teaspoon ground cumin

1/2 teaspoon hot sauce

1/2 teaspoon salt

2 kiwifruit, peeled and chopped

2 tablespoons chopped fresh cilantro

4 whole-wheat pita pockets

Heat grill. Rub chicken with oil, garlic, and pepper. Grill until cooked through, 15 to 20 minutes, turning once. Set aside. Raita: In a bowl, whisk yogurt, cumin, hot sauce, and salt until smooth. Add kiwi and cilantro; stir gently to combine. Set aside. Slice chicken; divide evenly among 4 pitas. Top each pita with 1/4 of the raita.

THE DISH 412 calories per serving, 9 g fat (2 g saturated), 34 g carbs, 5 g fiber, 44 g protein

Lentil and Roasted Broccoli Soup

SERVES 4

1½ pounds fresh broccoli, chopped

2 tablespoons olive oil

¼ teaspoon each salt and freshly ground black pepper

Vegetable oil cooking spray

2 cups chopped Vidalia onions

1 tablespoon dried thyme

¼ teaspoon red pepper flakes

6 cups chicken or vegetable broth

1 cup red or yellow lentils

2 tablespoons lemon juice

4 tablespoons shredded reduced-fat sharp Cheddar

4 whole-wheat dinner rolls

Heat oven to 400 degrees. Toss broccoli with oil, salt, and black pepper until coated. Place on a baking sheet coated with cooking spray; roast until browned and tender, 10 to 15 minutes. Set aside. Heat a large stockpot coated with cooking spray over medium heat. Cook onion until just tender, 3 to 4 minutes. Stir in broccoli, thyme, pepper flakes, broth, and lentils. Bring to a boil, reduce heat, and simmer until lentils are tender, 15 minutes. Puree in a blender or food processor until smooth (in batches, if necessary). Return to pot; stir in juice. Top each bowl with 1 tablespoon Cheddar before serving; serve with rolls.

THE DISH

373 calories per serving, 12 g fat (3 g saturated), 50 g carbs, 12 g fiber, 23 g protein

Sunny-side Up Lentil Salad
SERVES 4

1 can (14.5 ounces) diced tomatoes, with juices

1 cup chopped onion

$^3/_4$ cup lentils, rinsed

$^2/_3$ cup finely diced celery

$^1/_2$ cup finely diced carrot

1 tablespoon chopped fresh thyme

2$^1/_2$ tablespoons white wine vinegar, divided

2 tablespoons chopped fresh tarragon or parsley,
  divided

Salt and freshly ground black pepper

1 teaspoon Dijon mustard

2 teaspoons olive oil

Vegetable oil cooking spray

4 eggs

4 cups mixed baby lettuces

In a medium saucepan, boil 3 cups water, tomatoes, onion, lentils, celery, carrot, and thyme. Reduce heat to medium-low; simmer until lentils are tender, 20 to 25 minutes. Drain; reserve cooking liquid. Return liquid to pan; boil over high heat to reduce liquid to $^1/_4$ cup. Add 2 tablespoons vinegar and lentil mixture to liquid; stir over medium heat. Add 1 table-spoon tarragon; season with salt and pepper. Remove from heat but keep warm. In a bowl, whisk remaining $^1/_2$ tablespoon vinegar with mustard and oil; season with salt and pepper. Heat a medium skillet coated with cooking spray over medium heat. Carefully add eggs so yolks remain whole; cook until whites are set; season with salt and pepper. Toss lettuces with mustard dressing; divide evenly among 4 plates. Top each with $^1/_4$ of the lentil salad and 1 egg; sprinkle with remaining 1 tablespoon tarragon.

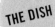
THE DISH

285 calories per serving, 8 g fat (2 g saturated), 37 g carbs, 15 g fiber, 18 g protein

Delicious Dinners

Chicken piccata, salmon cakes, seared steak, meatball minestrone—this list reads more like the menu at an upscale restaurant than a sampling of the so easy, so delectable recipes in a weight loss book, doesn't it? Restaurant entrées can contain twice as many calories as their home-cooked counterparts, so go ahead and indulge in these no-guilt, gourmet-caliber dishes. Whether you want to disclose just how nutritious and low in calories they are to your sure-to-be-impressed dining companions is up to you!

Sweet and Spicy Salmon

SERVES 4

4 dried Szechuan chiles (about 1 inch long), seeded
4 cloves garlic, finely chopped
1 teaspoon sesame oil
1 pint fresh blueberries
4 teaspoons apple cider vinegar
1 teaspoon sugar
$^1/_4$ teaspoon salt
4 wild salmon fillets (4 ounces each), grilled

Simmer chiles and $^1/_4$ cup water in a skillet until soft, 2 minutes. Add garlic and oil; cook until fragrant, 1 to 2 minutes. Stir in blueberries, vinegar, sugar, and salt. Bring to a boil and cook, mashing berries with a spoon until a thick sauce forms, 5 minutes. Remove from heat. Divide sauce over salmon.

 THE DISH 319 calories per serving, 12 g fat (2 g saturated), 17 g carbs, 3 g fiber, 35 g protein

Quinoa Stir-fry with Vegetables and Chicken
SERVES 4

$^3/_4$ cup quinoa, rinsed

$^1/_2$ teaspoon salt, divided

1 tablespoon vegetable oil

1 small carrot, peeled and thinly sliced

1 medium red bell pepper, chopped

2 teaspoons grated ginger

1 clove garlic, sliced

1 small red chile, chopped (optional)

2 cups snow peas, trimmed

$^1/_4$ teaspoon freshly ground black pepper

1 egg, beaten

4 ounces grilled boneless, skinless chicken breast, chopped

2 scallions, chopped

$^1/_2$ cup fresh cilantro

1 tablespoon soy sauce

In a small saucepan, bring quinoa to a boil with $^3/_4$ cup water and $^1/_4$ teaspoon salt. Reduce heat to low. Cover and cook, undisturbed, until quinoa absorbs water, 15 minutes. Remove from heat, fluff with a fork, and leave uncovered. Heat oil in a large skillet over medium-high heat. Cook carrot, stirring occasionally, until it softens, 1 minute. Add bell pepper, ginger, garlic, and chile (if desired); cook, stirring frequently, 2 minutes. Add peas, sprinkle with black pepper and remaining $^1/_4$ teaspoon salt, and cook, stirring frequently, 1 minute. Remove vegetables and return skillet to heat; add quinoa and egg. Cook, stirring constantly, until egg is evenly distributed, 2 minutes. Add vegetables, chicken, scallions, cilantro, and soy sauce; cook 1 minute more. Divide stir-fry among 4 bowls; serve warm.

THE DISH   254 calories per serving, 8 g fat (1 g saturated), 30 g carbs, 4 g fiber, 17 g protein

Artichoke-Chicken Piccata

SERVES 4

$\frac{1}{2}$ cup all-purpose flour

$\frac{1}{2}$ teaspoon Italian seasoning

$\frac{1}{4}$ teaspoon each salt and freshly ground black pepper

4 skinless, boneless chicken breasts (about 4 ounces each),
   pounded to $\frac{1}{2}$-inch thickness

2 tablespoons olive oil

2 cups chicken broth

1 can (13 ounces) artichoke hearts, drained

$\frac{1}{2}$ onion, chopped

$\frac{1}{2}$ cup dry white wine

$\frac{1}{4}$ cup capers or olives

2 tablespoons lemon juice

3 cloves garlic, chopped

2 cups cooked whole-wheat spaghetti or angel-hair pasta

Combine flour with Italian seasoning, salt, and pepper in a gallon-size resealable plastic bag. Add chicken, seal bag, and shake until coated. Remove chicken from bag. Heat oil in a large skillet over medium-high heat. Cook chicken until browned, 2 to 3 minutes. Flip and cook 2 minutes more. Add broth, artichokes, onion, wine, capers, juice, and garlic; cook until sauce reduces, getting slightly thick, 10 minutes. Serve over pasta.

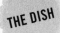

THE DISH

428 calories per serving, 11 g fat (2 g saturated), 45 g carbs, 10 g fiber, 34 g protein

Creamy Lemon Shrimp

SERVES 4

1/2 cup nonfat plain yogurt
1/4 cup reduced-fat sour cream
1/4 cup chopped fresh chives
1/4 cup chopped fresh tarragon
2 cloves garlic, finely chopped
2 teaspoons Dijon mustard
1 teaspoon olive oil
2 teaspoons sugar
1/2 teaspoon salt
1/4 teaspoon freshly ground black pepper
2 medium lemons
1 pound cooked shrimp (any size)
2 cups broccoli florets, cut into 1/2-inch pieces
2 cups arugula
8 ounces tofu noodles, rinsed and drained
    (found in the Asian section of grocery store)

In a bowl, mix yogurt with sour cream, chives, tarragon, garlic, mustard, oil, sugar, salt, and pepper. Zest lemons over bowl. Juice 1 lemon into bowl. Whisk until smooth. Add shrimp, broccoli, arugula, and noodles. Toss to coat.

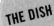 THE DISH 218 calories per serving 5 g fat (2 g saturated), 17 g carbs, 4 g fiber, 29 g protein

Udon Noodle Salad

SERVES 4

Dressing

1 medium carrot, peeled and grated

1 clove garlic, chopped

2 tablespoons white miso paste (found at health food stores)

1 tablespoon honey

1 tablespoon rice wine or apple cider vinegar

2 teaspoons sesame oil

Salad

Vegetable oil cooking spray

1 tablespoon canola oil, divided

8 ounces extra-firm tofu, drained well

4 scallions, sliced in 2-inch pieces

2 cups broccoli florets

1 cup frozen shelled edamame, thawed and rinsed

1/4 pound shiitake mushroom caps, sliced (about 1 cup)

1/4 pound cremini mushrooms, sliced (about 1 cup)

2 cups nonfat chicken broth

1/2 pound sugar snap peas

1/4 teaspoon each salt and freshly ground black pepper

8 ounces buckwheat udon noodles, cooked as directed
   on package and drained

In a blender, combine all dressing ingredients with $1/4$ cup water; set aside. Coat a large skillet or wok with cooking spray; heat $1^1/2$ teaspoons oil over high heat. Cook tofu and scallions 1 minute, then turn tofu once; cook 1 to 2 minutes more. Remove tofu, cut into $1/2$-inch cubes, and place in a bowl with scallions. Heat remaining $1^1/2$ teaspoons oil in same skillet over medium-high heat. Stir in broccoli, edamame, and mushrooms. Reduce heat to medium; cook, stirring often, 3 to 4 minutes. Add broth. Cover and cook until vegetables are tender, 3 to 4 minutes. Remove from heat; stir in peas, salt, and pepper. Add noodles and vegetable mixture to tofu mixture. Toss with dressing to coat.

THE DISH   438 calories per serving, 12 g fat (1 g saturated), 61 g carbs, 8 g fiber, 23 g protein

Salmon Cakes with Mixed Greens

SERVES 4

1/2 cup low-fat buttermilk

1/4 cup fat-free mayonnaise

1/4 cup plus 1 tablespoon chopped shallots, divided

2 teaspoons Dijon mustard, divided

1 1/2 teaspoons lemon juice

1 pound salmon fillet, skin removed, finely chopped

2 egg whites

1/2 cup plain bread crumbs

5 tablespoons capers

1/4 teaspoon each salt and freshly ground black pepper

2 teaspoons olive oil

8 cups mixed greens

In a bowl, combine buttermilk with mayonnaise, 1 tablespoon shallots, 1 teaspoon mustard, and juice. In another bowl, combine salmon with egg whites, remaining 1/4 cup shallots, bread crumbs, capers, remaining 1 teaspoon mustard, salt, and pepper; mix well; shape into eight 3-inch-round patties. Heat oil in a large nonstick skillet over medium heat. Cook salmon cakes until bottom is golden, 6 minutes; flip and cook until golden, 5 minutes more. Toss greens with half the buttermilk mixture, divide salad among 4 plates, and top each with 2 salmon cakes. Serve with remaining dressing on the side.

THE DISH 369 calories per 2 patties and 2 cups salad, 19 g fat (4 g saturated), 19 g carbs, 2 g fiber, 30 g protein

Vegetable Meat Loaf

SERVES 4

If you'd rather not spend time chopping the veggies superfine, you can coarsely chop, cook, and then puree them all together in a food processor.

Vegetable oil cooking spray

$1/2$ cup finely chopped onion

2 cloves garlic, chopped

$1/2$ cup finely chopped mushrooms

$1/4$ cup finely chopped carrot

2 tablespoons finely chopped green bell pepper

2 tablespoons finely chopped celery

$3/4$ cup canned pureed pumpkin or butternut squash

1 pound 90 percent lean ground beef

$1/2$ cup seasoned bread crumbs

1 egg, beaten

$1/4$ teaspoon each salt and freshly ground black pepper

$1/2$ teaspoon dried oregano

4 tablespoons canned tomato sauce, divided

Heat oven to 350 degrees. Coat a 9 x 5-inch loaf pan with cooking spray. Heat a medium skillet coated with cooking spray over medium heat. Cook onion until just tender, 2 minutes. Stir in garlic and mushrooms; cook, stirring occasionally, until soft, 5 minutes. Add carrot, bell pepper, and celery; cook 3 minutes more. Remove from heat; cool 5 minutes. Stir in pumpkin. In a bowl, combine beef with bread crumbs, egg, salt, pepper, oregano, and 2 tablespoons tomato sauce. Mix in vegetable mixture; stir until well combined. (It works best if done with wet hands.) Form into a loaf; place in prepared pan. Spoon remaining 2 tablespoons tomato sauce over top. Bake, uncovered, until meat is no longer pink, 45 to 50 minutes.

THE DISH

330 calories per serving, 14 g fat (5 g saturated), 23 g carbs, 4 g fiber, 28 g protein

Lentil Burgers

SERVES 4

3 tablespoons olive oil, divided
½ onion, chopped
3 cups cooked lentils
3 cloves garlic, finely chopped
1 egg, beaten
½ cup plain bread crumbs
1 teaspoon ground cumin
¼ teaspoon freshly ground black pepper
4 whole-wheat hamburger buns

Heat 1 tablespoon oil in a medium skillet over medium heat. Cook onion until just soft, 3 to 4 minutes. Remove from pan; set aside to cool slightly. In a bowl, combine lentils with garlic, egg, bread crumbs, cumin, and pepper. Mash until very well combined. (Mixture will be slightly lumpy.) Stir in onion. Form mixture into 4 patties (It works best if done with wet hands.) Heat remaining 2 tablespoons oil in same skillet over medium heat. Cook patties undisturbed until browned on bottom, 3 to 4 minutes. Flip patties; cook until browned, 3 to 4 minutes more. Remove from pan; place each patty on a bun. Serve immediately.

THE DISH 466 calories per burger, 15 g fat (2 g saturated), 66 g carbs, 16 g fiber, 21 g protein

Seared Steak with Asian Barbecue Sauce

SERVES 4

> 1 tablespoon plus 1 teaspoon sesame oil, divided
> 1 pound flank steak, cut into 4 pieces
> 8 ounces sliced mushrooms
> 2 cups broccoli florets
> 1 cup snow peas, trimmed
> 1/2 cup low-sodium ketchup
> 1/3 cup brown sugar
> 1/4 cup apple cider vinegar or rice wine vinegar
> 1/4 cup low-sodium soy sauce
> 1 tablespoon hot sauce
> 1 tablespoon sherry
> 1 teaspoon chopped ginger
> 2 cups cooked brown rice

Heat 1/2 tablespoon oil in a large skillet over medium-high heat; cook steak until browned and just cooked through, 3 to 4 minutes. Remove from skillet; set aside. Add 1/2 tablespoon oil to skillet; cook mushrooms 3 minutes, stirring frequently. Add broccoli and snow peas; cook until just tender, 5 minutes. Remove from skillet; keep warm. In a bowl, whisk ketchup, sugar, vinegar, soy sauce, hot sauce, sherry, ginger, and remaining 1 teaspoon oil until well combined; add to skillet. Bring to a boil, reduce heat, and simmer 5 minutes. To serve, spoon 1/2 cup rice onto each plate. Top with vegetables, then steak. Drizzle sauce evenly over each plate.

THE DISH

472 calories per serving, 17 g fat (5 g saturated), 56 g carbs, 4 g fiber, 25 g protein

Oatmeal-Meatball Minestrone

SERVES 6

1 pound lean ground beef or turkey

1/2 cup old-fashioned or quick-cooking oats

1 teaspoon Italian seasoning

1 teaspoon garlic powder

1/2 teaspoon onion powder

2 tablespoons olive oil

6 cups chicken or vegetable broth

1 can (28 ounces) chopped tomatoes, with juices

1 1/2 cups fresh or frozen green beans

3 carrots, peeled and sliced

2 celery stalks, sliced

1 leek, sliced

1 1/2 teaspoons dried thyme

1 1/2 teaspoons dried oregano

1 can (15 ounces) white beans (such as navy or cannellini),
    rinsed and drained

1/4 cup whole-wheat elbow macaroni

1/2 teaspoon salt

1/4 teaspoon freshly ground black pepper

1 zucchini, quartered and sliced

6 tablespoons grated Parmesan

In a bowl, mix beef, oats, Italian seasoning, garlic powder, and onion powder until well combined. Roll into 1-inch balls (about 24). Heat oil in a large stockpot over medium-high heat. Cook meatballs, turning occasionally, until browned. Add broth, tomatoes, green beans, carrots, celery, leek, thyme, and oregano. Bring to a boil, reduce heat, and simmer, covered, for 20 minutes. Remove lid; stir in white beans, macaroni, salt, and pepper; cook 10 minutes more. Add zucchini; cook 5 minutes more. Top each bowl with 1 tablespoon Parmesan before serving.

THE DISH 414 calories per serving, 15 g fat (5 g saturated), 41 g carbs, 9 g fiber, 31 g protein

Satisfying Snacks

Remember how much you looked forward to snack time when you were a kid? Get ready to feel that way again. Processed junk from the vending machine has got nothing on these speedy, fresh, hunger-silencing recipes. Make a big batch of your favorites on the weekend, then portion them out into individual servings and you'll be set—and set up to slim down—for the entire week.

Apple Chips

SERVES 4

2 tablespoons sugar
$1/8$ teaspoon cinnamon
4 apples, sliced crosswise into $1/8$-inch-thick rounds

Heat oven to 225 degrees. In a bowl, mix sugar with cinnamon. Arrange apple slices on two baking sheets lined with parchment paper; sprinkle with cinnamon sugar. Bake 1 hour. Peel apples off parchment and return to paper. Continue baking until golden and crisp, 30 minutes more. Store in an airtight container up to five days.

THE DISH 119 calories per cup, 0 g fat, 31 g carbs, 3 g fiber, 0 g protein

Edamame Hummus

SERVES 8

12 ounces frozen shelled edamame

3 whole-wheat pocket pitas, cut into 8 triangles each

2 cloves garlic

3 tablespoons lemon juice

2 tablespoons tahini

2 tablespoons olive oil

$3/4$ teaspoon salt

$1/2$ teaspoon ground cumin

$1/4$ teaspoon freshly ground black pepper

2 large red bell peppers, cut into 24 strips

Heat oven to 450 degrees. Bring edamame to a boil in a medium saucepan with enough water to cover; cook, stirring occasionally, 3 minutes. Drain in a colander and run under cold water. Bake pita triangles on a baking sheet until golden, 3 to 5 minutes. In a food processor, pulse edamame, garlic, juice, tahini, oil, salt, cumin, and black pepper until mixture is the consistency of guacamole; add water 1 tablespoon at a time if too thick. Cover; refrigerate until party time. Serve with pita toasts and bell peppers for dipping.

THE DISH 188 calories per $1/4$ cup hummus, 3 pita triangles, and 3 pepper strips, 8 g fat (1 g saturated), 22 g carbs, 5 g fiber, 8 g protein

Popcorn Trail Mix

SERVES 10

     3 ounces plain, unsalted microwave popcorn
        (or 3 cups air-popped popcorn)
     $1/4$ cup honey
     2 tablespoons olive oil
     2 bay leaves
     $1/2$ teaspoon salt
     1 cup dried cranberries
     $1/2$ cup chopped dried figs or pitted dates
     $1/2$ cup sliced almonds

Heat oven to 400 degrees. Pop popcorn as directed on bag; set aside. Combine honey with oil, bay leaves, and salt in a small saucepan over low heat, stirring frequently until fragrant, 5 minutes. Remove from heat. Remove bay leaves. In a bowl, toss warm popcorn with dried fruit and almonds. Drizzle trail mix with honey glaze, toss again, and spread evenly on a baking sheet. Bake until golden, 3 minutes. Turn off oven, remove sheet, and toss trail mix with a spatula; spread evenly on sheet and return to oven for 2 minutes more.

THE DISH   167 calories per serving, 6 g fat (1 g saturated), 29 g carbs, 3 g fiber, 2 g protein

Spiced Peanut Snacks

SERVES 8

1 pound green or raw peanuts, in the shell

1½ tablespoons kosher salt

¾ tablespoon cayenne pepper

Wash peanuts in cool water until water runs clear. Drain well. Add peanuts to a 12-quart pot along with salt, cayenne, and 3 gallons water. Stir well. Cover and cook on high for 3 hours. Test for doneness: Peanuts should be soft and not crunchy. Cook 1 hour more if needed. Cool before eating. Store boiled peanuts in an airtight container in the refrigerator for up to a week.

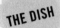

160 calories per serving, 14 g fat (2 g saturated), 5 g carbs, 2 g fiber, 7 g protein

Goji Berry Fruity Smoothie

SERVES 4

To rehydrate goji berries, place them in a bowl and cover with 1 to 2 cups hot water for 20 minutes. Drain before using.

> 2 cups nonfat plain Greek yogurt
> 1 cup coconut water
> 1 cup fresh or frozen sliced peaches
> 1 cup fresh or frozen cubed mango
> 1/2 cup goji berries, rehydrated
> 1/3 cup orange juice
> 2 tablespoons lemon juice

In a blender or food processor, blend all ingredients until smooth, adding ice if desired.

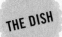 155 calories per serving, 0 g fat, 31 g carbs, 4 g fiber, 5 g protein

Spiced Trail Mix with Pumpkin Seeds

SERVES 10

>Vegetable oil cooking spray
>
>2 tablespoons unsalted butter
>
>1/4 cup brown sugar
>
>3/4 teaspoon cinnamon
>
>3/4 teaspoon ground cumin
>
>1 cup roasted shelled pumpkin seeds
>
>1 cup dried cranberries
>
>1 cup chopped walnuts or almonds
>
>2/3 cup dried apricots, chopped
>
>1/2 cup bite-size pretzels

Heat oven to 350 degrees. Coat a cookie sheet or jelly roll pan with cooking spray. Melt butter and sugar in a large saucepan over medium heat. Stir in cinnamon and cumin. Add pumpkin seeds, cranberries, walnuts, apricots, and pretzels, stirring well until coated. Spread onto prepared sheet. Bake until crunchy and lightly browned, 15 minutes. Cool. Store in an airtight container for up to two weeks.

THE DISH   166 calories per serving, 7 g fat (2 g saturated), 26 g carbs, 3 g fiber, 2 g protein

Cherry-Berry Ice Pops
SERVES 12

$1^{1}/_{2}$ pounds fresh or frozen cherries
(pitted if fresh, thawed if frozen)
$1^{1}/_{2}$ pounds frozen mixed berries, thawed
2 cups nonfat plain Greek yogurt
$^{1}/_{2}$ cup orange juice
$^{1}/_{4}$ cup honey

In a blender or food processor, process all ingredients until smooth. Spoon mixture into twelve 4-ounce paper cups; freeze 1 hour. Remove from freezer, insert a wooden ice-pop stick into each cup, and return to freezer until hard, at least 4 hours. Remove from freezer; tear off cups before serving. You can also make these in ice-pop molds. Store in the freezer for up to one month.

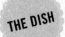 THE DISH 122 calories per serving, 0 g fat, 19 g carbs, 2 g fiber, 10 g protein

Cranberry-Peanut-Chocolate Treats
SERVES 4

4 tablespoons dark chocolate, broken into pieces
⅓ cup dried cranberries
1 tablespoon roasted peanuts, chopped

Microwave chocolate in a microwavable bowl on high for 20 seconds. Stir well, and microwave again, in 20-second increments, until chocolate melts, 1 minute. Stir cranberries into chocolate with a small rubber spatula. Spread mixture onto a cookie sheet covered with waxed paper, shaping it into a 4-inch square. Sprinkle top with peanuts and press lightly into chocolate. Refrigerate until the chocolate is firm, 10 minutes. Break into 4 pieces.

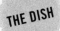 **THE DISH** 151 calories per serving, 9 g fat (4 g saturated), 16 g carbs, 2 g fiber, 3 g protein

Warm Almond-Fruit Wraps

SERVES 4

4 corn tortillas (6 inches each)
4 tablespoons almond butter
2 cups sliced or diced peaches or pears
1 teaspoon cinnamon
Vegetable oil cooking spray

Spread each tortilla with 1 tablespoon almond butter. Divide fruit evenly among tortillas (1/2 cup each). Top each with 1/4 teaspoon cinnamon. Roll up tortillas burrito-style. Heat a skillet coated with cooking spray over medium heat. Cook rolled tortillas until lightly browned and warm, 3 to 4 minutes.

 THE DISH 180 calories per serving, 10 g fat (1 g saturated), 21 g carbs, 4 g fiber, 5 g protein

Pomegranate Fruit Salad with Mint and Lime

SERVES 6

1 pineapple, peeled, cored, and chopped

1 cantaloupe, peeled, seeded, and chopped

$^1/_2$ honeydew melon, peeled, seeded, and chopped

$^1/_2$ cup pomegranate seeds

$^1/_2$ cup lime juice

$^1/_4$ cup chopped fresh mint

$^1/_8$ teaspoon salt

In a bowl, combine all ingredients; toss to coat. Refrigerate 1 hour before serving.

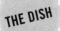

THE DISH 154 calories per serving, 1 g fat (0 g saturated), 39 g carbs, 4 g fiber, 2 g protein

drop 10 inspiration

"I'm shrinking all over!"

NAME: Grace Mendez

AGE: 33

OCCUPATION: Special events planner

FAMILY STATUS: Single, one son

HEIGHT: 5 feet 7 inches

STARTING WEIGHT: 175

DROP 10 WEIGHT: 156

LOST: 19 pounds in thirteen weeks

My story: "In 2007, I lost 50 pounds and felt amazing. A few years later, I became depressed—I stopped exercising and started eating fast food and gained the weight back. I tried diet pills to help me take it off, but they didn't work and gave me horrible mood swings. I was exhausted and tired of feeling sorry for myself. My body was begging to be healthy."

Biggest challenge to losing weight: "Emotional eating, fear of failure, and lack of motivation."

Why Drop 10 clicked: "I saw results in two weeks, which motivated me to continue. And I love the freebie calories! They help me stay on track. If I don't do well one day, I can redeem myself the next. And if I have a social event coming up, I can save up my freebies and not feel guilty for indulging."

How my body changed: "I went from a size 12 or 14 to an 8! I lost 6 inches from my waist and 2 inches from my bust. Best of all, I have a better attitude at work and my relationships are even healthier. I want to lose 16 more pounds, and I know I can do it!"

Success tip: "Consistency is key. When I go a few days without doing any exercise, I feel like dead weight, like I'm headed in a bad direction again. I pick myself up and get going!"

Treat Tracking:
How Your Favorite Foods Fit into the Drop 10 Diet

Cheesy pizza, warm cookies, cold beer—is your mouth watering yet? Good! Whatever your can't-live-without-it food or drink may be, there's room for it and scores of other lip-smacking treats in the Drop 10 diet. Asking you to surrender the things you've been eating (and love to eat) isn't only cruel, it sets you up to feel deprived and crave-y. That's the fast track to giving up. Forget that! The Drop 10 diet helps you splurge the smart way.

That's because along with the satisfying, fat-burning superfood meals and snacks in the previous chapter, you get an additional 200 "happy" calories a day to play with. Spend them on whatever makes you happy each day, or save up two, three, or four days' worth (400, 600, or 800 calories) for a bigger indulgence; the only guideline is to keep track of everything that goes down the hatch. (Limit your rollovers to four days, or 800 calories, so you don't become overly hungry or have cravings on the days you forgo your treat.) What's more, because the superfood dishes at the heart of the Drop 10 diet are naturally satiating and help tame wild cravings, when you do spend your happy calories on salty, sweet, or savory treats, you're less likely to creep into binge territory. That keeps you on course and steadily melting off inches.

How it works: We collected data on more than 300 splurge-worthy items. Use the calorie tallies to plan and track how you spend your happy calories.* You may want to find and mark your favorites now to get an idea of their calorie counts. Plan ahead when you can. For example, if you're going to a cocktail party this weekend, check out the entries on pages 316–317, decide what you want to eat and drink, then figure how many happy calories you need to save up. It's that easy!

You'll also find bigger, meal-type splurges in this chapter—Chinese takeout dishes, a cheeseburger, and the like—because, well, that's life! We know you may not want to eat every single meal from the Drop 10 meal plan, and that's okay. The important thing is that you follow it and incorporate superfoods into your diet on most days to yield the best fat-melting, crave-busting results. But if on occasion you want to save your happy calories to spend on one dinner, go ahead. You'll still lose. Happy eating!

Splurge with the Superfoods!

Spend your happy calories indulging in any of the following delectable, quickie superfood recipes and you'll gain an extra, slimming edge on weight loss. Each comes in at around 200 calories.

Goji-Vanilla Shake
Blend 3 tablespoons goji berries with ⅓ cup low-fat vanilla ice cream and ¼ cup skim milk.

Broiled Banana with Oat Topping
Cut a medium banana lengthwise. Top with 1 tablespoon oats mixed with 1 teaspoon brown sugar and 2 teaspoons trans-fat-free margarine. Broil until it bubbles.

Micro Baked Apple
Microwave a small cored apple filled with 1 tablespoon raisins until tender, 3 to 5 minutes. Top with ½ cup low-fat vanilla ice cream.

---

* If you don't see a personal favorite here, look up the calorie counts at NutritionData .Self.com and jot them down at the end of this chapter for handy reference.

Faux Fondue

Spear ½ cup blueberries and ½ cup sliced strawberries on kebab sticks. Dip into a 100-calorie dark chocolate pudding cup.

Pomegranate Sundae

Top ½ cup low-fat vanilla ice cream with ¼ cup pomegranate seeds and 2 tablespoons light chocolate syrup.

Dark Chocolate and Fruit

Have 1 ounce dark chocolate with 1 serving of fruit (such as 1 kiwifruit, ¼ cup pomegranate seeds, or ½ cup cherries).

Banana Pop

Melt ½ ounce dark chocolate and drizzle over 1 small banana. Freeze until chocolate hardens and banana is firm.

Cream Cheese Dippers

Mix 1½ ounces room temperature low-fat cream cheese with 1 teaspoon honey and a few shakes of cinnamon. Serve with 1 small sliced apple.

Maple Baked Apple

Quarter an apple, then remove and discard core and stem; place quarters in a nonstick baking dish. Drizzle with 1 tablespoon maple syrup; sprinkle with 1 tablespoon chopped walnuts and a few shakes of cinnamon. Bake at 350 degrees until apple is tender, 25 to 30 minutes.

Baked Sweet Potato

Place 1¼ cups cubed sweet potato on a baking sheet coated with cooking spray. Drizzle with 1 tablespoon honey, then sprinkle with cinnamon. Bake at 425 degrees until tender, about 25 minutes.

Almond Butter Fondue

Mix 1 tablespoon almond butter with 1 teaspoon honey in a bowl. Nuke 20 seconds, then stir. Serve with ½ banana, sliced, and ½ pear, sliced.

Sweet and Salty Toast

Spread ½ teaspoon almond butter and 1 teaspoon honey on 1 slice whole-grain toast; serve with 10 cherries.

Berry-Yogurt Pops

Blend ½ cup nonfat vanilla yogurt with ½ cup blueberries and ⅓ cup pomegranate juice. Pour mixture into ice pop molds and freeze.

Dark Chocolate Yogurt

Stir 2 teaspoons honey and 1 teaspoon unsweetened dark cocoa powder into 1 cup of 2 percent plain Greek yogurt.

Apple-Caramel Shortcake

Top 1 cup cubed trans-fat-free angel food cake with ½ cup grated apple, 1½ tablespoons caramel sauce, and 2 tablespoons nonfat whipped cream.

Pear with Creamy Peanut Dip

Stir 1 tablespoon all-natural peanut butter into ½ cup nonfat plain yogurt. Serve with ½ pear, sliced.

Chocolate-Nut Pudding

Top 1 cup dark chocolate pudding with 1 tablespoon chopped peanuts.

Strawberries and Cream

Mix ¾ cup sliced strawberries and 2 teaspoons maple syrup or honey into 8 ounces nonfat plain Greek yogurt.

Cherry, Ricotta, and Cinnamon Sundae

Combine ½ cup part-skim ricotta cheese with ⅓ cup chopped cherries and a sprinkle of cinnamon.

Banana Roll

Roll a whole banana in 1 tablespoon chopped peanuts. Serve with 1 cup tea with 1 teaspoon honey and 2 tablespoons warmed skim milk.

Cocoa Berries

Mix 2 tablespoons dark-chocolate-covered blueberries and 2 tablespoons goji berries.

Sweet Toast

Spread 1 tablespoon almond butter on 1 slice whole-wheat cinnamon-raisin toast; top with ½ pear, sliced.

Nutty Caramel Sundae

Top ½ cup light vanilla ice cream (such as Edy's Slow Churned Light Vanilla Ice Cream) with 2 teaspoons caramel sauce, 2 teaspoons chopped peanuts, and 1 tablespoon whipped cream.

Hot Apple "Pie"

Top a thinly sliced apple with 1 tablespoon chopped pecans, 1 teaspoon honey, and a sprinkle of cinnamon. Microwave until warm, 30 seconds.

Grab-and-Go Snacks

Got a sweet tooth? Or are you feeling salty? Either way, most of these packaged treats come in under or around your 200 happy calories allowance per serving. (Make your happy calories go even further by having, say, a single cookie or one "fun size" piece of candy.) If you think you're at risk for gobbling up an entire box of cookies or bag of chips, buy single-serving packages on an as-needed basis, or dole out your helping and then put the bag out of sight in a cabinet before digging in to your portion.

Sweet Treats

Cookies

1 Nabisco SnackWell's Devil's Food Cookie Cake
    50 calories
1 Keebler Chips Deluxe Soft 'N Chewy Cookie
    70 calories

1 Keebler Chips Deluxe Rainbow Chocolate Chip Cookie
   80 calories

2 Fig Newtons
   110 calories

3 Pepperidge Farm Chessmen Cookies
   120 calories

2 LU Le Petit Écolier Extra-Dark Chocolate Cookies
   130 calories

1 Pepperidge Farm Sausalito Crispy Milk Chocolate Macadamia Nut
   Cookie
   130 calories

1 Kashi TLC Oatmeal Dark Chocolate Cookie
   130 calories

2 Carr's Ginger Lemon Cremes
   130 calories

2 Nabisco Nutter Butter Sandwich Cookies
   130 calories

8 Nabisco Nilla Wafers
   140 calories

1 Pepperidge Farm Soft Baked Nantucket Dark Chocolate Cookie
   140 calories

8 Nabisco Sugar Wafers
   140 calories

3 Keebler FudgeShoppe Fudge Stripes Cookies
   150 calories

2 Keebler Vienna Fingers Cookies
   150 calories

3 Nabisco Oreo Cookies
   160 calories

3 Chips Ahoy! Chocolate Chip Cookies
   160 calories

8 Keebler Animals Frosted Cookies
   160 calories

3 Pepperidge Farm Milano Cookies
   180 calories

Candy

Sun-Maid Chocolate Yogurt Raisins (¼ cup)
  120 calories
York Peppermint Patty (1.4-ounce package)
  140 calories
Jelly Belly (35 jelly beans)
  140 calories
2 Milky Way Fun Size Bars (34 g)
  160 calories
2 Snickers Fun Size Bars (34 g)
  160 calories
Hershey's Kisses (9 Kisses)
  200 calories
Hershey Bar (1.51-ounce bar)
  210 calories
Reese's Peanut Butter Cups (1.5-ounce package)
  210 calories
Kit Kat Bar (1.5-ounce package)
  210 calories
Heath Toffee Bar (1.4-ounce bar)
  210 calories
Almond Joy (1.61-ounce package)
  220 calories
PayDay (1.83-ounce bar)
  240 calories
Starburst (2.07-ounce package)
  240 calories
M&M's (1.69-ounce package)
  240 calories
M&M's Peanut Butter Chocolate Candies (1.63-ounce package)
  240 calories
Skittles (2.17-ounce package)
  240 calories
M&M's Peanut Chocolate Candies (1.74-ounce package)
  250 calories

3 Musketeers (2.13-ounce bar)
260 calories

Milky Way (2.05-ounce bar)
260 calories

Butterfinger (2.1-ounce bar)
270 calories

Other Sweet Treats

Fruit by the Foot (1 roll)
80 calories

Sunkist Mixed Fruit Snacks (1 package)
80 calories

Fruit Gushers Watermelon Blast (1 package)
90 calories

Kellogg's Rice Krispies Treats (1 treat)
90 calories

Jell-O Chocolate Pudding Cup (1 cup)
120 calories

Kozy Shack Rice Pudding Cup (1 cup)
130 calories

Hostess Twinkies (1 cake)
150 calories

Hostess Ding Dongs (1 package)
180 calories

Luna Bar Blueberry Bliss Flavor (1 bar)
180 calories

Nature Valley Crunchy Granola Oats 'n Dark Chocolate Bars
(1 package—2 bars)
190 calories

Lärabar Cherry Pie Flavor (1 bar)
190 calories

Kellogg's Pop-Tarts Frosted Strawberry (1 pastry)
200 calories

Kind Bar Peanut Butter Dark Chocolate + Protein Flavor (1 bar)
200 calories

Kellogg's Pop-Tarts Frosted Apple Strudel (1 pastry)
200 calories

Clif Bar Oatmeal Raisin Walnut Flavor (1 bar)
240 calories

Savory Snacks

Chips (All 1 Ounce)

Popchips Sour Cream & Onion
100 calories

Terra Yukon Gold Salt & Pepper Potato Chips
130 calories

Stacy's Pita Chips
130 calories

Sunchips Harvest Cheddar Flavored Multigrain Snacks
140 calories

Garden of Eatin' Blue Corn Tortilla Chips
140 calories

Food Should Taste Good Sweet Potato Tortilla Chips
140 calories

Hawaiian Luau BBQ Kettle Style Potato Chips Crispy
& Crunchy
140 calories

Kettle Honey Dijon Potato Chips
150 calories

Doritos
150 calories

Kettle Potato Chips Sea Salt
150 calories

Terra Original Exotic Vegetable Chips
150 calories

Lay's Barbecue Flavored Potato Chips
160 calories

Cheetos
160 calories

Cheetos Puffs
>160 calories

Ruffles Potato Chips
>160 calories

Fritos Corn Chips
>160 calories

Pretzels and Crackers (All 1 Ounce)

Health Valley Organic Garden Herb Crackers
>70 calories

Keebler Club Crackers
>70 calories

Ritz Crackers
>80 calories

Carr's Whole Wheat Crackers
>80 calories

Rold Gold Honey Wheat Braided Twists
>110 calories

Rold Gold Tiny Twists Pretzels
>110 calories

Dare Breton Crackers
>110 calories

Snack Factory Pretzel Crisps Deli Style
>110 calories

Snyder's of Hanover Sourdough Nibblers Pretzels
>120 calories

Triscuit
>120 calories

Kashi TLC Original 7 Grain Crackers
>120 calories

Wheat Thins Honey Wheat Crunch Stix Crackers
>130 calories

Snyder's of Hanover Honey Mustard & Onion Pretzel Pieces
>140 calories

Wheat Thins
> 140 calories

Wheat Thins Sundried Tomato & Basil
> 140 calories

Wheat Thins Parmesan & Basil
> 140 calories

Goldfish Crackers
> 150 calories

Good Health Natural Foods Peanut Butter Filled Pretzels
> 150 calories

Cheese Nips
> 150 calories

Ice Cream and Frozen Treats

You scream, I scream, it's no dream—you *can* eat ice cream! And you've got plenty of options, too. Hit up the ice-cream parlor, or buy your favorites at the supermarket to enjoy at home. Once you know the calorie counts, you decide whether to save up for a big splurge (Dairy Queen Blizzard, anyone?) or chill out every night with a lower-calorie cool treat (mmm, a Skinny Cow Fudge Bar).

At the Ice-Cream Parlor

Baskin-Robbins Fat-Free Vanilla Frozen Yogurt (2.5-ounce scoop)
> 90 calories

Baskin-Robbins Mint Chocolate Chip Ice Cream (4-ounce scoop)
> 260 calories

Baskin-Robbins Chocolate Chip Cookie Dough Ice Cream (4-ounce scoop)
> 310 calories

→ **Trim-Down Tip:** When scooping up ice cream, if you opt for one flavor rather than two, you may be less inclined to want seconds. A study in *Physiology & Behavior* reports that switching flavors midmeal sends your brain the signal to eat more of the new food—in some cases, nearly twice as much.

Dairy Queen Chocolate Dipped Cone (small)
> 330 calories

Dairy Queen Double Fudge Cookie Dough Blizzard (mini)
> 450 calories

Dairy Queen Banana Split
> 520 calories

→ **Trim-Down Tip:** Ice cream, yum! Order yours in a cup, not a cone, and you can take your time enjoying each spoonful rather than having to gobble it up to thwart drippage. Skipping the sugar cone also saves you 40 calories.

At-Home Frozen Treats

Edy's/Dreyer's Slow Churned Fudge Tracks (½ cup)
> 120 calories

Edy's/Dreyer's Grand Real Strawberry (½ cup)
> 120 calories

Edy's/Dreyer's Chocolate Chip (½ cup)
> 150 calories

Ben & Jerry's FroYo Half Baked (½ cup)
> 180 calories

Häagen-Dazs Chocolate Almond Frozen Yogurt (½ cup)
> 190 calories

Ben & Jerry's Cherry Garcia (½ cup)
> 240 calories

Ben & Jerry's Chunky Monkey (½ cup)
> 290 calories

Dairy Queen Caramel Sundae (small)
> 300 calories

Häagen-Dazs Rocky Road (½ cup)
> 300 calories

Häagen-Dazs Mint Chip (½ cup)
> 300 calories

➡ **Trim-Down Tip:** At the grocery store, look for ice cream, fro yo, ice pops, and other frozen treats with no added sugar.

1 Ciao Bella Fat Free Blood Orange Sorbet Bar
   60 calories
1 Edy's All Natural Strawberry Fruit Bar
   80 calories
1 Fudgsicle Fudge Bar
   100 calories
1 Skinny Cow Fudge Bar
   100 calories
Ciao Bella Sorbet Banana Mango (½ cup)
   110 calories
Ciao Bella Sorbet Passion Fruit (½ cup)
   120 calories
1 Tofutti Dairy-Free Vanilla Cuties Sandwich
   130 calories
1 Skinny Cow Vanilla Ice Cream Sandwich
   140 calories
1 Skinny Cow Chocolate with Fudge Cone
   150 calories
1 Breyers Vanilla Fudge Brownie Sandwich
   160 calories
Ciao Bella Sorbet Dark Chocolate (½ cup)
   200 calories
15 Almond Dream Dessert Bites
   230 calories
1 Good Humor Classic Strawberry Shortcake Bar
   230 calories
1 Klondike Bar
   250 calories
1 Nestlé Drumstick Simply Dipped Vanilla Ice Cream
   270 calories
1 Ciao Bella Key Lime Graham All Natural Gelato Square
   280 calories

SUPERFOOD ICE POPS

Want to really banish that extra fat? Whip up a batch of these tasty pops to keep in your freezer. They're just as delish as ice cream and sorbet but boast superfood powers and use up a fraction of your day's happy calories. Pretty cool!

Break the Mold

You'll find ready-made molds at home-goods stores for around $12. If you'd prefer to make your own, though, you don't need any special gear. Simply fill 3-ounce paper cups with your favorite mix, then place a craft stick in each when the pop is partially frozen.

Wild-Berry Pops

The blueberries give you fiber, and yogurt's satiating protein and flab-burning calcium help you give fat the cold shoulder.

MAKES 16 POPS, 3 OUNCES EACH; 38 CALORIES EACH

1½ cups fresh blackberries, divided
1½ cups fresh blueberries, divided
1 cup low-fat plain yogurt
1 cup prepared blueberry juice
2 tablespoons honey
2 tablespoons fresh lemon juice

Blend ¾ cup blackberries and ¾ cup blueberries with yogurt, blueberry juice, honey, and lemon juice in a blender until smooth. Stir in remaining berries. Pour into molds and add sticks. Freeze 6 hours.

Strawberry and Seed Pops

Protein-packed, chewy pumpkin seeds are a nice surprise amid the vitamin C–rich fruit, helping turn this treat into a filling snack.

MAKES 16 POPS, 3 OUNCES EACH; 51 CALORIES EACH

¹/₃ cup shelled pumpkin seeds

3 cups hulled and halved strawberries

³/₄ cup strawberry juice

³/₄ cup pineapple juice

3 tablespoons sugar

1 ripe banana

Heat oven to 300 degrees. Roast pumpkin seeds in a shallow pan for 6 minutes; stir and roast 4 minutes more. Simmer berries, juices, and sugar in a medium saucepan for 5 minutes. Let cool. Transfer mixture to a blender; add banana and blend until smooth. Stir in seeds. Fill molds and add sticks. Freeze 6 hours.

1 Häagen-Dazs Chocolate & Dark Chocolate Ice Cream Bar
   290 calories
1 Häagen-Dazs Vanilla & Almonds Ice Cream Bar
   310 calories
5 Dove Miniatures Milk Chocolate and Vanilla Ice Cream Bars
   340 calories

Coffee and Bakery Sweets

Coffee breaks won't break your diet if you splurge the smart way by saving up and using your happy calories for those must-have specialty sips and fave pastries. (Yup, even though coffee is a superfood for weight loss, coffee drinks with added flavoring, sweeteners, and whole milk sneak into the treat category.)

Coffee

Starbucks Grande Skinny Latte
   130 calories
Starbucks Venti Skinny Caramel Macchiato
   160 calories

Starbucks Grande Caffè Vanilla Frappuccino Light Blended Beverage
170 calories
Starbucks Grande Caffè Mocha (with 2 percent milk and whipped cream)
330 calories

→ **Trim-Down Tip:** Order your drinks "skinny" at Starbucks or other coffee shops. Sugar-free syrups and skim milk can save you serious calories—for example, if you sip a Starbucks Grande Skinny Caramel Macchiato instead of a regular Grande Caramel Macchiato, you automatically shave 130 calories off your coffee break. Also consider this rule of thumb: The longer the coffee order, the more calories it typically contains. How many more? A 16-ounce Iced Peppermint White Chocolate Mocha with whipped cream tops out at 520 calories and 20 grams of fat—and that's with 2 percent milk!

Dunkin' Donuts Medium Vanilla Latte (with skim milk)
130 calories
Dunkin' Donuts Small Coffee Coolatta (with skim milk)
200 calories
Dunkin' Donuts Small Dunkaccino
240 calories
Dunkin' Donuts Medium Caramel Mocha Latte (with skim milk)
260 calories

Brownies

Mrs. Fields Butterscotch Blondie Brownie Bite
67 calories
Mrs. Fields Double Fudge Brownie
260 calories
Panera Double Fudge Chocolate Brownie with Icing
480 calories

→ **Trim-Down Tip:** When scanning the pastry or doughnut case, look for items without icing, caramel, sprinkles, filling, or other add-ons unless those extras truly will make you happier. For example, a doughnut minus the frosting can save you around 140 calories.

Croissants

Au Bon Pain Plain Croissant
240 calories
Starbucks Chocolate Croissant
300 calories
Panera French Croissant
310 calories

Cakes and Muffins

Starbucks Peanut Butter Mini Cupcake
180 calories
Starbucks Carrot Cake Mini Cupcake
190 calories
Au Bon Pain Double Chocolate Cupcake
320 calories
Starbucks Reduced-Fat Cinnamon Swirl Coffee Cake
340 calories
Starbucks Blueberry Streusel Muffin
360 calories
Au Bon Pain Red Velvet Cupcake
400 calories
Panera Wild Blueberry Muffin
440 calories
Au Bon Pain Carrot Walnut Muffin
560 calories

→ **Trim-Down Tip:** Mini cupcakes aren't the only petite treats Starbucks sells. You'll find a range of treats that don't use up more than a day's worth of happy calories. At any coffee chain, look around for mini versions of your favorites. (Doughnut holes come to mind.) Sometimes two bites are all you need to satisfy your sweet tooth.

Cinnamon Rolls

Au Bon Pain Iced Cinnamon Roll
  410 calories
Panera Cinnamon Roll
  620 calories

Scones

Starbucks Petite Vanilla Bean Scone
  140 calories
Starbucks Blueberry Scone
  460 calories
Au Bon Pain Orange Scone
  480 calories
Panera Cinnamon Chip Scone
  600 calories

Doughnuts

Krispy Kreme Original Glazed Doughnut Holes
  50 calories each
Dunkin' Donuts Glazed Munchkins
  70 calories each

→ **Trim-Down Tip:** Mulling over whether to splurge on a doughnut or a bagel and schmear? Glazed doughnuts actually have fewer calories. A medium bagel with 2 tablespoons cream cheese clocks in at nearly 400 calories.

Dunkin' Donuts Jelly Filled Munchkins
  80 calories each
Starbucks Double Fudge Mini Doughnut
  130 calories
Kripy Kreme Original Glazed Doughnut
  190 calories

Dunkin' Donuts Glazed Donut
 260 calories
Dunkin' Donuts Chocolate Frosted Donut
 270 calories
Krispy Kreme Glazed Raspberry Filled Doughnut
 290 calories
Krispy Kreme Glazed Chocolate Cake
 300 calories

→ **Trim-Down Tip:** Don't waste your happy calories on things that, well, don't make you happy. It sounds obvious, but knee-jerk mindless noshing can be a tough habit to break, and doing so takes awareness. Before you reach for a doughnut at your morning meeting just because it's there, ask yourself whether you truly want it (were you thinking about doughnuts before you saw them?) and whether eating one would be worth the calories. If not, skip it and save those calories for something that will really make you smile later.

Cookies

Mrs. Fields Peanut Butter Bite-Size Nibbler Cookies
 57 calories each
Panera Chocolate Chipper Petites
 110 calories each
Mrs. Fields Oatmeal, Raisins and Walnuts Cookie
 200 calories
Mrs. Fields Cinnamon Sugar Cookie
 210 calories
Mrs. Fields Semi-Sweet Chocolate Cookie
 210 calories

→ **Trim-Down Tip:** Why not eat sweets that fill you up with more than just sugar? For a supersatisfying cookie, choose one made with oats (a superfood!), dried fruit, or nuts, all of which add fiber.

Dunkin' Donuts Oatmeal Raisin Cookie
   290 calories
Starbucks Chocolate Chunk Cookie
   380 calories

→ **Trim-Down Tip:** At some places, cookies, muffins, doughnuts, and other pastries look as if they were made for giants. Split yours with a friend and save tomorrow's happy calories for another treat.

Happy Hour Indulgences

Cocktails, wine, and other alcoholic drinks, as well as platters of cheese and bread, are prime sources for sneaky calories. But if you make room for them in your diet, you will be toasting to your new, slimmer body in no time. If you don't see your favorite drinks here, keep in mind that the simplest sips (think gin and tonic) are typically made with 1.5 to 2 ounces of liquor, but drinks with several different liquors (Long Island Iced Teas, for instance) may contain much more alcohol.

Light beer (12 ounces)
   103 calories
Red or white wine (5 ounces)
   125 calories
Rum and cola (5 ounces)
   136 calories
Gin and tonic (5 ounces)
   145 calories
Regular beer (12 ounces)
   153 calories
Vodka and cranberry (5 ounces)
   157 calories
Whiskey sour (5 ounces, made with sour mix)
   203 calories
Cosmo (6 ounces)
   218 calories

Margarita on the rocks (5 ounces)
    250 calories
Frozen margarita (8 ounces)
    312 calories
Martini, gin or vodka (6 ounces)
    374 calories

→ **Trim-Down Tip:** Decide how you'll spend your happy calories and exactly how many you'll use before heading to happy hour, then vow to follow through no matter what. Also have a filling snack beforehand so you're not starved. Researchers at Princeton University found that alcohol triggers an increase in galanin, a compound that makes you crave fatty food. Cocktails are also notorious for turning diet determination into "a double-bacon cheeseburger isn't that many calories, right?" Having a strategy in place can help you resist.

→ **Trim-Down Tip:** Want to make your happy calories last longer during happy hour? You can have two wine spritzers for about the same calorie cost as one glass of vino. Or, swap zero-calorie soda water for tonic, cola, or ginger ale in mixed drinks to shave about 35 calories off each drink. Sipping nonalcoholic seltzer between each alcohol-containing drink also helps control your intake.

Brie (2 ounces)
    189 calories
Blue cheese (2 ounces)
    200 calories
Swiss (2 ounces)
    215 calories
Cheddar (2 ounces)
    229 calories
Gruyère (2 ounces)
    234 calories

→ **Trim-Down Tip:** Cheese provides a dose of fat-fighting calcium, but it's easy to overdo it. A 2-ounce serving is about the size of eight dice.

Water crackers (5 crackers)
    70 calories
Dried fruit (¼ cup)
    100 calories
Mixed nuts (¼ cup)
    203 calories

Slim-ify Your Cocktail

Happy hour doesn't have to obliterate several days' worth of happy calories. Use these recipes to lighten up your favorite sips.

COSMOPOLITAN

This twist on the classic saves you about 75 calories per serving. Serves 4

8 ounces light cranberry juice
6 ounces vodka
5 ice cubes
2 ounces fresh lime juice
1 tablespoon grated orange zest, plus 4 zest slices for garnish

In a cocktail shaker, combine cranberry juice, vodka, ice, lime juice, and grated zest; close and shake well. Strain liquid into 4 chilled martini glasses; garnish each with 1 zest slice.

✳ **THE DISH:** 110 calories per serving, 0 g fat, 4 g carbs, 0 g fiber,
      0 g protein

MALIBU BAY BREEZE

A serving of cranberry juice contains 39 percent of your daily recommended amount of vitamin C, a potent fat-fighter. Serves 4

8 ounces light cranberry juice
8 ounces pineapple juice

6 ounces coconut-flavored rum
10 ounces sparkling water
Ice cubes
4 wedges pineapple (optional)
8 pineapple leaves (optional)

In a pitcher, combine cranberry juice, pineapple juice, and rum. Stir in sparkling water. Divide evenly among 4 glasses filled with ice; garnish each with 1 pineapple wedge and 2 leaves, if desired.

❊ **THE DISH:** 139 calories per serving, 0 g fat, 11 g carbs, 0 g fiber, 0 g protein

PINK TOM COLLINS

Pomegranate juice adds fat-torching vitamin C to this otherwise old-school cocktail, and the fresh pom seeds provide belly-slimming fiber. Serves 4

2 ounces fresh lemon juice
2 tablespoons confectioners' sugar
8 ounces pomegranate juice
6 ounces gin
4 ounces sparkling water
Ice cubes
4 black cherries (optional)
4 lemon slices, halved (optional)
1 tablespoon fresh pomegranate seeds (optional)

In a pitcher, whisk lemon juice and sugar until sugar dissolves. Add pomegranate juice, gin, and sparkling water; stir until well combined. Divide evenly among 4 glasses filled with ice; garnish each with 1 cherry, 2 halved lemon slices, and ¾ teaspoon pomegranate seeds, if desired.

❊ **THE DISH:** 148 calories per serving, 0 g fat, 13 g carbs, 0 g fiber, 0 g protein

MOJITO

Lime zest and sparkling water add zing for few calories. Bonus: Whiffs of mint may help ease cravings. Serves 4

4 limes, cut into wedges
½ cup packed mint, plus 4 sprigs for garnish
¼ cup sugar
2 teaspoons grated lime zest
16 ounces lime sparkling water
6 ounces white rum
Ice cubes

In a pitcher, place lime wedges, mint, sugar, and zest. Mash mint, sugar, and zest into limes with a muddler or wooden spoon to release juice and blend flavors. Stir in sparkling water and rum. Divide evenly among 4 glasses filled with ice; garnish with mint sprigs.

❄ **THE DISH:** 151 calories per serving, 0 g fat, 14 g carbs, 0 g fiber, 0 g protein

STRAWBERRY DAIQUIRI

Strawberries and raspberries deliver vitamin C, which helps block fat absorption. Berry cool! Serves 4

10 ice cubes
1 cup strawberries, plus 2 halved for garnish (optional)
1 cup raspberries
6 ounces white rum
2 ounces fresh lime juice
¼ cup confectioners' sugar

In a food processor, blend ice, 1 cup of strawberries, raspberries, rum, juice, and sugar until smooth. Divide evenly among 4 glasses; garnish with 1 strawberry half, if desired.

❋ **THE DISH:** 160 calories per serving, 0 g fat, 14 g carbs, 3 g fiber,
1 g protein

DARK AND STORMY

Snaps to ginger, which helps soothe aching muscles. Why not reward yourself with this cocktail the evening after an intense, calorie-torching workout? Serves 4

Ice cubes
24 ounces ginger beer, chilled
6 ounces dark rum
2 ounces fresh lime juice
1 tablespoon grated ginger, plus 4 slices for garnish (optional)
2 lime slices, halved (optional)

Fill a large pitcher with ice. Stir in ginger beer, rum, juice, and grated ginger. Divide evenly among 4 glasses; garnish each with 1 slice ginger and 1 slice lime, if desired.

❋ **THE DISH:** 164 calories per serving, 0 g fat, 18 g carbs, 0 g fiber,
0 g protein

SANGRIA BLANCA

Fresh fruit, not sugar, gives this sip its sweetness. Munch a few pieces between sips to take in waist-whittling fiber. Serves 8

Ice cubes
10 green grapes, halved
4 strawberries, hulled and sliced
1 peach, pitted and sliced, plus 8 slices for garnish (optional)
1 bottle (750 milliliters) cava (or dry sparkling wine)
12 ounces white grape juice
4 ounces Licor 43 (found at liquor stores)

2 sprigs fresh mint
1 peach, sliced (optional)

Fill a large glass pitcher halfway with ice; add fruit, except garnish. Tilt pitcher and pour cava very slowly down side (to preserve bubbles). Add juice and Licor; stir gently. Stir in mint. Divide evenly among 8 glasses; garnish each with 1 peach slice, if desired.

✻ **THE DISH:** 167 calories per serving, 0 g fat, 18 g carbs, 1 g fiber, 0 g protein

AMARETTO SOUR

Swap the store-bought sweet-and-sour mix for this lower-sugar version to save about 40 calories per serving. Serves 4

¼ cup confectioners' sugar
2 ounces each fresh lemon and lime juice
Ice cubes
6 ounces almond liqueur, divided
12 black cherries (optional)
1 teaspoon grated lemon zest (optional)

In a bowl, whisk sugar, juices, and 1 cup water until sugar dissolves. Chill at least 1 hour. Divide evenly among 4 glasses filled with ice. Divide almond liqueur evenly among glasses and stir. Garnish each with 3 cherries and ¼ teaspoon lemon zest, if desired.

✻ **THE DISH:** 197 calories per serving, 0 g fat, 9 g carbs, 0 g fiber, 0 g protein

FROZEN LIME MARGARITA

This 'rita saves you more than 120 calories per serving compared with many store-bought mixes. Serves 4

16 ice cubes

6 ounces tequila

4 ounces fresh lime juice

3 ounces triple sec

3 tablespoons confectioners' sugar

4 lime slices (optional)

In a food processor, blend first five ingredients until smooth. Divide evenly among 4 chilled margarita glasses; garnish each with 1 lime slice, if desired.

❊ **THE DISH:** 199 calories per serving, 0 g fat, 16 g carbs, 0 g fiber, 0 g protein

SEX ON THE BEACH

Slash around 120 calories per serving by skipping the peach schnapps and using light instead of full-calorie juices. Serves 4

Ice cubes

8 ounces vodka

8 ounces each light plum juice, light cranberry juice, and orange juice

1 teaspoon almond extract

2 orange slices, halved (optional)

Fill a large pitcher with ice. Stir in vodka, juices, and almond extract. Divide evenly among 4 glasses; garnish each with 1 halved orange slice, if desired.

❊ **THE DISH:** 201 calories per serving, 1 g fat (0 g saturated), 15 g carbs, 1 g fiber, 1 g protein

PIÑA COLADA

If you like piña coladas—and flat abs—you'll love this tipple: Yogurt promotes the growth of good bacteria in your gut, which crowds out belly-bloating bugs. Serves 4

16 ice cubes
2 cups low-fat plain yogurt
½ cup confectioners' sugar
4 ounces coconut water (plain or pineapple-flavored)
4 ounces coconut-flavored rum
1 teaspoon coconut extract
4 wedges fresh pineapple (optional)
12 coconut shavings (optional)

In a food processor, blend first six ingredients. Divide evenly among 4 glasses; garnish each with 1 pineapple wedge and 3 coconut shavings, if desired.

✳ **THE DISH:** 202 calories per serving, 4 g fat (3 g saturated), 22 g carbs, 0 g fiber, 4 g protein

APPLETINI

The superfood kiwifruit gives this 'tini slimming superpowers: It's loaded with fat-burning vitamin C! Serves 4

4 kiwifruit, peeled, plus 2 slices, halved, for garnish (optional)
¼ cup confectioners' sugar
8 ounces green apple vodka
Ice cubes

In a food processor, blend whole kiwifruit, sugar, and ½ cup water until smooth. Drain mixture through a fine strainer, reserving liquid. (This takes about 10 minutes.) Transfer liquid to a cocktail shaker, add vodka and ice, then close and shake. Strain into 4 chilled martini glasses; garnish each with 1 halved kiwi slice, if desired.

✳ **THE DISH:** 204 calories per serving glass, 0 g fat, 18 g carbs, 2 g fiber,
1 g protein

MAI TAI

Almond joy! Swapping crème d'amande for almond extract trims more
than 100 calories per serving. Serves 4

Ice cubes
8 ounces orange juice
6 ounces white rum
4 ounces pineapple juice
4 ounces light plum juice
2 ounces triple sec
1 teaspoon almond extract
4 plum slices (optional)
2 orange slices, halved (optional)

Fill a large pitcher with ice. Stir in the next six ingredients. Divide evenly
among 4 glasses; garnish each with 1 plum slice and 1 halved orange
slice, if desired.

✳ **THE DISH:** 205 calories per serving, 0 g fat, 18 g carbs, 1 g fiber,
1 g protein

TEQUILA SUNRISE

The orange juice in this libation helps fuel fat burning. Serves 4

Ice cubes
8 ounces tequila, divided
12 ounces orange juice, divided
4 ounces carrot juice, divided
4 tablespoons grenadine syrup, divided
2 orange slices, halved (optional)
2 baby carrots, halved (optional)

Fill 4 glasses with ice. Divide tequila and juices evenly among glasses. Slightly tilt 1 glass and pour 1 tablespoon grenadine down side. (It will settle on bottom.) Repeat with remaining glasses and grenadine. Garnish each with 1 halved orange slice and 1 halved carrot, if desired.

❊ **THE DISH:** 236 calories per serving, 0 g fat, 26 g carbs, 0 g fiber, 1 g protein

Nonalcoholic Drinks

Sometimes there's nothing better than an icy cold soft drink, and as long as you make room for the calories, you can go ahead and gulp your favorites. Do keep in mind, however, that liquid calories can be extra dangerous for your diet. Sodas, bottled teas, energy drinks, and even some juices are loaded with sugar and little else. As a result, they don't fill you up like solid food, so it's incredibly easy to swallow hundreds of calories in a sitting, then forget all about them—until weigh-in day, that is. Don't fall for the trap: Log the liquid calories as you do any others.

Ocean Spray Cran-Grape (8 ounces)
      120 calories
Seagram's Ginger Ale (12-ounce can)
      130 calories
Coca-Cola (12-ounce can)
      140 calories
Sprite (12-ounce can)
      140 calories
Minute Maid Lemonade (12-ounce can)
      150 calories
Fanta Orange (12-ounce can)
      160 calories
Hansen's Cherry Vanilla Créme Soda (12-ounce can)
      160 calories
Minute Maid Orange Juice (12-ounce bottle)
      170 calories

Simply Apple Juice (13.5-ounce bottle)
    180 calories
Original Gatorade (32-ounce bottle)
    200 calories
Lemon AriZona Iced Tea (20-ounce bottle)
    225 calories

➡ **Trim-Down Tip:** Instead of drinking a full glass of juice (and its full calorie load), pour out an ounce and top it off with soda water or seltzer for a refreshing spritzer that costs you a mere 15 calories or so.

Red Bull (8.4-ounce can)
    110 calories
Rockstar Energy Drink (8 ounces)
    140 calories

Fast-Food Favorites

Can't break your drive-through habit? No problem! You've got several finger-licking options that won't necessarily break your diet as long as you stay within your day's limit for base calories (or happy calories) and indulge no more than once a week. If you don't see your favorites listed here, look online at the chain's website, or ask at the counter. (For smarter, superfood-containing picks, turn to chapter 14.)

McDonald's

French Fries (small)
    230 calories
Chipotle Grilled BBQ Snack Wrap
    250 calories
Six Chicken McNuggets
    280 calories
Cheeseburger
    300 calories

Premium Grilled Chicken Sandwich
    350 calories

→ **Trim-Down Tip:** In fast-food speak, "crispy" is synonymous with fried. Clucking for a chicken sandwich? Order yours grilled, and voilà!—you'll cut about 150 calories. Trade out the mayo and add ketchup and you'll save another 50. Together, that's about a day's worth of happy calories!

Burger King

Six-Piece BK Chicken Fries
    250 calories
French Fries (small)
    340 calories
Whopper Jr.
    340 calories
BK Single Stacker
    380 calories
Tendergrill Chicken Sandwich
    470 calories

Wendy's

Chili (small)
    210 calories
Value Fries
    230 calories
Jr. Cheeseburger
    270 calories
Homestyle Chicken Go Wrap
    320 calories
Ultimate Chicken Grill Sandwich
    360 calories

Taco Bell

Fresco Crunchy Taco
  150 calories
Cheese Roll-Up
  190 calories
Fresco Burrito Supreme Chicken
  350 calories
Bean Burrito
  370 calories
Chalupa Baja Beef
  410 calories
Nachos Supreme
  440 calories

Arby's

Kids Curly Fries
  270 calories
Prime-Cut Chicken Tenders (3)
  360 calories
Roast Beef Classic
  360 calories
Cravin' Roast Chicken Sandwich
  370 calories

KFC

Original Chicken Drumstick
  120 calories
Biscuit
  180 calories
KFC Snacker with Crispy Strip
  310 calories
Crispy Strips (3)
  390 calories

Popcorn Chicken
    400 calories

Special Occasion Splurging

Spending your happy calories on everyday indulgences such as cookies and potato chips is a good way to head off feelings of deprivation, but there will probably come a time when you find yourself faced with (or longing for) an indulgence that's more—how shall we put it?—major. Whether it's sizzling glazed ribs at a backyard barbecue, Chinese take-out after a long day, or something else, you can enjoy it without feeling as if you're cheating or doing something "bad." All it takes is a little planning. Scroll through these categories to find your favorite eats. Then see how many happy calories you need to save to have exactly what you want, minus the guilt.

Movie-Night Snacks

Popcorn at AMC Theatres (small)
    370 calories
Popcorn at Cinemark Theatres (small)
    420 calories
Popcorn at Regal Entertainment Group theaters (small)
    670 calories

→ **Trim-Down Tip:** Yes, popcorn is a superfood, but popping it in oil, drenching it in buttery topping, and gobbling up a giant bucket of it is like turning it into kryptonite—a body-busting treat. Check out page 119 for ways you can munch on popcorn at the movies without having to save up several days' worth of happy calories.

Milk Duds (3-ounce box)
    370 calories
Sno-Caps (3.1-ounce box)
    400 calories

Raisinets (3.5-ounce box)
   380 calories
Twizzlers (5-ounce bag)
   460 calories
Sour Patch Kids (5-ounce box)
   490 calories

→ **Trim-Down Tip:** The boxes of candy available at movie theaters are substantially bigger than regular-size bags. Why not spread the love over two days? Portion out a single serving, then stash the rest in your purse for another time.

Soda at Cinemark (small)
   150 calories
Soda at AMC (small)
   200 calories
Soda at Regal (small)
   300 calories

→ **Trim-Down Tip:** Don't want to drink away your happy calories? Order soda water to get all the bubbles but none of the calories. If that doesn't cut it, and you've got a strong hankering for soda, sip diet flavors sparingly; research suggests that downing more than one diet soft drink a day increases your risk for obesity.

Pizza Party

1 slice vegetable pizza (medium-size pie)
   230 calories

→ **Trim-down Tip:** That old trick of using a napkin to sop up extra grease from a slice really works! It's tough to say exactly how many calories you'll save, but every little bit counts. Another slim-eating idea: If your favorite pizza joint uses tons of cheese, ask for only half and you'll cut another small chunk off your bottom line.

1 slice cheese pizza
  240 calories
1 slice pepperoni pizza (medium-size pie)
  250 calories

→ **Trim-Down Tip:** Veggie pizza may save you only a handful of calories over pepperoni, but it tends to be more filling thanks to the fiber. You'll also take in more vitamins and minerals and lose a gram of saturated fat.

Italian Eats

1 breadstick
  140 calories
Olives (20)
  150 calories
Caesar salad
  220 calories
Caprese salad
  480 calories
Tiramisu
  690 calories
Eggplant parmigiana (2½ cups)
  800 calories
Spaghetti marinara (3½ cups)
  850 calories
Lasagna (2 cups)
  960 calories
Fettuccine Alfredo (2½ cups)
  1,500 calories

→ **Trim-Down Tip:** Alfredo serves up serious fat and calories. If it's your all-time favorite, fill up first on a big salad, then spoon up a small portion.

Chinese Takeout

1 pan-fried vegetable dumpling
  60 calories
1 spring roll
  156 calories
1 egg roll
  215 calories
Shrimp lo mein (7 ounces)
  227 calories
Beef with broccoli (7 ounces)
  290 calories

→ **Trim-Down Tip:** Split your order or save some for another day: The calories listed here for entrées are for one serving, not the entire plateful or pint container.

Kung Pao chicken (5 ounces)
  383 calories
Sweet-and-sour pork (10 ounces)
  460 calories

→ **Trim-Down Tip:** Veggie-loaded dishes are a great splurge because they help you fill up on fewer calories. Ask how any meat is prepared, however. In some Chinese dishes, particularly sweet-and-sour items, the meat is deep-fried, which adds extra calories. Opt for grilled, stir-fried, or pan-fried meat when you can.

Plain white rice (6 ounces)
  220 calories
Combo fried rice (8 ounces)
  363 calories

→ **Trim-Down Tip:** Swap white for brown rice whenever possible; the latter is a whole grain and delivers more filling, hunger-curbing fiber.

Mexican Fiesta

Margarita on the rocks (5 ounces)
    250 calories
Frozen margarita (8 ounces)
    312 calories

. . . .

→ **Trim-Down Tip:** Always order your 'rita on the rocks—frozen versions tend to pack more calories because the serving sizes are usually bigger. If you're shaking up your drinks at home, also skip the premade, bottled mixers, which are usually loaded with sugar. Check the recipes for healthier cocktails starting on page 314.

. . . .

Soft chicken taco (6 ounces)
    210 calories
Crispy chicken taco (5 ounces)
    220 calories
Cheese enchilada (5 ounces)
    370 calories
Cheese nachos (7 ounces)
    810 calories
Beef burrito (14 ounces)
    830 calories
Cheese quesadilla (11½ ounces)
    900 calories

Pub Fare

French fries
    590 calories
Hamburger (with mustard, lettuce, tomato, and onion)
    660 calories
Buffalo wings (12 wings without dressing)
    700 calories
Mozzarella sticks, appetizer (9 sticks)
    830 calories

Southern Barbecue

Grilled chicken leg (no skin)
  90 calories
Fried drumstick
  120 calories
Coleslaw (¼ pound)
  150 calories
Corn on the cob (with butter)
  155 calories
Potato salad (4.5 ounces)
  210 calories
Grilled chicken breast (no skin)
  220 calories
Hot dog
  297 calories
Fried chicken breast
  360 calories
Ribs (¼ slab)
  459 calories

Holiday Meals

Ham
  104 calories per 3 ounces
Turkey (white meat without skin)
  119 calories per 3 ounces
Green bean casserole
  148 calories per cup
Latkes
  150 calories each
Turkey (dark meat with skin)
  155 calories per 3 ounces
Bread crumb stuffing
  176 calories per ½ cup
Mashed potatoes
  237 calories per cup

→ **Trim-Down Tip:** Pick the leaner cuts of breast meat and leave off the skin to save around 40 calories compared with the same portion of dark meat with skin.

Pumpkin pie
   316 calories per slice ($^1/_8$ of 9-inch pie)
Eggnog
   440 calories per ½ cup
Pecan pie
   503 calories per slice

LOG YOUR FAVORITES!

If you don't see your go-to foods in this chapter, look up the nutritional information at NutritionData.Self.com (or on the food manufacturer's website), then write them here for easy reference.

drop 10 inspiration

"I've stopped snacking all the time—and don't feel hungry!"

NAME: Jennifer Kremer

AGE: 38

OCCUPATION: Health care software designer

FAMILY STATUS: Married, one child

HEIGHT: 5 feet 5 inches

STARTING WEIGHT: 170

DROP 10 WEIGHT: 160

LOST: 10 pounds in five weeks

My story: "I always thought that if I ate too much, I could just exercise it off the next day. But this wasn't a good long-term solution. I wasn't happy with my weight, and I wasn't seeing results."

Biggest challenge to losing weight: "Portion size and snacking. I used to snack a lot."

Why Drop 10 clicked: "I really focused on my food intake. I'd never realized how much impact my food choices had. I always thought exercise was the most important factor. The plan gave me many good options of high-energy, high-protein foods to eat in the right amounts. I do not feel hungry, so I'm less likely to snack. The plan really helped me be more mindful and creative about what I put in my body."

How my body changed: "I went down one size and am very close to going down another one. I'm motivated now to get down to 150 pounds. I follow a running schedule and am even training for a half-marathon."

Success tip: "Diet and exercise work together—you need to focus on both."

Superworkouts to Zap Fat Even Faster

Batman had Robin, James Bond had Q, even Erin Brockovich had her crotchety lawyer boss. Sure, maybe each of the top-billed names could have succeeded alone, but the duos were unstoppable: stronger, smarter, and dangerously more effective than either half solo. That is exactly what you get by teaming up the superfood-fueled Drop 10 eating plan with its super sidekick, exercise. If it's your mission to take down fat, the diet and workout plan together will make it easier than ever to get there, erasing a full 2 pounds per week!

For those of you who just groaned or grew anxious at the mention of exercise, relax! Working out doesn't have to mean dragging yourself to a gym, logging endless hours on a treadmill, or grunting in a stinky weight room, any more than dieting means giving up Oreos. Research shows that the trick to melting serious fat and inches with fitness isn't necessarily working out longer or following a strict plan. If you work out smarter, you can do it in less time and you might even start enjoying it. Really!

In order for exercise to be your EZ Pass on the road to weight loss, your workout plan must include a few different things. First, you need a routine that combines strength training and cardio. You know about the calorie-cooking power of the latter; the former builds and sculpts lean muscle, which not only helps you look firm and toned, but also stokes your metabolism. The more fat you replace with lean muscle, the more calories your body burns doing everyday activities (say, sitting at your computer). And as you'll see from our weight-free workout later in this chapter, you can strength train at home without picking up a single dumbbell. Activities that get your heart rate up and blood pumping count as cardio, the type of exercise that torches the most fat and calories for fuel. If you infuse your weekly workouts with a little of both types, any grumbles about exercise will quickly turn into aahs as you notice your jeans getting looser.

The second secret to exercising smarter: doing intervals, or short bursts of high-intensity activity followed by a slower period or short rest phase. Among trainers, fitness insiders, and other experts, intervals are known as weight loss magic—the superfood of the fitness world. Even a few minutes of go-all-out bouts per session will increase the size and number of your muscles' mitochondria, key subunits of cells that use oxygen to burn calories and fat. The more mitochondria you've got and the bigger they are, the better your results will be and the less time you'll need to spend working out to get in amazing shape. Bonus: Intervals keep your metabolism cranking post-workout, too. That could mean burning up to an extra 120 calories after you've hit the shower. And intervals are even fun: You don't have time to zone out while alternating between high-intensity bursts and recovery time, so you don't get bored during a long cardio session.

And that leads us to the final piece of the exercise-smarter puzzle: A workout is only as good as its appeal to the person doing it. (That would be you!) Tedious or time-consuming sessions, complicated programs, and activities you plain don't like won't help you lose weight—they only make it easier to find excuses for why you should put on slippers instead of sneakers. On the other hand, a workout plan that incorporates interesting moves, short but effective sessions, and the option to exercise when you want and do activities you enjoy will seal the deal on your smaller-size future. Such workouts feel easier, so the minutes speed by; and they are tailored to your needs and schedule and thus excuse-proof.

The easy, flexible, and fun Drop 10 plan you'll see on the next few pages incorporates all these smart strategies, and we've carefully designed it to maximize both fat burning and your time. But if you want to do other strength, cardio, and interval workouts, that's okay, too. The important thing is to find something you like and do it consistently. Then there will be no stopping you!

The Amazing Proof

- An overview of weight loss studies published in *The Cochrane Library* finds that people who followed a low-cal eating plan and also worked out lost an average of 23 pounds, but those who either dieted or exercised struggled to slim down.
- Almost 90 percent of adults in the National Weight Control Registry (a database of people who have lost at least 30 pounds and kept it off for a year) count regular exercise as part of their successful weight loss strategy.
- Women who did three strength-training sessions per week weighed less and had a lower percentage of body fat after twenty-four weeks than those who didn't train, a study in the *Journal of Aging and Health* reports.
- Women who mixed sprints with jogging for twenty minutes dropped three times as much fat from their legs and butt as those who jogged steadily for forty minutes, according to a study from the University of New South Wales in Sydney, Australia.

The Drop 10 Workout Plan

Part 1: The Burn-and-Firm Superworkout

As you probably guessed, strength training, cardio, and intervals are the three pillars of the Drop 10 workout plan. But we've taken things a key step further by combining all three fitness elements into one wildly effective and outrageously efficient fat-flaying superworkout. You can bank on obliterating up to 400 calories with every thirty-two-minute session! (Want to skip ahead to the workout? The moves start on page 343.)

How did we fit three workouts into one? Simple: Several of the eight moves that make up the Drop 10 superworkout are strength-cardio hybrids that help you build lean, metabolism-revving muscle and blast burn-baby-burn calories in a big way. Plus, instead of doing the standard two sets of ten reps of each move, you'll be doing something called Tabata intervals, which are based on the work of Japanese researcher Izumi Tabata, PhD. Here's the deal: You perform a move for 20 seconds, then rest for 10 seconds. Repeat that 20/10 cycle eight times before moving on to the next exercise. Easy, right? (You can do practically anything for 20 seconds!) This stellar combo helps you melt maximum calories, tone muscles, and blast more fat than ever. (That's thanks not only to the fat-fighting intervals: Moves that call on several muscle groups at once, such as the ones in the Drop 10 plan, trigger your cells to release more fat, which you then burn for energy.) Do this workout three times per week, and even if you're a fitness newbie, you'll be zipping through the moves like a pro and watching the pounds fly off in no time.

Part 2: Choose-How-You-Lose Fat Burning

Just as you've got options and flexibility in the diet portion of the Drop 10 plan, this is the place in the workout where you call the shots. You decide not only what you'll do, but when and for how long. The only guideline: Sizzle 700 additional calories per week with any activity or activities you like, in addition to doing your three superworkouts. For example, you could jog for as little as ten minutes every day to reach your 700-calorie quota or scorch them all in one Saturday session.

If you hate jogging, don't worry—it's far from your only choice. Use the flowchart on page 352 to ID activities that best fit your fitness style, then find out how many calories each fries per minute to help you plan your week's burn-athon. Or, if you like to mix up your workouts and already know what floats your exercise boat, jump straight to the exercise list to scope your favorites and see how long it will take to crush your 700-calorie-per-week goal. Any way you burn 'em, you lose inches and flab.

Part 1: The Burn-and-Firm Superworkout

- What you need: A light- to medium-resistance band with or without handles (you can get one online or at a sporting goods store) and a timer. If you'd rather go low-tech to time yourself, use the old "one-one hundred, two-one hundred" counting trick.

- What to do: Do the first move for 20 seconds, then rest for 10 seconds. Repeat eight times, then continue with the second move, and so on until you've done all eight moves for eight intervals each. Complete the workout three times per week.

1. **Tap Out Fat**

WORKS SHOULDERS, TRICEPS, CHEST, ABS, OBLIQUES

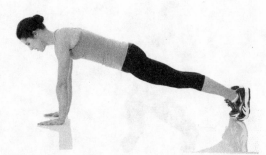

Start in a plank with wrists directly under shoulders (as shown).

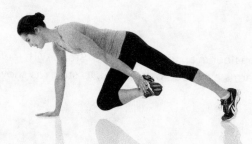

Bring right knee toward chest and tap right foot with left hand (as shown). Return to plank. Repeat on opposite side. Continue alternating taps for 20 seconds.

2. **Jump Squat**
WORKS BUTT, THIGHS, HAMSTRINGS, CALVES

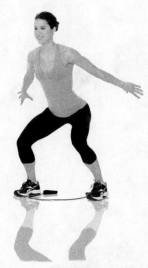

Place band on floor in an upside-down U. Stand with feet outside handles. Squat, arms extended behind you, to start (as shown).

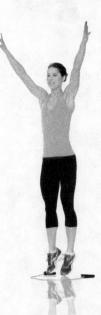

Jump, raising arms overhead (as shown), landing inside band, then jump back to start. Continue jumping in and out for 20 seconds.

3. **Freeze Firmer**

WORKS SHOULDERS, BICEPS, TRICEPS, CHEST, ABS

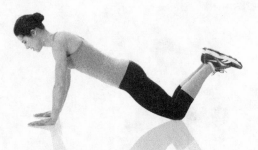

Start in a modified push-up position on knees, hands under shoulders (as shown).

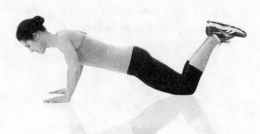

Bend elbows 90 degrees (as shown) and hold for the entire 20-second interval, keeping abs engaged.

4. Slimming Swing

WORKS SHOULDERS, TRICEPS, UPPER BACK, ABS, BUTT,
THIGHS

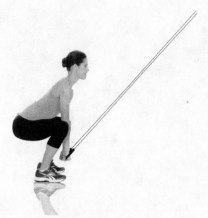

Anchor band at chest level in front of you (try looping it around a banister, railing, or pole); grip an end in each hand. Stand with feet hip-width apart; extend arms forward at shoulder level with band taut. Squat, lowering hands between legs (as shown).

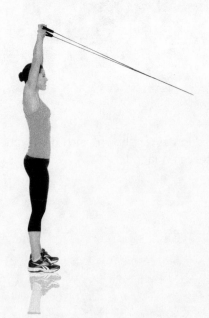

Stand tall with abs engaged as you quickly raise arms overhead (as shown). Repeat for 20 seconds.

5. Sit Tight

WORKS ABS, BICEPS, CHEST

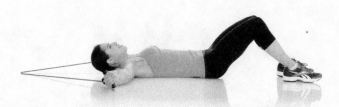

Lie faceup with knees bent, feet flat; anchor center of band securely about a foot behind head and hold an end in each hand, arms extended to sides at shoulder level (as shown), to start.

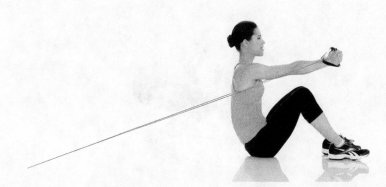

Engage abs and sit up, bringing hands forward and together at chest level with arms straight but not locked (as shown). Return to start. Repeat for 20 seconds.

6. Bulge-Blasting Burpee

WORKS SHOULDERS, BACK, ABS, BUTT, THIGHS

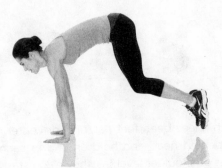

Stand with feet hip-width apart. Crouch down; place hands on floor under shoulders. With hands planted, jump feet behind you (as shown), landing in a plank.

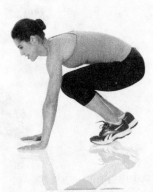

Hop feet back to hands (as shown), then quickly jump up to return to standing. Repeat for 20 seconds.

7. **Twist and Tone**

WORKS SHOULDERS, TRICEPS, ABS, OBLIQUES, BUTT, THIGHS

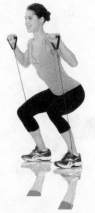

Stand on band with feet hip-width apart, an end in each hand, elbows bent, hands at shoulders; squat (as shown).

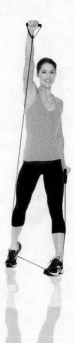

Stand as you rotate right foot and torso to left, extending right arm overhead (as shown). Return to squat. Repeat, rotating to right. Continue, alternating sides, for 20 seconds.

8. Get-Lean Leap
WORKS ABS, BUTT, THIGHS

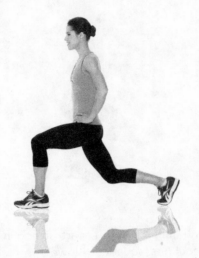

Start in a lunge with left foot forward, knee directly over ankle, hands on hips (as shown).

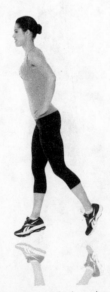

Push off feet and switch legs in air (as shown), landing in a lunge with right foot forward. Repeat on opposite side. Continue, alternating sides, for 20 seconds.

If you're sweating, you need to be swigging—it's the best way to replace lost fluids and keep your system functioning optimally. Once you've got your workout down and are exercising at a higher intensity, you may need to down 8 to 16 ounces of water for every thirty minutes you're losing it through your pores. If you exercise intensely for more than an hour, electrolyte-infused H_2O can help replenish the potassium, calcium, and magnesium depleted through sweat, but it's not any more hydrating than what comes from your faucet. (And you can replace electrolytes with food, too.) But unless you're running a long race or working out for hours at a time, avoid flavored sport drinks. Most contain lots of added sugar, causing you to gulp back the calories you worked so hard to burn off.

Choose-How-You-Lose Fat Burning

In addition to doing the burn-and-firm superworkout three times per week, aim to torch an extra 700 calories weekly doing, well, just about anything. You can burn off a few every day or sweat them all out in one or two days. Likewise, you can stick with one activity or have a rotating list of go-tos—you pick! If you're not sure which workouts best suit you, use this get-fit personality chart, then check out the activities and the number of calories that each burns per minute.* You'll also find at-home options throughout. Yep, you can get slim without setting foot in the gym!

* Calculations are based on a 135-pound woman.

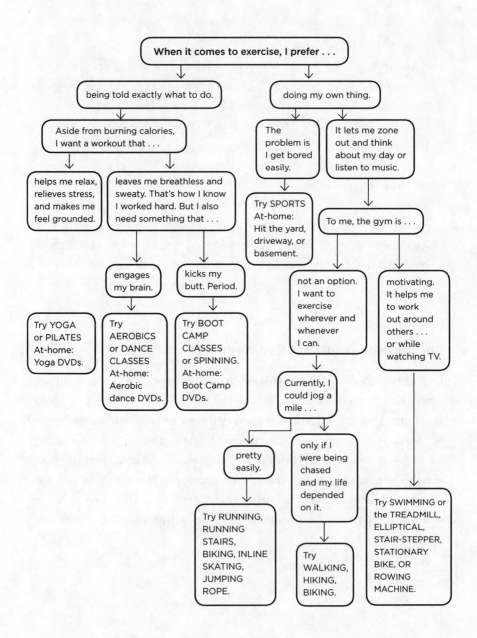

When it comes to exercise, I prefer . . .

being told exactly what to do.

doing my own thing.

Aside from burning calories, I want a workout that . . .

helps me relax, relieves stress, and makes me feel grounded.

leaves me breathless and sweaty. That's how I know I worked hard. But I also need something that . . .

The problem is I get bored easily.

It lets me zone out and think about my day or listen to music.

Try SPORTS At-home: Hit the yard, driveway, or basement.

To me, the gym is . . .

engages my brain.

kicks my butt. Period.

Try YOGA or PILATES At-home: Yoga DVDs.

Try AEROBICS or DANCE CLASSES At-home: Aerobic dance DVDs.

Try BOOT CAMP CLASSES or SPINNING. At-home: Boot Camp DVDs.

not an option. I want to exercise wherever and whenever I can.

motivating. It helps me to work out around others . . . or while watching TV.

Currently, I could jog a mile . . .

pretty easily.

only if I were being chased and my life depended on it.

Try RUNNING, RUNNING STAIRS, BIKING, INLINE SKATING, JUMPING ROPE.

Try WALKING, HIKING, BIKING.

Try SWIMMING or the TREADMILL, ELLIPTICAL, STAIR-STEPPER, STATIONARY BIKE, OR ROWING MACHINE.

On the following pages, you'll find the best exercises to help you sizzle away your 700 calories-per-week quota. ⟶

Yoga or Pilates. You can get Zen and slim from the same workout. Both yoga and Pilates incorporate low-impact moves best known for toning, improving posture, enhancing flexibility, and helping you chill out. But—surprise!—you'll also burn calories, especially doing the more vigorous forms of yoga such as Vinyasa (aka power or flow yoga). Look for Vinyasa yoga or Pilates DVDs for use at home.

Calories burned per minute:

> Yoga (Vinyasa) = 7.1
> Pilates = 3.2

Aerobics, step aerobics, boxing/kickboxing, or dance classes. Following an instructor and learning new steps and moves keep your brain busy and you focused on something other than how much you're sweating. What else helps: The classes are fun and challenging, and there are tons of types and hybrids to choose from. Go to a few different classes until you find one you love. At home, opt for DVDs. A good, old-fashioned dance party also counts. Move the coffee table and bring on the Beyoncé!

Calories burned per minute:

> Kickboxing = 10.7
> Step = 10.7
> Boxing = 9.6
> Aerobics:
>   high-impact (lots of jumping and hopping) = 7.5
>   low-impact (no jumping) = 5.3
> Zumba (Latin-inspired dance workout) = 6.9
> Dance (various styles) = 5.1

Boot camp or spinning classes. Drop and give us 20 (calories)! If you're looking for a no-nonsense, challenging workout that will have you sweating buckets and burning serious calories, you're in the right place. Boot camp fitness instructors lead you through fast-paced, multitasking drills; Spinning teachers push you to crank your way up imaginary hills and sprint past make-believe opponents. There's also something to be said for doing intense workouts in a group, where you can feed off your classmates' energy (and high-five afterward). At home: You'll find plenty of boot camp DVDs, or search online for drop-in classes that meet at local parks.

Calories burned per minute:

> Spinning = 12.3
> Boot camp = 8.6

Sports. Whether you want to join a team or prefer going one-on-one with an opponent, get in the game and you'll never be bored. The combination of sweating, socializing, and healthy competition keeps things fun and incredibly motivating. There's also plenty of variety for different tastes and fitness levels, putting you in charge of your workouts. At home: Shoot hoops in the driveway, play Ping-Pong in the basement, or go for volleyball or badminton in the backyard—anything that gets your heart rate up can count toward your 700-calorie-per-week goal.

Calories burned per minute:

> Beach volleyball = 8.6
> Volleyball = 8.6
> Lacrosse = 8.5
> Racquetball = 7.5
> Soccer = 7.5
> Tennis = 7.5
> Basketball = 6.4
> Badminton = 4.8
> Golf = 4.8
> Ping-Pong = 4.3

Swimming, treadmill running, elliptical training, stair stepping, or rowing-machine workouts. Gyms often get a bad rap, but for some people a gym is the perfect place to sweat, a spot devoted solely to helping you reach your exercise goals, where you can do something different nearly every day of the week. Plus, swimming and machine-assisted workouts are efficient, allowing you to get in and out quickly minus a few hundred calories. Gyms also offer plenty of distractions if you need them, whether you watch people or the latest episode of your favorite reality show.

Calories burned per minute:

Swimming:
   butterfly = 11.8
   breaststroke = 10.7
   freestyle = 10.7
   backstroke = 7.5
Treadmill walking/running:
   7 mph = 12.3
   6 mph = 10.7
   5 mph = 8.5
   4 mph = 5.3
   3 mph = 3.5
Elliptical:
   vigorous = 8.2
   moderate = 6.9
Stair-stepper = 9.6
Stationary biking:
   vigorous = 11.3
   moderate = 7.5
Rowing = 12.8

Jogging, running, running stairs, biking, inline skating, or jumping rope. Fitness minimalists and those with hectic schedules who need total flexibility still have a slew of options that require little or no gear and that you can do just about anywhere, anytime, for free. Exercising outdoors can also be a real bonus; the fresh air and scenery may be an extra motivator that boosts your mood, energy, and drive.

Calories burned per minute:

> Biking:
>> racing = 17.1
>> leisure = 6.4
>
> Running stairs = 16
> Inline skating = 13.4
> Jumping rope = 12.8
> Running:
>> 7 mph = 12.3
>> 6 mph = 10.7
>> 5 mph = 8.5

Walking, hiking, or biking. These options are among the simplest ways to burn extra calories and ultimately drop pounds, especially for exercise novices and those who dislike formal workouts. Low-impact (on both body and wallet) and easy to do anywhere, they're perfect gateway activities that will help you realize how amazing you look and feel when you move more. Why not start right now? Get out and take a walk or bike to do your next errand.

Supercharge Fat Burning with Intervals

If you run, walk, bike, swim, or use the elliptical or stair-stepper, crank up your speed for even faster results. Incorporating short, high-intensity bursts into your choose-how-you-lose activities helps you burn bonus calories and fat. Try it: Simply push your pace for 30 to 60 seconds, then reduce your speed back to when you started. After that, you make the rules: Set a goal for how many sprints you want to do in a session—start with only one or try for six! Also feel free to vary your sprint and recovery speeds depending on how you're doing, and take as long to recover between intervals as you need. Every sprint gets you that much closer to a trimmer, healthier you.

> **. . . . .**
> ## FLEX APPEAL
> **. . . . .**
>
> Feeling tight? Can't touch your toes? Stretching can improve flexi-
> bility and help you get lean. Broadening your joint range of motion
> can make exercise seem less challenging, which leads you to do
> more of it! But guess what? Stretching cold muscles preworkout
> isn't the ticket. (One exception: If you've been exercising regularly
> and usually stretch beforehand, don't stop now; changing your rou-
> tine could up your risk for injury.) Instead, it's best to warm up your
> muscles with 3 minutes of cardio before you stretch, or to get
> bendy after your usual workout. Also ban bouncing, which may
> cause muscles to contract rather than extend. You want to ease
> into a stretch until you feel a light strain, then hold for 30 seconds
> while breathing deeply.

Calories burned per minute:

> Biking = 6.4
> Hiking = 6.4
> Walking:
> 　4 mph = 5.3
> 　3 mph = 3.5

Ten Get-Moving Motivators

Unless you have a personal trainer who hollers at you until you move,
you might need some help from time to time mustering the mojo to
keep up with your exercise routine. These ten tips will help you stay inspired for the long haul.

1. *Put the fun in fitness.* The more you enjoy an activity, the less it
   feels like a workout and the easier it will be to stick with it. If you
   picked a specific exercise from the chart in this chapter that
   you're not loving, change it up! Sports, hiking, biking, inline

skating, and other outdoor activities keep your mind occupied on things other than sweat. But remember that discovering your perfect workout match can be like dating: You might have to meet a few duds until you find true love.

2. *Embrace Lycra.* Think about how you feel in a ratty, oversize T-shirt and shorts versus a sleek, body-flattering outfit. Working out in clothes that encourage lounging on the couch won't help you. On the other hand, the right gear can motivate you by upping your body confidence and helping you feel comfortable throughout your workout. Investing in a few fitness-specific pieces (such as tanks, tees, shorts, or workout pants) in bright colors, fun patterns, and flattering cuts will make you more jazzed to start sweating. Exercise wear moves with you (no wedgies, no chafing), and sweat-wicking materials keep you dry—exactly what you need to go that extra mile.

3. *Groove while you move.* Here's research that will be music to your ears: Pressing "play" on your iPod or stereo at the beginning of a workout can make whatever you're doing feel easier and keep you motivated to exercise longer. Music also boosts your mood and can even prompt you to push your pace and stay strong. When the tempo of music was increased by only 10 percent without study subjects knowing, they cycled farther and pedaled with more power, according to a study in the *Scandinavian Journal of Medicine & Science in Sports.* Pick upbeat, steady songs with a driving beat (think hip-hop, rock, or fast pop) that will encourage you to move in time with the tunes.

4. *Buddy up.* Friends make everything more fun, including exercise. But mixing sweat and social hour does more than help the time fly by. You're less likely to blow off a workout if you know a pal (or a whole team!) is counting on you to show. And don't forget the power of a little healthy competition. People who worked out with a virtual video-game partner that was programmed to always be fitter than they were stuck it out 24 percent longer than when they sweated alone, a study from Michigan State University suggests. Even if you don't have a friend around to egg you on, take a group aerobics or Spin class and aim to be

the strongest pupil. Or spot a superfit runner on one of the other treadmills or running track and try to keep up.

5. *Plan to succeed.* Schedule your workouts a week ahead of time—thinking about when and how long you'll exercise makes you move more, a study in the *Journal of Consumer Research* shows. In fact, people who asked themselves the simple question "How much will I work out?" increased their activity by 138 percent! Why not schedule your calorie-burning plans on the same calendar as your calorie-burning meals? Jot down exactly what you'll do and for how long. And no lowballing! Give yourself something to strive for, then rise to the occasion.

6. *Mix it up.* If you get bored easily, make sure you've got a few different calorie-torching activities in your weekly arsenal. For example, take a yoga class on Tuesdays, set a standing gym date with a friend every Thursday, and hit the bike trail on Saturdays. Not only will you stay engaged, but your body will as well. By never getting the chance to adapt to one activity, your calorie burn stays sky-high.

7. *Set microgoals.* Yes, trimming your tummy before your sister's wedding might be your end game, but supplementing big-picture goals with smaller ones that you can work toward—and achieve—during each session helps propel you through a tough workout and leaves you eager to come back for more. (What's better than crushing a new challenge day in and day out?) While lacing up your sneakers, decide what your goal for that day's workout will be. Maybe it's mastering Crow pose in yoga, perfecting your tennis backhand, jogging faster or longer than last week, or even getting through all eight intervals of the burn-and-firm superworkout without extra rest time.

8. *Be your own cheerleader.* The little voices in your head are a lot more powerful than you think. If you're consumed by self-doubts (as in, Ugh, this is so hard, I'm not sure I can finish), you're more apt to throw in the towel. But pumping yourself up with confidence-building cues (I'm strong, I can do it, I'm getting better, let's go!) might actually improve your performance, a review in *Perspectives on Psychological Science* suggests. You don't need

to sugarcoat a tough session; simply spin the truth. Acknowledge that what you're doing is difficult, then focus on how you can succeed anyway and how you're getting fitter with every step or move you make. Mind over muscles!

9. *Bargain with yourself.* If you're having a hard time finding the get-up-and-go to exercise after a long day or to get out from under a warm comforter in the a.m., tell yourself that if you put on your workout clothes and do something for only five or ten minutes, you can call it quits right after. Some days you might do exactly that, and that's okay; but more often than not, you'll keep moving and end up logging a full session.

10. *Listen to your body.* When you're really struggling to keep your drive alive, whether before or during a workout, your body could be telling you it's time to take a day off. Be honest with yourself: If you've been at it regularly for a few weeks and feel like you truly need a break, take it! Don't exercise at all, or go for a leisurely walk or an easy bike ride instead of your usual sessions. Trust your instincts, then let them lead you back to the gym in another day or two.

Does Your Workout Need a Sandwich?

After following the Drop 10 workout plan for about two weeks, review your food journal entries and think back on whether your appetite has changed. Are you hungry all the time? Have you been indulging more often? The fitness-food connection can be a complicated one: For some people, it's as if exercising flips their stomach's feed-me switch to the on position—suddenly they want to hoover up anything and everything in sight. Others may not technically be hungrier, but exercising regularly causes them to feel more deserving of extra helpings and treats. As a result, they find themselves sweating but not slimming. Then there are those for whom an intense workout acts as a temporary appetite suppressant.

Obviously, if exercise makes you less hungry, you're in good shape. But regardless of which group you fall into, have a meal or snack within an hour or so of finishing a workout. That's when muscles are primed to soak up the most nutrients and your body can best replenish its energy stores. Also, drink water to replace lost fluids. If you are one of those people who tend to think, Hmm, I just worked out and I can have that extra [fill in the blank], be careful: People often overestimate the number of calories they burn and underestimate the calorie cost of brownies and other treats. Resist the "it all evens out" mentality, and remember that exercise and diet work together to create the calorie deficit that leads to weight loss success. If you do decide to indulge over and above your 200 freebie calories per day, take a look at the calorie counts for your chosen treat in chapter 12, then calculate how many minutes of exercise it takes to burn off that item. If it adds up to more calories and more minutes on the elliptical than you bargained for, rethink your bite. Better yet, indulge in a calorie-free goody instead. What do you really love doing that has nothing to do with food? Start rewarding yourself for tough workouts with that.

For those whose tummies truly have been growling more since beginning regular workouts, know that it could be your body's way of adjusting to fewer calories coming in and more going out—as if it's saying, "Whoa, Nelly! I think I need those!" Also, take a look at what you're eating before your workouts—it may affect how hungry you are after. Your appetite should level off within a few weeks.

Keep in mind that you never want to exercise immediately following a big meal. In order to digest food, your body pumps blood to your gut, but during a sweat session, blood gets diverted to muscles. That could cause stomach cramps or leave you feeling sluggish (and snackish). But hitting the gym with a belly that's been empty for several hours is no good either—hello, energy crisis! What's ideal: picking a snack from the meal plan or having a piece of whole fruit or something equally small and low in calories an hour or two prior to lacing up your sneakers. Doing so will fuel your body, steady your appetite, and help you stay within your day's calorie limits.

drop 10 inspiration

"This plan gave me back my confidence."

NAME: Kat Chalensouk

AGE: 28

OCCUPATION: Telecommunications project manager

FAMILY STATUS: Single

HEIGHT: 5 feet 2 inches

STARTING WEIGHT: 143

DROP 10 WEIGHT: 134

LOST: 9 pounds in five weeks

My story: "I've tried to slim down in the past, but I didn't see much success. I wasn't motivated, nor was I living in the right environment. When I moved to the beach, I was determined to lose weight and set a goal to become a runner and do a charity run once a month."

Biggest challenge to losing weight: "Balancing diet and exercise with my busy travel schedule for work. Traveling takes a toll on the body and mind. I would always go with the best intentions but end up overindulging and never unpack my sneakers."

Why Drop 10 clicked: "This plan showed me that I can travel and still make healthy choices about what I eat and drink and what activities I can do. Now at business dinners, I order my meal first so I'm not influenced by others. I also walk instead of taking a cab if I'm going eight blocks or fewer. As far as exercising goes in general, I realized I don't need to be in a gym—I go running with my running group or bike riding instead."

How my body changed: "I went from a size 10 to a 6! Seeing results week after week motivated me to continue."

Success tip: "I kept a food diary and a workout journal to track my progress and emotions. Early in the program, I came back from a client lunch and there was a huge plate of cookies in the break room. I had no problem walking right by it because I'd had a filling meal and didn't want to add a cookie to my list. I also told my friends and co-workers about my goals, so they could help me be accountable. Now I feel much more confident, full of energy, and all-around healthier."

14

Superfood Swaps When Dining Out:
How to Tap the Fat-Melting Powers of Superfoods Anywhere

Dinner with friends, a client lunch, breakfast on the road—for many of you, eating out a few times a week is as much a part of life as whipping up meals in your own kitchen. That's why with the Drop 10 diet you don't have to swear off restaurants, delis, or even fast-food drive-throughs. Nor must you stick to picking at dinky side salads while your tablemates tuck into tasty entrées. With this plan, you can order up delicious food and still lose weight. It's true that the chips at restaurants— not to mention the fries, sauces, sides, portion sizes, and a slew of other things—are stacked against you. Among all the diet-busting dishes on menus, though, you will find gems that fill you up on fewer calories, contain superfoods to rev fat burning, and keep you within your day's 1,600-calorie limit. All you have to do is know what to order and how it fits into your regular Drop 10 routine.

The charts in this chapter list the healthier superfood options at America's most popular restaurant chains. You can swap any of them for the meals in the Drop 10 plan as needed. Does that mean you can have a fast-food lunch every day and expect the same results that you'd get eat-

Disclaimer: Nutrition information and menu items accurate as of press time. If an item is no longer available, check that restaurant's website for nutrition information for similar items.

NOT EATING AT A CHAIN RESTAURANT?

If you don't see the restaurant where you're going to eat listed in the following pages, don't panic: Look for items on the menu that are similar to those listed here. Pizza stats, for example, aren't likely to differ that much among restaurants. If you are eating at a unique spot, however, do your homework. Look up the restaurant's menu online, then use these tips to help you decide what to order and how to estimate calories:

1. Scan for superfoods. Obviously! If wild salmon, steak, sardines, eggs, lentils, or others are the centerpiece of a dish, you're headed in the right direction.

2. Think simple. Lighter dishes (a fillet of grilled fish and roasted vegetables, for example) tend to be prepared in basic, straight-forward ways. Also, more calories than you can imagine hide in sauces, so ask for yours on the side and add only a little.

3. Know the lingo. Red-light anything with descriptions that include "crispy" or "battered" (translation: fried); "au gratin," "scalloped," or "creamed" (laden with saturated fat); and "glazed" or "sweet" (probably coated in sugar). But you can green-light items dubbed "grilled," "blackened," "baked," "broiled," and "roasted"; these descriptions typically signal healthier preparations.

4. Tally your calories. Once you decide on a dish, use the descriptions and information at NutritionData.Self.com to estimate its calorie count. Whatever you come up with, add about 300 calories to account for oil, butter, or other items chefs tend to pour on during prep. Bear in mind that although the total number you arrive at will doubtless sound high, it's probably still a low estimate for the entire dish—restaurant servings tend to be gargantuan! Plan to eat only about half your entrée, and start with a green salad dressed with a little olive oil and vinegar to take the edge off your appetite and prevent overeating.

5. Run interference. When you are seated, use the general rules starting on page 405 to help you shave even more calories off your meal.

ing mostly from our menu? No way. Are the eating-out grabs as effective as ours when it comes to curbing hunger and helping you lose weight? Nope. But for those times when you can't or don't want to make meals at home, the items we highlight here are more diet-friendly than many of the other selections. Simply order from this pared-down menu the next time you're out, and you'll be served weight loss results rather than an extra helping of fat.

What to do: Before you head out to eat, review the restaurant's menu options in this chapter, note the calorie and nutrition stats, then decide what you'll order. Your goal is to stay within your day's 1,600-calorie limit, give or take whatever happy calories you want to save or use. As a starting point, remember that on the Drop 10 plan, breakfasts are 350 calories, lunches and dinners are 450, and snacks are 150. When ordering, try to stick close to those amounts, but if you want to go over, do it—that's what your 200 happy calories per day, plus rollovers, are there for. Similarly, if you need to steal a few dozen calories from your day's snack or another meal to round out your plate, that's okay. As long as you don't leave yourself so little at those other meals that you end up starving, feel free to make minor caloric trade-offs. Pretty simple, huh? Now, what are you having?

Fast Food That Fights Fat

Kudos to our drive-through friends: Several spots now offer multiple menu items that boast superfood ingredients and won't break your calorie bank.

Item	Superfood(s)	Calories	Fat (g)	Saturated fat (g)	Fiber (g)	Carbs (g)	Protein (g)
MCDONALD'S							
Breakfast							
Fruit & Maple Oatmeal	Oats, apples	290	4.5	2	5	57	5
Egg McMuffin	Eggs	300	12	5	2	30	18
Lunch/dinner							
Premium Caesar Salad (With Grilled Chicken and Newman's Own Creamy Caesar Dressing)	Parmesan	410	24	6.5	3	16	32
Premium Caesar Salad (Without Chicken, With Newman's Own Creamy Caesar Dressing)	Parmesan	280	22	6	3	13	9
Snacks/desserts/extras							
Fruit 'n Yogurt Parfait	Yogurt, blueberries	160	2	1	1	3	14
Small Strawberry Banana Smoothie	Yogurt	210	0.5	0	2	49	2

Item	Superfood(s)	Calories	Fat (g)	Saturated fat (g)	Fiber (g)	Carbs (g)	Protein (g)
Small Wild Berry Smoothie	Yogurt	210	0.5	0	3	48	2
Snack Size Fruit & Walnut Salad	Apples, yogurt	210	8	1.5	2	31	4
Baked Hot Apple Pie	Apples	250	13	7	4	32	2
Apple Dippers With Low Fat Caramel Dip	Apples	100	0.5	0	0	23	0

BURGER KING

Item	Superfood(s)	Calories	Fat (g)	Saturated fat (g)	Fiber (g)	Carbs (g)	Protein (g)
Breakfast							
BK Kids Breakfast Muffin Sandwich	Eggs	240	11	4	N/A	23	9
BK Breakfast Burrito (With Potato, Egg, Cheese & Salsa)	Eggs	320	17	6	N/A	29	13
BK Breakfast Burrito (With Bacon, Egg, Cheese & Salsa)	Eggs	300	16	6	N/A	24	15
Snacks/desserts/extras							
BK Fresh Apple Fries	Apples	70	0.5	0	N/A	16	0

WENDY'S

Lunch/dinner

	Superfood						
Half of an Apple Pecan Chicken Salad (With Pomegranate Vinaigrette Dressing)	Apples, pomegranate	340	18	4.5	4	28	19
Berry Almond Chicken Salad (With Fat Free Raspberry Vinaigrette Dressing)	Blueberries	450	16	6	7	42	38
Broccoli and Cheese Potato	Brocoli	330	2	1	69	11	20

ARBY'S

Lunch/dinner

	Superfood						
Jr. Roast Beef Sandwich	Steak	210	8	3	1	24	12

Snacks/desserts/extras

Applesauce	Apples	80	0	0	2	21	12

Item	Superfood(s)	Calories	Fat (g)	Saturated fat (g)	Fiber (g)	Carbs (g)	Protein (g)
Lunch/dinner							
			PIZZA HUT				
1 Slice of Thin Crust Pepperoni and Mushroom Pizza	Mushrooms	180	8	3.5	1	22	9
1 Slice of Fit 'n Delicious Pizza with Chicken, Mushroom, and Jalapeño	Mushrooms	170	4.5	1.5	1	22	11
1 Slice of Fit 'n Delicious Pizza with Diced Red Tomato, Mushroom, and Jalapeño	Mushrooms	150	4	1.5	2	23	6
1 Slice of Pepperoni and Mushroom Pizza (12" Medium Pan Pizza)	Mushrooms	240	10	4	1	27	10
1 Slice of Supreme Pizza (12" Medium Pan Pizza)	Mushrooms	290	14	5	2	27	12
1 Slice of Veggie Lover's Pizza (12" Medium Pan Pizza)	Mushrooms	230	9	3.5	2	28	9

1 Slice of Supreme Pizza (12" Medium Thin 'N Crispy Pizza)	Mushrooms	240	12	5	1	23	10
1 Slice of Pepperoni and Mushroom Pizza (12" Medium Thin 'N Crispy Pizza)	Mushrooms	180	8	3.5	1	22	9
1 Slice of Veggie Lover's Pizza (12" Medium Thin 'N Crispy Pizza)	Mushrooms	180	6	3	1	23	8
1 Slice of Supreme Pizza (12" Medium Hand-Tossed Style Pizza)	Mushrooms	260	12	5	1	26	12
1 Slice of Pepperoni and Mushroom Pizza (12" Medium Hand-Tossed Style Pizza)	Mushrooms	210	8	3.5	1	26	10
1 Slice of Veggie Lover's Pizza (12" Medium Hand-Tossed Style Pizza)	Mushrooms	200	6	3	1	26	14

Item	Superfood(s)	Calories	Fat (g)	Saturated fat (g)	Fiber (g)	Carbs (g)	Protein (g)
Veggie Lover's Pizza (6" Personal Pan Pizza)	Mushrooms	550	20	8	70	4	22
TACO BELL							
Lunch/dinner							
Fresco Grilled Steak Soft Taco	Steak	150	4	2	2	19	9
Fresco Burrito Supreme—Steak	Steak	340	8	2.5	7	50	15
Fresco Soft Taco—Beef	Steak	180	7	3	3	20	8
Gordita Baja—Steak	Steak	310	15	3.5	3	28	14
Gordita Nacho Cheese—Steak	Steak	260	11	2	2	29	12
Gordita Supreme—Steak	Steak	270	11	4	2	29	14
Chalupa Baja—Steak	Steak	380	23	4	3	28	13
Chalupa Nacho Cheese—Steak	Steak	330	19	2.5	3	30	12
CHIPOTLE							
Lunch/dinner							
Kid's Flour Tortilla Taco (with Steak, Cilantro-Lime Rice, Corn Salsa, and Lettuce)	Steak	220	6	1.5	1	28	14

Kid's Soft Corn Tortilla Taco (with Steak, Black Beans, Tomato Salsa, Guacamole, and Lettuce)	Steak, avocado	220	7.5	1	7	28	14.5
Steak Salad (with Lettuce, Black Beans, Steak, Fajita Vegetables, and Tomato Salsa)	Steak	360	8	2	13	35	42
Flour Tortilla Taco (with Cilantro-Lime Rice, Black Beans, Lettuce, Guacamole, and Green Tomatillo Salsa)	Avocados	505	19.5	3.5	19	70	14

DUNKIN' DONUTS

Breakfast

Blueberry Bagel	Blueberries	330	3	1	5	65	11
Egg White Turkey Sausage Flatbread	Eggs	280	8	3	3	32	19

Item	Superfood(s)	Calories	Fat (g)	Saturated fat (g)	Fiber (g)	Carbs (g)	Protein (g)
Egg White Turkey Sausage Wake-Up Wrap	Eggs	150	5	2.5	1	14	11
Egg White Veggie Wake-Up Wrap	Eggs	150	6	3	1	14	10
Egg & Cheese on English Muffin	Eggs	320	15	5	1	34	14
Egg White Veggie Flatbread	Eggs	280	10	4	3	32	16
Egg & Cheese Wake-Up Wrap	Eggs	180	11	4	1	14	8
Ham, Egg & Cheese Wake-Up Wrap	Eggs	200	11	4.5	1	14	11

PANDA EXPRESS

Lunch/dinner

Item	Superfood(s)	Calories	Fat (g)	Saturated fat (g)	Fiber (g)	Carbs (g)	Protein (g)
Entrée of Mixed Veggies	Broccoli	35	0	0	3	7	2
Broccoli Beef	Broccoli, steak	130	4	1	3	13	10
Kobari Beef	Mushrooms, steak	210	7	1.5	2	20	15

Mushroom Chicken	Mushrooms	220	13	3	1	9	17
Kung Pao Chicken	Peanuts	280	18	3.5	2	12	18
Hot and Sour Soup	Eggs, mushrooms	100	3.5	0.5	1	12	4

CHICK-FIL-A

Breakfast

Yogurt Parfait	Yogurt	230	3	2	0	44	6
Yogurt Parfait with Granola	Yogurt	290	6	2	1	53	7

Lunch/dinner

Chargrilled & Fruit Salad (with Reduced-Fat Berry Balsamic Vinaigrette Dressing)	Apples	290	8	4	4	34	22
Chargrilled Chicken Garden Salad (with Light Italian Dressing)	Broccoli	195	7	4	4	13	23

Snacks/sides

Fruit Cup	Apples	70	0	0	2	17	1

Item	Superfood(s)	Calories	Fat (g)	Saturated fat (g)	Fiber (g)	Carbs (g)	Protein (g)
WHITE CASTLE							
Breakfast							
Egg and Cheese Slider	Eggs	160	8	3	1	13	10
Egg Slider	Eggs	140	6	2	1	12	9
Bacon, Egg, and Cheese Slider	Eggs	190	11	4	1	13	12
Bacon and Egg Slider	Eggs	200	11	3.5	1	12	12
Hamburger and Egg Slider	Eggs	200	11	4	1	12	13
SONIC							
Snacks/sides/desserts							
Apple Slices and Fat-Free Caramel Dipping Sauce	Apples	110	0	0	2	28	0

Lighter Deli Delights

Sandwich shops net you a variety of fresh, flab-obliterating options, but there are still some calorie cows hiding between (and near) the fresh-baked rolls. Stick with these picks to stay on track.

Item	Superfood(s)	Calories	Fat (g)	Saturated fat (g)	Fiber (g)	Carbs (g)	Protein (g)
PANERA BREAD							
Breakfast							
Blueberry Bagel	Blueberries	330	1.5	0	2	68	10
Whole-Grain Bagel	Oats	340	2.5	0	6	67	13
Breakfast Power Sandwich	Eggs, oats	340	14	7	4	31	23
Pumpkin Muffie	Pumpkin	300	11	2	1	45	3
Grilled Egg & Cheese Sandwich on Ciabatta	Eggs	390	15	7	2	43	19
Strawberry Granola Parfait	Yogurt, oats	310	11	4	3	44	9
Lunch/dinner							
Half of a Steak & White Cheddar Panini (with Caramelized Onions and Horseradish Sauce on a French Baguette)	Steak	480	18	7	2	56	21

Half of a Turkey Artichoke Panini (with Spinach Artichoke Spread, Asiago Parmesan Blend, Tomatoes, and Caramelized Onions on Focaccia)	Artichoke, Parmesan	370	13	4	2	43	21
Half of an Asiago Roast Beef Sandwich (with Smoked Cheddar, Lettuce, Tomatoes, Red Onions, and Horseradish Sauce on Asiago Cheese Demi-Baguette)	Steak	350	14	7	2	32	24
Half of a Chicken Caesar Sandwich (with Asiago Parmesan Blend, Lettuce, Tomatoes, Red Onions, and Caesar Dressing on Three Cheese Miche)	Parmesan	360	16	5	2	35	22

Item	Superfood(s)	Calories	Fat (g)	Saturated fat (g)	Fiber (g)	Carbs (g)	Protein (g)
Full Strawberry, Poppyseed & Chicken Salad (with Fat-Free Poppyseed Dressing)	Blueberries	340	13	1.5	6	34	29
Full Thai Chopped Chicken Salad (with Low-Fat Thai Chili Vinaigrette)	Edamame	390	15	2.5	5	36	34
Half of a Chopped Chicken Cobb Salad (with Greek Dressing)	Eggs	250	18	4.5	2	6	19
Half of a Caesar Salad (with Caesar Dressing)	Parmesan	200	14	4	1	13	6
Half of a Grilled Chicken Caesar Salad (with Caesar Dressing)	Parmesan	260	15	4.5	1	14	18
Half of a Fuji Apple Chicken Salad (with White Balsamic Fuji Apple Vinaigrette)	Apples	280	17	3.5	3	18	16
Drinks							
Organic Apple Juice (9 fluid ounces)	Apples	120	0	0	0	29	0

Sides/extras

Oatmeal Raisin Cookie	Oats	370	14	8	2	57	5
Apple	Apple	80	0	0	4	21	0

QUIZNOS

Lunch/dinner

Small Veggie Classic Sub (with Guacamole, Black Olives, Lettuce, Tomatoes, Onions, Mushrooms, Mozzarella, Cheddar, and Red Wine Vinaigrette on Wheat Bread)	Mushrooms, olive oil, avocado	510	28	9	7	43	17
Small Harvest Chicken Salad (with Acai Vinaigrette)	Apples, pumpkin seeds	240	13	2.5	2	27	6
Regular Harvest Chicken Salad (with Acai Vinaigrette)	Apples, pumpkin seeds	450	23	4.5	4	48	12
Pesto Turkey Toasty Bullet (with Turkey, Mozzarella, Lettuce, Tomatoes, Basil Pesto, and Red Wine Vinaigrette on a Baguette)	Olive oil	340	12.5	2	2	42	15

Item	Superfood(s)	Calories	Fat (g)	Saturated fat (g)	Fiber (g)	Carbs (g)	Protein (g)
Bistro Steak Melt Flatbread Sammy (with Roast Beef, Mozzarella, Lettuce, Tomatoes, and Mild Peppercorn Sauce on a Flatbread)	Steak	410	22.5	6	1	31	17
Veggie Flatbread Sammy (with Guacamole, Black Olives, Lettuce, Tomatoes, Red Onions, Mozzarella, Cheddar, Mushrooms, and Red Wine Vinaigrette on a Flatbread)	Mushrooms, olive oil, avocado	340	20	4.5	3	29	14
Cantina Chicken Flatbread Sammy (with Chicken, Tomatoes, Sautéed Onions, Mushrooms, and Honey Bourbon Mustard on a Flatbread)	Mushrooms	280	7	2	2	36	12

Roadhouse Steak Flatbread Sammy (with Roast Beef, Sautéed Onions, Mushrooms, and Sweet & Spicy Steak Sauce on a Flatbread)	Steak, mushrooms	270	6	1	1	39	14

SUBWAY

Breakfast

Egg White & Cheese Muffin Melt	Egg	150	3.5	1.5	5	24	12
Egg White & Cheese (with Ham) Muffin Melt	Egg	170	4	1.5	5	24	14
Breakfast B.M.T. (with Egg Whites)	Egg	220	8	3	5	25	16
Bacon, Egg (White) & Cheese Muffin Melt	Egg	180	5	2	5	24	13
Steak, Egg (White) & Cheese Muffin Melt	Egg, steak	180	4	1.5	5	25	15
Sunrise Melt (with Egg Whites)	Egg	210	6	2.5	5	26	18
Egg & Cheese Muffin Melt	Egg	170	6	2	6	24	12

Item	Superfood(s)	Calories	Fat (g)	Saturated fat (g)	Fiber (g)	Carbs (g)	Protein (g)
Egg & Cheese (with Ham) Muffin Melt	Egg	190	6	2	6	24	14
Breakfast B.M.T. (with Whole Egg)	Egg	240	10	4	6	25	16
Bacon, Egg & Cheese Muffin Melt	Egg	200	7	3	6	24	13
Steak, Egg & Cheese Muffin Melt	Egg, steak	200	6	2.5	6	25	15
Sunrise Melt (with Whole Egg)	Egg	230	8	3	6	26	18
Egg White & Cheese on Mornin' Flatbread	Egg	170	5	1.5	1	21	9
Egg White & Cheese (with Ham) on Mornin' Flatbread	Egg	180	5	2	1	22	12
Breakfast B.M.T. (with Whole Egg)	Egg	250	12	4	1	22	14
Bacon, Egg & Cheese on Mornin' Flatbread	Egg	210	9	3.5	1	21	11
Steak, Egg & Cheese on Mornin' Flatbread	Steak, egg	210	8	3	1	22	13

Item							
Sunrise Melt on Mornin' Flatbread (with Whole Egg)	Egg	240	10	3.5	1	23	16
Egg & Cheese on Mornin' Flatbread	Egg	190	1	2.5	1	21	9
Egg & Cheese (with Ham) on Mornin' Flatbread	Egg	200	8	2.5	1	22	12
Breakfast B.M.T on Mornin' Flatbread (with Egg Whites)	Egg	230	10	3.5	1	22	14
Bacon, Egg White & Cheese on Mornin' Flatbread	Egg	190	7	2.5	1	21	11
Steak, Egg White & Cheese on Mornin' Flatbread	Steak, egg	190	6	2	7	22	13
Sunrise Melt on Mornin' Flatbread (with Egg White)	Egg	220	8	3	1	23	16
6" Egg White & Cheese Omelet Sandwich	Egg	320	8	3	4	44	19
6" Egg White & Cheese (with Ham) Omelet Sandwich	Egg	350	9	3.5	4	45	24

Item	Superfood(s)	Calories	Fat (g)	Saturated fat (g)	Fiber (g)	Carbs (g)	Protein (g)
6" Bacon, Egg White & Cheese Omelet Sandwich	Egg	370	11	4.5	4	45	23
6" Egg & Cheese Sandwich	Egg	360	12	4.5	5	44	19
6" Egg & Cheese (with Ham) Sandwich	Egg	390	13	5	5	45	24
Egg White & Cheese Omelet on 6" Flatbread	Egg	330	10	3.5	2	42	19
Egg White & Cheese (with Ham) Omelet on 6" Flatbread	Egg	360	11	3.5	2	43	23
Dannon Light & Fit Yogurt	Yogurt	80	0	0	0	16	5
Yogurt Parfait	Yogurt	160	2	1	2	30	6

Lunch/dinner
All sandwiches and salads include lettuce, tomato, onions, cucumbers, and green peppers; salads also include olives.

Item	Superfood(s)	Calories	Fat (g)	Saturated fat (g)	Fiber (g)	Carbs (g)	Protein (g)
6" Roast Beef Sandwich on 9-Grain Wheat	Steak	320	5	1.5	5	45	24

6" Subway Club on 9-Grain Wheat	Steak	310	4.5	1.5	5	46	23
6" Roast Beef on Flatbread	Steak	330	7	2	3	43	23
6" Subway Club on Flatbread	Steak	320	7	2	3	44	22
6" Steak & Cheese Sandwich on 9-Grain Wheat Bread	Steak	380	10	4.5	5	48	26
Subway Club Salad (with Fat-Free Italian dressing)	Steak	175	3.5	1	4	18	18
Roast Beef Salad (with Fat-Free Italian dressing)	Steak	175	3.5	1	4	17	19
Bowl of Vegetable Beef Soup	Steak	100	2	0.5	3	17	5
Snacks							
Oatmeal Raisin Cookie	Oats	200	8	4	1	30	3
Apple Pie	Apples	250	10	2	1	37	0
Apple Slices (1 package)	Apples	35	0	0	2	9	0
Drinks							
Apple Juice Box	Apples	100	0	0	0	24	0

STARBUCKS

Item	Superfood(s)	Calories	Fat (g)	Saturated fat (g)	Fiber (g)	Carbs (g)	Protein (g)
Breakfast							
Starbucks Perfect Oatmeal	Oats	140	2.5	0.5	4	25	5
Reduced-Fat Turkey Bacon, White Cheddar & Cage-Free Egg White Classic Breakfast Sandwich	Egg	320	7	2	3	43	18
Spinach, Feta & Cage-Free Egg White Breakfast Wrap	Egg	280	10	3.5	6	33	18
Apple Bran Muffin	Apple	350	9	2.5	7	64	6
Pumpkin Bread	Pumpkin seeds	390	15	2.5	2	60	6
Multigrain Bagel	Oats	320	4	0	4	62	12
Dark Cherry Yogurt Parfait	Yogurt, cherries	310	4	0.5	3	61	10
Greek Yogurt Honey Parfait	Yogurt, pumpkin seeds	300	12	6	<1	44	8
Strawberry & Blueberry Yogurt Parfait	Yogurt, blueberries	300	3.5	0	3	60	7

Lunch

Chicken Lettuce Wraps Bistro Box	Chocolate, peanuts	360	19	4	4	32	17
Sesame Noodles Bistro Box	Broccoli, chocolate, peanuts	350	11	3	6	50	15

Snacks

Protein Bistro Box	Egg, apple	380	19	6	5	37	13

BOSTON MARKET

Lunch/dinner

Regular Beef Brisket Meal	Steak	230	13	3.5	0	0	28
Fresh Steamed Vegetables	Broccoli, olive oil	60	2	0	3	8	2
Sweet Potato Casserole	Sweet potatoes, oats	460	16	4.5	3	77	4
Half of a Caesar Salad (with Dressing)	Parmesan	280	21	5	2	16	16

Item	Superfood(s)	Calories	Fat (g)	Saturated fat (g)	Fiber (g)	Carbs (g)	Protein (g)
Half of a Hand-Carved Roasted Turkey Carver Sandwich (with Turkey Breast, Parmesan Dill Sauce, Swiss Cheese, Tomatoes, and Greens on a Multi-Grain Roll)	Olive oil, Parmesan	395	17.5	4.5	1	33	25
Half of a Brisket Dip Carver Sandwich (with Beef Brisket, Swiss Cheese, and Mayo on a Whole-Grain Roll)	Steak	420	23	6	2	31	23
Half of a Turkey BLT (with Lettuce, Dill Parmesan Sauce, and Vinaigrette on Multi-Grain Bread)	Parmesan, olive oil	515	29	6	6	45	24
Meatloaf Sliders (choose three Mini Sliders served on a bun)	Steak	270	11	3.5	2	34	11
Half of a Caesar Salad (with Chicken and with Caesar Dressing)	Parmesan, olive oil, egg	330	21	5	1	16	19

Snacks

Cinnamon Apples	Apple	210	3	0	3	47	0

Breakfast

AU BON PAIN

Egg on a Bagel	Egg	430	12	4	2	58	22
Small Apple Cinnamon Oatmeal	Apple, oats	190	3	0	4	37	6
Small Oatmeal	Oats	170	3	0	4	32	6
Blueberry Yogurt with Blueberries	Blueberries, yogurt	250	3	2	0	50	8
Strawberry Yogurt with Blueberries	Yogurt, blueberries	250	2	2	0	50	7
Vanilla Yogurt with Blueberries	Yogurt, blueberries	220	3	2	0	41	9
Honey 9-Grain Bagel	Oats	310	2	0	6	63	11
Low-Fat Triple Berry Muffin	Apple, blueberries	300	3	0	2	65	4

Lunch/dinner

Black Bean Burger	Avocado, oats	560	18	4	14	76	29
Roast Beef on Baguette	Steak	500	12	3	3	65	33

Item	Superfood(s)	Calories	Fat (g)	Saturated fat (g)	Fiber (g)	Carbs (g)	Protein (g)
Thai Peanut Chicken Wrap	Peanuts	560	17	5	8	68	34
Small Butternut Squash and Apple Soup	Apple, pumpkin	160	6	2	2	27	3
Small Curried Rice and Lentil Soup	Lentils	130	2	0	6	22	6
Small French Moroccan Tomato Lentil Soup	Lentils	140	2	0	8	24	7
Small Garden Vegetable Soup	Broccoli	50	1	0	2	9	2
Small Harvest Pumpkin Soup	Pumpkin	180	10	5	2	21	3
Small Italian Wedding Soup	Steak	120	7	3	1	11	5
Small Mediterranean Pepper Soup	Lentils	120	4	0	5	19	5
Small Pasta E Fagioli Soup	Parmesan, olive oil	190	6	2	7	26	8
Small Portuguese Kale Soup	Kale	90	4	1	2	11	4

Small Tuscan Vegetable Soup	Mushrooms, olive oil	120	4	2	2	16	5
Small Tuscan White Bean Soup	Olive oil	120	3	0	4	19	6
Small Vegetable Beef Barley Soup	Steak	100	2	1	3	15	6
Small Vegetarian Lentil Soup	Lentils	130	1	0	8	22	7
Small Wild Mushroom Bisque	Mushrooms	130	7	2	2	16	3
Small BBQ Chicken and Beef Stew	Steak	200	7	3	2	24	13
Small Beef and Vegetable Stew	Steak	220	11	2	2	18	13
Small Beef Chili (Gluten-Free)	Steak	200	9	3	4	19	12
Small Chicken and Vegetable Stew	Mushrooms	210	12	3	2	18	8
Snacks							
Dark Chocolate Covered Raisins	Dark chocolate	180	8	5	2	26	2
Apples, Bleu Cheese, and Cranberries	Apples	200	10	4	3	27	4

Item	Superfood(s)	Calories	Fat (g)	Saturated fat (g)	Fiber (g)	Carbs (g)	Protein (g)
Mixed Nuts	Peanuts	180	16	3	1	7	5
The 19th Hole Snack Mix	Peanuts	160	10	2	2	15	4
Mini Oatmeal Raisin Cookie	Oats	60	3	1	1	10	1
Oatmeal Raisin Cookie	Oats	250	9	5	2	40	4
Drinks							
Medium Peach Smoothie	Yogurt	310	1	0	4	69	4
Medium Strawberry Smoothie	Yogurt	310	1	0	3	66	4

No-Weight Restaurant Meals

Sit-down spots offer a ton of healthier choices, but you'll also get a ton of food—restaurant portions can be up to eight times the size of a single serving! Because of that, consider splitting your dish with a pal, eating only half and taking the rest home, or, if possible, ordering a half portion. (For certain marked options below, the calorie information listed is for only a portion of the dish.)

APPLEBEE'S

Item	Superfood(s)	Calories	Fat (g)	Saturated fat (g)	Fiber (g)	Carbs (g)	Protein (g)
Lunch/dinner							
Asiago Peppercorn Steak (with Steamed Herb Potatoes and Seasonal Vegetables)	Steak, broccoli	380	14	6	5	25	44
Signature Sirloin with Garlic Herb Shrimp (with Steamed Herb Potatoes and Seasonal Vegetables)	Steak, almonds	500	21	8	6	31	51
Grilled Dijon Chicken & Portobellos (with Herb Potatoes and Seasonal Vegetables)	Mushrooms, broccoli	470	16	7	5	30	55
7-ounce House Sirloin (with Fried Red Potatoes and Seasonal Vegetables)	Steak	435	17	6	6	29	42
Half of an Orange-Glazed Salmon	Salmon	365	8.5	1.75	3	49	23
Half of a Garlic Herb Salmon	Salmon	345	14.5	4	2.5	30.5	23

Item	Superfood(s)	Calories	Fat (g)	Saturated fat (g)	Fiber (g)	Carbs (g)	Protein (g)
Teriyaki Shrimp Pasta	Mushrooms, broccoli	440	8	2	10	74	30
Teriyaki Chicken Pasta	Mushrooms	450	8	2	10	73	34
CHILI'S							
Lunch/dinner							
Half of a Cobb Salad (with Dressing)	Eggs, avocado	355	26	7.5	5.5	11	23
Half of a Caribbean Salad (with Grilled Chicken and Dressing)	Cherries	305	12.5	2	3	32.5	16.5
Half of a Caribbean Salad (with Grilled Shrimp and Dressing)	Cherries	310	15.5	3	3	33	9.5
Guiltless Grill Salmon (with Garlic & Herbs, Sides of Rice and Broccoli)	Salmon, broccoli	480	17	5	5	37	49
Half of a Classic Sirloin (with Mashed Potatoes, Gravy, and Broccoli)	Steak, broccoli	505	30	12	4	30	31

Item	Superfood(s)	Calories	Fat (g)	Saturated fat (g)	Fiber (g)	Carbs (g)	Protein (g)
Half of a Regular Grilled Salmon (with Garlic & Herbs, Sides of Rice and Broccoli)	Salmon, broccoli	290	14	5	2.5	19	24.5
Guiltless Grill Classic Sirloin with Salmon, Broccoli	Steak, salmon, broccoli	370	9	4	6	20	53
OLIVE GARDEN							
Lunch/dinner							
Half of a lunch-size Raviolo di Portobello	Mushrooms	225	9.5	5.5	4	26.5	9
Half of a dinner-size Chicken Marsala (with Tuscan Potatoes and Bell Peppers)	Mushrooms	385	18.5	2.5	8	29.5	26
Lunch-size Venetian Apricot Chicken (with Broccoli, Asparagus, and Tomatoes)	Broccoli	290	5	2	6	34	29
Dinner-size Venetian Apricot Chicken	Broccoli	400	7	2	6	34	51

Lunch-size Shrimp Primavera on Penne Pasta	Mushrooms	510	9	1.5	12	79	30
Dinner-size Herb-Grilled Salmon (with Broccoli)	Salmon, broccoli	510	26	6	2	5	64
Dinner-size Seafood Brodetto (with Bread Side)	Mushrooms	480	16	3	7	35	47
Half of a dinner-size Shrimp Primavera in Penne Pasta	Mushrooms	365	6	1	7	55	23

OUTBACK STEAKHOUSE

Lunch/dinner

Half of a New York Strip, 14 ounces (with Sweet Potato)	Steak, sweet potato	541	27	11	9	32	44
Norwegian Salmon (with Fresh Seasonal Veggies)	Salmon	483	27	7	7	14	43

RUBY TUESDAY

Lunch/dinner

Fit & Trim Petite Sliced Sirloin (with Mashed Potatoes and Broccoli)	Steak, broccoli	399	24	n/a	5	20	27

Item	Superfood(s)	Calories	Fat (g)	Saturated fat (g)	Fiber (g)	Carbs (g)	Protein (g)
Chicken Bella	Parmesan, mushrooms, artichoke	405	18	n/a	9	8	54
Asian Glazed Salmon	Salmon	417	24	n/a	3	12	40
Light & Fit Petite Grilled Salmon (with Broccoli and White Cheddar Mashed Potatoes)	Salmon, broccoli	470	32	n/a	7	25	25
Half of an Avocado Turkey Burger (without Fries)	Avocado	479	30	n/a	3	28	25
P.F. CHANG'S							
Appetizers							
Chang's Chicken Lettuce Wraps (one serving)	Mushrooms	160	7	1	2	17	8
Wonton Soup (34-ounce bowl)	Mushrooms	92	3	1	0	9	7
Hot and Sour Soup (34-ounce bowl)	Mushrooms	80	3	1	0	9	5

Egg Drop Soup (7-ounce cup)	Eggs	60	3	0	0	8	1
Lunch/dinner							
Half of a lunch-size Pepper Steak (with Brown Rice)	Steak	395	13	3	3	47	22
Lunch-size Almond and Cashew Chicken (with Brown Rice)	Mushrooms, almonds	535	22	4	5	59	25
Lunch-size Beef with Broccoli (with Brown Rice)	Steak, broccoli	420	13	3	4	52	23
Lunch-size Asian Grilled Norwegian Salmon (with Brown Rice)	Salmon	320	6	1	3	44	22
Lunch-size Mandarin Chicken	Broccoli	360	15	2	3	29	33
Norwegian Salmon Steamed with Ginger	Salmon	330	19	3	12	31	31

Item	Superfood(s)	Calories	Fat (g)	Saturated fat (g)	Fiber (g)	Carbs (g)	Protein (g)
CALIFORNIA PIZZA KITCHEN							
Lunch/dinner							
Full Roasted Vegetable Salad (with Dressing)	Artichoke, avocado, olive oil	597	n/a	6	16	48	11
Half of a Roasted Vegetable Salad (with Sautéed Salmon and Dressing)	Artichoke, avocado, olive oil, salmon	528	n/a	6	8	24	26
Half of a Miso Shrimp Salad (with dressing)	Edamame, avocado	436	n/a	4	8	33	24
Half of a Miso Shrimp Salad (with Dressing; substitute Chicken for Shrimp)	Edamame, avocado	420	n/a	4	8	33	20
Pizza							
Wild Mushroom Pizza (1/3 of Pizza)	Mushroom	378	n/a	7	2	40	13.6
Vegetarian Pizza with Japanese Eggplant (on Honey Wheat with Whole-Grain Crust, 1/3 of Pizza)	Mushroom, broccoli	368	n/a	6	5.7	44.6	17

Thin crust pizza

Roasted Artichoke and Spinach Pizza (1/3 of Pizza)	Artichoke	318	n/a	6.3	3	35.7	15.3
Roasted Artichoke and Spinach Pizza (with Chicken, 1/3 of Pizza)	Artichoke	343	n/a	6.3	3	35.7	20
Four Seasons Pizza (1/3 of Pizza)	Artichoke, mushroom, Parmesan	331	n/a	6.7	2.7	35.3	15.7

Pasta and specialties

Half of a Broccoli Sun-Dried Tomato Fusilli	Broccoli	508	n/a	5	5	56	18
Half of a Norwegian Atlantic Salmon (with Wok-Stirred Vegetables)	Salmon	373	n/a	3.5	4	12.5	26

Tacos

Half of a Carnitas Tacos (with Avocado)	Avocado	454	n/a	4.5	5.5	39	26
Half of a Baja Fish Tacos (with Avocado)	Avocado	492	n/a	5.5	5	44.5	18

Item	Superfood(s)	Calories	Fat (g)	Saturated fat (g)	Fiber (g)	Carbs (g)	Protein (g)
Snacks							
Non-Fat Yogurt Strawberry Smoothie	Yogurt	220	n/a	0	2	52	2
Non-Fat Yogurt Strawberry Banana Smoothie	Yogurt	223	n/a	0	3	52	2
Non-Fat Yogurt Mango Smoothie	Yogurt	200	n/a	0	4	50	2
Non-Fat Yogurt Mango Banana Smoothie	Yogurt	208	n/a	0	5	51	2
Non-Fat Yogurt Peach Smoothie	Yogurt	200	n/a	0	4	50	2

TEN WAYS TO SLIM YOUR RESTAURANT MEAL

Whether or not you're following the Drop 10 plan, these ten tenets will help you order lighter meals, cut out sneaky extra calories, and resist the temptation to overindulge.

1. *Snack first.* You're more likely to order fattening dishes and gorge on everything in sight if you arrive at the table famished. If your dinner reservations are more than four hours after your last meal, eat something rich in protein and fiber and that contains a little fat at the four-hour mark, such as $\frac{1}{2}$ cup of low-fat yogurt with fresh blueberries, or an apple and 1 tablespoon of almond butter.

2. *Know what you're getting into.* People who dined at restaurants they believed were healthy estimated that they ate a full 52 percent fewer calories than they actually did, according to research from Cornell University. As a result, many rewarded themselves with soda and dessert. Meals aren't low in calories just because you're dining at, say, a vegetarian or organic restaurant. Check out the menu online beforehand and consider the calories of everything that goes into a dish when doing your mental tally—it's easy to forget about extras such as mayo, sour cream, cheese, and salad dressings.

3. *Make friends with your waiter.* Servers are your best allies. Kindly explain your mission up front and ask for their help. If you approach it this way, they'll probably be more patient and willing when you request substitutions and quiz them on how meals are prepared.

4. *Wait to order a drink.* Sip a cocktail or glass of wine on a near empty stomach and your diet resolve may suddenly dissolve. Before you know it, cheese sticks and fried chicken are on the way to your table. Don't let alcohol cloud your judgment; sip water as you peruse the menu, then order a drink with the rest of your food. This also helps reduce your drinking, saving you liquid calories.

5. *Be the boss.* Now that your server's on your side, don't be afraid to ask that the kitchen go easy on the oil, skip the butter, and swap high-calorie sides such as coleslaw and fries for salad or veggies, or make other substitutions. Scan the entire menu: If you see a healthy side or addition to another dish, ask for it on the one you're ordering. Don't need the bacon, mayo, or special (aka dripping-with-fat) sauce but would rather have the whole-wheat bread? You're the one paying, so it's worth asking—most places will accommodate you.

6. Hold the freebies. If you know you'll be tempted to dive into the bread basket or chips and salsa once they appear on your table, head them off at the pass: Tell your server right away to keep 'em in the kitchen.

7. Start with soup or salad. Fresh greens and vegetarian or bean-based soups fill you up on few calories, so you're less apt to shovel in your entire entrée once it arrives. When ordering your salad, skip the cheese and creamy dressing, opting instead for 1 tablespoon of vinaigrette or olive oil and vinegar (ask for it on the side and drizzle it on yourself).

8. Order two appetizers as your main course. Not only will you get to try two different dishes, but the calorie total is typically lower than that of one entrée. If the apps don't interest you, ask for half a portion of an entrée or that your server wrap up half to go before you even see it on the plate.

9. *Stop eating when you're full.* You're probably thinking, "Duh!" But gauging your appetite is actually trickier than you might think. Eat fast and you'll probably take in more food because you don't give your stomach enough time (about twenty minutes) to send the all-full sign. Plus, it's human nature to eat everything that's in front of us, and seeing food on the plate can lead you to fork in more than your body needs or wants. When blindfolded, people ate up to 24 percent less but felt as satisfied as when they could see their food, a study in *Obesity* reports. Likewise, you may unconsciously take cues from your dining

companions' shovel-it-in habits. To shut out such visual signals, regularly close your eyes during your meal to check in with your stomach and determine how hungry you truly are; when you're full, call your server over and have him take your plate regardless of what's still on it.

10. *Watch for sales pitches.* Your waitress may be your pal, but she still needs to make money, and that means selling you on more food and drinks by suggesting appetizers, talking up the bartender's special margaritas, suggesting a bottle of wine rather than a glass, and bringing around the dessert tray so you can "take a look." If you're aware of it, you won't be caught off guard.

Acknowledgments

These People Love to Eat!

I knew the Drop 10 concept—shed pounds with delicious, naturally slimming foods without giving up a single favorite treat—was weight loss gold. Who doesn't want to eat what they love and get healthier doing it? My hunch bloomed into this scientifically proven plan with the high-energy help of the best nutrition experts and brilliant editors in the business. Together, we mixed great research, entertaining writing, and tasty menus into a whole new way to get—and stay—forever thin. With this crew, deprivation is permanently off the menu! My deepest thanks to . . .

The Editorial Team:

Carla Rohlfing Levy, *SELF*'s special projects director, print, whose veteran calm and dedicated editing took this project from a bright idea to the best diet book in the business;

Beth Janes, whose rich knowledge of nutrition, science, and service brought every word to inspiring life;

Heather K. Jones, R.D., for her nutrition expertise and for overseeing the creation of menus and recipes that make eating the right thing easy;

Tamara Goldis, R.D., for her invaluable recipe development;

Kate Winner Muller, R.D., who helped infuse the meal plans with deliciousness;

Wendy Marcus, *SELF*'s copy director, who weaves a quiet magic in blue ink;

Pat Singer, *SELF*'s research director, who keeps us all honest;

Mark Leydorf and Molly Powell, our keen-eyed copy editors;

Marjorie Korn, Sara Vigneri, Trang Chuong, Maura Corrigan, and Carlene Bauer, members of *SELF*'s crack research team;

Allison Baker, *SELF*'s associate nutrition editor, who acted as cheerleader to dozens of real-life Drop 10 testers;

Marnie Cochran, my talented, speedy, and enthusiastic editor at Random House. You make a fun lunch date, too!

The Scientists:

Bahram H. Arjmandi, Ph.D.
Margaret A. Sitton Professor and Chair
Director, Center for Advancing Exercise and Nutrition Research on Aging
Department of Nutrition, Food & Exercise Sciences
The Florida State University in Tallahassee

Maira Bes-Rastrollo, Ph.D.
Associate Professor of Preventative Medicine and Public Health
University of Navarra in Pamplona, Spain

Jon Buckley, Ph.D.
Associate Professor
Director, Nutritional Physiology Research Centre
Sansom Institute for Health Research
University of South Australia in Adelaide

Lawrence J. Cheskin, M.D.
Director, Johns Hopkins Weight Management Center
Associate Professor of Health, Behavior and Society
Johns Hopkins University School of Public Health

Ka He, M.D., Sc.D.
Associate Professor of Nutrition and Epidemiology
University of North Carolina in Chapel Hill

Janine A. Higgins, Ph.D.
Nutrition Research Director, Clinical Translational Research Center
Assistant Professor of Pediatrics
University of Colorado in Denver, Anschutz Medical Campus

Leena A. Hilakivi-Clarke, Ph.D.
Professor of Oncology
Georgetown University

Carol S. Johnston, Ph.D.
Professor and Associate Director, Nutrition Program at the School of
    Nutrition and Health Promotion
Arizona State University in Phoenix

Michael J. Keenan, Ph.D.
Associate Professor, Human Nutrition and Food Division, School of
    Human Ecology
Louisiana State University Agricultural Center

Penny Kris-Etherton, Ph.D.
Distinguished Professor of Nutrition
The Pennsylvania State University in University Park

Keith R. Martin, Ph.D.
Assistant Professor of Nutrition
Arizona State University in Phoenix

Richard D. Mattes, Ph.D.
Distinguished Professor of Nutrition Science
Purdue University

Muraleedharan Nair, Ph.D.
Professor of Natural Products Chemistry
Senior Associate to the Dean of the College of Agriculture and Natural
    Resources
Michigan State University

Shibu Poulose, Ph.D.
Molecular Biologist, Human Nutrition Research Center on Aging
Tufts University.

Barbara J. Rolls, Ph.D.
Director, Laboratory for the Study of Human Ingestive Behavior
Professor and Helen A. Guthrie Chair in Nutritional Sciences
The Pennsylvania State University in College Park

Thomas B. Shea, Ph.D.
Director, Center for Cellular Neurobiology and Neurodegeneration
    Research
Professor of Biological Sciences
University of Massachusetts in Lowell

E. Mitchell Seymour, Ph.D.
Manager, Cardioprotection Research Laboratory
University of Michigan Medical School

Mario J. Soares, M.D.
Associate Professor, Program of Nutrition/Faculty of Health Sciences
Curtin University in Perth, Australia

Larry Tucker, Ph.D.
Professor of Exercise Sciences
Brigham Young University in Provo, Utah

Taylor C. Wallace, Ph.D.
Senior Director, Scientific & Regulatory Affairs
Council for Responsible Nutrition

Michael B. Zemel, Ph.D.
Director, The Nutrition Institute
Professor of Nutrition and Medicine
University of Tennessee in Knoxville

Notes

Chapter 1: Welcome to the Last Weight Loss Program You'll Ever Need

4   **dieters end up gaining back the** Kraschnewski, JL, et al. "Long-term weight loss maintenance in the United States." *International Journal of Obesity.* 2010 November; 34(11):1644–54.

7   **more than two-thirds of Americans** Obesity and Overweight, FastStats Homepage Website. Centers for Disease Control and Prevention. http://www.cdc.gov/nchs/fasstats/overwt.htm. Updated June 18, 2010.

7   **a weight loss diet who ate** Zemel, MB, et al. "Effects of calcium and dairy on body composition and weight loss in African-American adults." *Obesity Research.* 2005 July; 13(7):1218–25.

9   **Researchers at the Karolinska Institute** Larsson, SC, et al. "Whole grain consumption and risk of colorectal cancer: A population-based cohort of 60,000 women." *British Journal of Cancer.* 2005 May 9;92(9):1803–37.

10 **Yet fewer than 1 in 10** Kimmons, J, et al. "Fruit and vegetable intake among adolescents and adults in the United States: Percentage meeting individualized recommendations." *Medscape Journal of Medicine.* 2009; 11(1):26.

10 **We consume only about half** "Increasing fiber intake." University of California San Francisco Medical Center Patient Education Website. http://www.ucsfhealth.org/education/increasing_fiber_intake. Updated August 17, 2011.

10 **only about 10 percent** Usual Intake of Total Fish & Other Seafood. Risk Factor Monitoring and Methods Branch Website. Applied Research

Program, National Cancer Institute. http://riskfactor.cancer.gov/diet/
usualintakes/pop/fish_all.html. Updated August 25, 2010.

10 **Heart disease is now** "February is American Heart Month." CDC Features Website. Centers for Disease Control and Prevention. http://www
.cdc.gov/features/heartmonth. Updated January 31, 2011.

10 **diabetes rates** "Number of Americans with diabetes projected to double
or triple by 2050." Press release, October 22, 2010. Centers for Disease
Control and Prevention. http://www.cdc.gov/media/pressrel/2010/r101022
.html.

10 **Being overweight or obese is linked** Must, A, et al. "The disease burden
associated with overweight and obesity." *Journal of the American Medical
Association.* 1999 October 27;282(16):1523–29.

10 **Diabetes. Losing a scant 2 pounds** Hamman, RF, et al. "Effect of weight
loss with lifestyle intervention on risk of diabetes." *Diabetes Care.* 2006
September;29(9):2102–27.

10 **High blood pressure. Overweight people** Moore, LL, et al. "Weight loss
in overweight adults and the long-term risk of hypertension: The Framingham Study." *Archives of Internal Medicine.* 2005 June 13;165(11):
1298–303.

10 **Inflammation. A modest weight loss** Viardot, A, et al. "The effects of
weight loss and gastric banding on the innate and adaptive immune system
in type 2 diabetes and prediabetes." *The Journal of Clinical Endocrinology
and Metabolism.* 2010 June;95(6):2845–50.

11 **Back pain** Kotowski, SE, et al. "Influence of weight loss on musculo-
skeletal pain: Potential short-term relevance." *Work.* 2010;36(3):295–304.

11 **Self-confidence** Kolotkin, RL, et al. "One-year health-related quality of
life outcomes in weight loss trial participants: Comparison of three measures." *Health and Quality of Life Outcomes.* 2009 June 9;7:53.

29 **Dieters who have support** Gorin, A, et al. "Involving support partners in
obesity treatment." *Journal of Consulting and Clinical Psychology.*
2005;73(2):341–43.

30 **One study in the *American Journal of Preventive Medicine*** Hollis, JF, et
al. "Weight loss during the intensive intervention phase of the weight-loss
maintenance trial." *American Journal of Preventive Medicine.* 2008 August;35(2):118–26.

31 **This type of internal, personal motivation** Webber, KH, et al. "Motivation and its relationship to adherence to self-monitoring and weight loss in
a 16-week Internet behavioral weight loss intervention." *Journal of Nutrition Education and Behavior.* 2010 May–June;42(3):161–67.

Chapter 2: Super Fruits

34 **People who ate an apple** Flood-Obbagy, JE, et al. "The effect of fruit in different forms on energy intake and satiety at a meal." *Appetite.* 2009 April;52(2):416–22.

34 **Women who ate about a cup** Arjmandi, B, et al. Florida State University. Study presented at Experimental Biology 2011 conference, Washington, DC, April 12, 2011 (unpublished).

34 **In a similar study** de Oliveira, MC, et al. "A low-energy-dense diet adding fruit reduces weight and energy intake in women." *Appetite.* 2008 September;51(2):291–95.

35 **In 2008, researchers working** Fulgoni, VL, et al. "Apple consumption is associated with increased nutrient intakes and reduced risk of metabolic syndrome in adults from the National Health and Nutrition Examination Survey (1999–2004)." Study presented at Experimental Biology 2008 conference, San Diego, California, April 5, 2008 (unpublished).

35 **They fight cancer** Jedrychowski, W, et al. "Case-control study on beneficial effect of regular consumption of apples on colorectal cancer risk in a population with relatively low intake of fruits and vegetables." *European Journal of Cancer Prevention.* 2010 January;19(1):42–47.

35 **Your ticker hearts apples** Mink, PJ, et al. "Flavonoid intake and cardiovascular disease mortality: A prospective study in postmenopausal women." *The American Journal of Clinical Nutrition.* 2007; 85:895–909.

36 **You might breathe easier** Shaheen, SO, et al. "Dietary antioxidants and asthma in adults population-based case-control study." *American Journal of Respiratory and Critical Care Medicine.* 2001 November;164:1823–28.

36 **It's smart for your brain** Shea, Thomas. Interview with Beth Janes.

37 **although Fuji, Red Delicious** Boyer, J, et al. "Apple phytochemicals and their health benefits." *Nutrition Journal.* 2004 May;3(5).

37 **know that only 3 to 4 percent** "Pesticide Monitoring Program FY 2007." U.S. Food and Drug Administration. http:www.fda.gov/Food/FoodSafety/FoodContaminantsAdulteration/Pesticides/ResidueMonitoringReports/ucm169577.htm

38 **Men who eat at least** Baer, DJ, et al. "Dietary fiber decreases the metabolizable energy content and nutrient digestibility of mixed diets fed to humans." *The Journal of Nutrition.* 2007 April;127(4):579–86.

40 **Apple nutrition by the numbers** USDA National Nutrient Database for Standard Reference, USDA Agriculture Research Service, Nutrient Data Laboratory. http://www.nal.usda.gov/fnic/foodcomp/search.

41 **Preliminary research in animals** Seymour, Mitchell. Interview by author.

41 **After researchers at the University of Michigan** Ibid.

42 **Reams of research** Rolls, Barbara J. Interview with Beth Janes.

42 **You'll score brain benefits** Krikorian, Robert. Email to Beth Janes. April 23, 2011.

42 **Antioxidants in blueberries** Pagán, Camille Noe. "20 superfoods for weight loss." *SELF*. August 2008, p. 128.

42 **Your heart loves blueberries** Wallace, TC. "Anthocyanins in cardiovascular disease." *Advances in Nutrition*. 2011; 2:1–7.

43 **The fiber and antioxidants in blueberries** Håkansson, A, et al. "Blueberry husks, rye bran and multi-strain probiotics affect the severity of colitis induced by dextran sulphate sodium." *Scandinavian Journal of Gastroenterology*. 2009;44(10):1213–25.

43 **When it comes to UTIs** Howell, Amy. Email to Beth Janes. July 5, 2011.

43 **The waist of a breakfast eater** Smith, KJ, et al. "Skipping breakfast: Longitudinal associations with cardiometabolic risk factors in the childhood determinants of adult health study." *The American Journal of Clinical Nutrition*. 2010 December;92(6):1316–25.

44 **Fight weight creep by eating** Drapeau, V, et al. "Modifications in food-group consumption are related to long-term body-weight changes." *The American Journal of Clinical Nutrition*. (2004) July;80(1):29–37.

45 **Blueberry nutrition by the numbers** USDA National Nutrient Database for Standard Reference, USDA Agriculture Research Service, Nutrient Data Laboratory. http://www.nal.usda.gov/fnic/foodcomp/search.

46 **antioxidants that may jump-start** Seymour, Mitchell. Interview with Beth Janes.

47 **Obese rats** Ibid.

47 **study from Michigan State University** Jayapraksam, B, et al. "Amelioration of obesity and glucose intolerance in high-fat-fed C57BL/6 mice by anthocyanins and ursolic acid in cornelian cherry (*Cornus mas*)." *Journal of Agricultural and Food Chemistry*. 2006 January;54(1):243–48.

47 **Women with diabetes** Ataie-Jafari, A, et al. "Effects of sour cherry juice on blood glucose and some cardiovascular risk factors improvements in diabetic women: A pilot study." *Nutrition & Food Science*. 2008;38(4):355–60.

48 **Cherries' potent concentration** Nair, Muraleedharan. Interview with Beth Janes.

48 **Cherries are a treat** Kelly, DS, et al. "Consumption of bing sweet cherries lowers circulating concentrations of inflammation markers in healthy men and women." *The Journal of Nutrition*. (2006) April;136(4):981–86.

48 **You could help ward off cancer** McCune, LM, et al. "Cherries and health: A review." *Critical Reviews in Food Science and Nutrition*. 2011 January;51(1):1–12.

48 **cherries' compounds fight the oxidative damage** Shea, Thomas. Interview with Beth Jones.

48 **Tart cherries are** McCune, LM, et al. "Cherries and health: A review." *Critical Reviews in Food Science and Nutrition*. 2011 January;51(1):1–12.

48 **Tart cherries are highly acidic** Nair, Muraleedharan. Interview with Beth Janes.

50 **Cherry nutrition by the numbers** USDA National Nutrient Database for Standard Reference, USDA Agriculture Research Service, Nutrient Data Laboratory. http://www.nal.usda.gov/fnic/foodcomp/search.

51 **a staple of traditional Chinese medicine** Potterat, O. "Goji (*Lycium barbarum* and *L. chinense*): Phytochemistry, pharmacology and safety in the perspective of traditional uses and recent popularity." *Planta Medica*. 2010 January;76(1):7–19.

51 **In a study from Purdue** Leidy, HJ, et al. "Higher protein intake preserves lean mass and satiety with weight loss in pre-obese and obese women." *Obesity*. 2007 February;15(2):421–29.

52 **In a similar twelve-week trial** Leidy, HJ, et al. "The effects of consuming frequent, higher protein meals on appetite and satiety during weight loss in overweight/obese men." *Obesity*. 2011 April;19(4):818–24.

52 **Studies show that the lower** Johnston, Carol. Email to Beth Janes. May 2, 2011.

52 **You'll reap all the health** Potterat, O. "Goji (*Lycium barbarum* and *L. chinense*): Phytochemistry, pharmacology and safety in the perspective of traditional uses and recent popularity." *Planta Medica*. 2010 January;76(1):7–19.

53 **Goji berries may bolster skin's** Reeve, VE, et al. "Mice drinking goji berry juice (*Lycium barbarum*) are protected from UV radiation-induced skin damage via antioxidant pathways." *Photochemical & Photobiological Sciences*. 2010 April;9(4):601–7.

53 **Compounds in goji berries** Potterat, O. "Goji (*Lycium barbarum* and *L. chinense*): Phytochemistry, pharmacology and safety in the perspective of traditional uses and recent popularity." *Planta Medica*. 2010 January;76(1):7–19.

53 **You could see benefits** Hammond, Billy. Email to Beth Janes. May 11, 2011.

54 **Goji berry nutrition by the numbers** "Organic Goji Berries Nutritional Information." Navitas Naturals Website. http://www.navitasnaturals.com/products/goji/goji-berries.html.

55 **Vitamin C may increase** Johnston, Carol. Email to Beth Janes. May 2, 2011.

55 **People with marginal levels** Johnston, Carol. Email to Beth Janes. May 2, 2011. "Marginal vitamin C status is associated with reduced fat oxidation during submaximal exercise in young adults." *Nutrition & Metabolism*. 2006 August 31; 3:35.

56 **Kiwis pack more nutrition** Lachance, PA, et al. "Fruits in preventative health and disease treatment: Nutritional ranking and patient recommendations." Paper presented at annual meeting of the American College of Nutrition, New York, New York, September 27, 1997.

56 **They're a green light** Duttaroy, AK, et al. "Effects of kiwi fruit consumption on platelet aggregation and plasma lipids in healthy human volunteers." *Platelets.* 2004 August;15(5):287–92.

56 **Once known as a gooseberry** "History of Kiwifruit." California Kiwifruit Commission Website. http://www.kiwifruit.org/about/history.aspx.

57 **people who eat plenty of C-rich foods** Cosgrove, MC, et al. "Dietary nutrient intakes and skin-aging appearance among middle-aged American women." *The American Journal of Clinical Nutrition.* (2007 October;86(4): 1225–31.

57 **You'll boost your immunity** McLaughlin, Leah. "Eat to beat." *SELF.* April 2010, p. 122.

58 **The fruit may calm** Chang, C, et al. "Kiwifruit improves bowel function in patients with irritable bowel syndrome with constipation." *Asia Pacific Journal of Clinical Nutrition.* 2010 December;19(4):451–57.

59 **Kiwifruit nutrition by the numbers** USDA National Nutrient Database for Standard Reference, USDA Agriculture Research Service, Nutrient Data Laboratory. http://www.nal.usda.gov/fnic/foodcomp/search.

60 **One especially worth noting** Epstein, LH, et al. "Increasing fruit and vegetable intake and decreasing fat and sugar intake in families at risk for childhood obesity." *Obesity Research.* 2001 March;9(3):171–78.

61 **eating more fruits and veggies** Bes-Rastrollo, M, et al. "Association of fiber intake and fruit/vegetable consumption with weight gain in a Mediterranean population." *Nutrition.* 2006 May;22(5):504–11.

62 **They're a red-letter fruit** Ross, SM. "Pomegranate: Its role in cardiovascular health." *Holistic Nursing Practice.* 2009 May–June;23(3):195–97.

62 **People with carotid artery disease** Aviram, M, et al. "Pomegranate juice consumption for 3 years by patients with carotid artery stenosis reduces common carotid intima-media thickness, blood pressure and oxidation." *Clinical Nutrition.* 2004 June 23(3):423–33.

62 **Poms are promising cancer fighters** Adhami, VM, et al. "Cancer chemoprevention by pomegranate: Laboratory and clinical evidence." *Nutrition and Cancer.* 2009;61(6):811–15.

63 **a protective effect on joint** Rasheed, Z, et al. "Pomegranate extract inhibits the interleukin-1induced activation of MKK-3, p38-MAPK and transcription factor RUNX-2 in human osteoarthritis chondrocytes." *Arthritis Research & Therapy.* 2010;12(5):R195.

63 **help shield the brain** Hartman, RE, et al. "Pomegranate juice decreases amyloid load and improves behavior in a mouse model of Alzheimer's disease." *Neurobiology of Disease.* 2006 December;24(3):506–15.

64 **Pomegranate nutrition by the numbers** USDA National Nutrient Database for Standard Reference, USDA Agriculture Research Service, Nutrient Data Laboratory. http://www.nal.usda.gov/fnic/foodcomp/search.

Chapter 3: Super Vegetables

66 **Researchers from the Institute of Neuroscience** Fantini, N, et al. "Evidence of glycemia-lowering effect by a *Cynara scolymus L.* extract in normal and obese rats." *Phytotherapy Research.* 2011 March;25(3):463–66.

67 **research suggests may increase fat burning** Higgins, JA. "Resistant starch: Metabolic effects and potential health benefits." *Journal of AOAC International.* 2004 May–June;87(3):761–68.

67 **stimulate the hormones in your gut** Keenan, Michael. Interview with Beth Janes.

67 **Over the course of twenty months** Tucker, LA, et al. "Increasing total fiber intake reduces risk of weight and fat gains in women." *The Journal of Nutrition.* 2009 March;139(3):576–81.

67 **In a study of more than** Beunza, J, et al. "Adherence to the Mediterranean diet, long-term weight change, and incident overweight or obesity: The Seguimiento Universidad de Navarra (SUN) cohort." *The American Journal of Clinical Nutrition.* 2010 December;92(6):1–8.

68 **Research from the Molecular Pathology** Miccadei, S, et al. "Antioxidative and apoptotic properties of polyphenolic extracts from edible part of artichoke (*Cynara scolymus L.*) on cultured rat hepatocytes and on human hepatoma cells." *Nutrition and Cancer.* 2008;60(2):276–83.

70 **Resistant starch acts the same** Higgins, JA. "Resistant starch: Metabolic effects and potential health benefits." *Journal of AOAC International.* 2004 May–June;87(3):761–68.

70 **increase the production of GLP-1 and PYY** Keenan, Michael. Interview with Beth Janes.

70 **After eating a meal** Higgins, JA, et al. "Resistant starch consumption promotes lipid oxidation." *Nutrition & Metabolism.* 2004 October;1(1):8.

70 **Animal research from Louisiana State University** Shen, L, et al. "Dietary resistant starch increases hypothalamic POMC expression in rats." *Obesity.* 2009 January;17(1):40–45.

70 **RS may help prevent the production** Higgins, JA, et al. "Consumption of resistant starch decreases postprandial lipogenesis in white adipose tissue of the rat." *Nutrition Journal.* 2006 September;20(5):25.

71 **temperature can alter the amount of RS** Higgins, Janine. Email to Beth Janes. May 31, 2011.

72 **Artichoke nutrition by the numbers** USDA National Nutrient Database for Standard Reference, USDA Agriculture Research Service, Nutrient Data Laboratory. http://www.nal.usda.gov/fnic/foodcomp/search.

73 **Compared with carbs and protein** Little, TJ, et al. "Modulation by high-fat diets of gastrointestinal function and hormones associated with the regulation of energy intake: Implications for the pathophysiology of

obesity." *The American Journal of Clinical Nutrition.* 2007 September;86(3):531–41.

74 **Over the course of an eighteen-month** McManus, K, et al. "A randomized controlled trial of a moderate-fat, low-energy diet compared with a low-fat, low-energy diet for weight loss in overweight adults." *International Journal of Obesity.* 2001 October;25(10):1503–11.

74 **In a study published** Pelkman, CL, et al. "Effects of moderate-fat (from monounsaturated fat) and low-fat weight-loss diets on the serum lipid profile in overweight and obese men and women." *The American Journal of Clinical Nutrition.* (2004) February;79(12):204–12.

75 **You'll shrink your risk** Jenkins, DJA, et al. "Adding monounsaturated fatty acids to a dietary portfolio of cholesterol-lowering foods in hypercholesterolemia." *Canadian Medical Association Journal.* 2010 December;182(18):1961–67.

75 **Researchers from Rovira i Virgili University** Salas-Salvado, J, et al. "Reduction in the incidence of type 2 diabetes with the Mediterranean diet: Results of the PREDIMED-Reus nutrition intervention randomized trial." *Diabetes Care.* 2011 January;34(1):14–19.

76 **Pairing foods rich in fat-soluble vitamins** Unlu, NZ, et al. "Carotenoid absorption from salad and salsa by humans is enhanced by the addition of avocado or avocado oil." *The Journal of Nutrition.* 2005 March;135(3):431–36.

77 **Avocado nutrition by the numbers** USDA National Nutrient Database for Standard Reference, USDA Agriculture Research Service, Nutrient Data Laboratory. http://www.nal.usda.gov/fnic/foodcomp/search.

79 **In a study of 658 dieters** Ledikwe, JH, et al. "Reductions in dietary energy density are associated with weight loss in overweight and obese participants in the PREMIER trial." *The American Journal of Clinical Nutrition.* 2007 May;85(5):1212–21.

79 **When subjects ate a 3-cup** Rolls, BJ, et al. "Salad and satiety: Energy density and portion size of a first-course salad affect energy intake at lunch." *Journal of the American Dietetic Association.* 2004 October;104(10):1570–76.

79 **It could slash your cancer risk** Vasanthi, HR, et al. "Potential health benefits of broccoli: A chemico-biological overview." *Mini-Reviews in Medicinal Chemistry.* 2009 June;9(6):749–59.

79 **Broccoli keeps your heart healthy** Yochum, L, et al. "Dietary flavonoid intake and risk of cardiovascular disease in postmenopausal women." *American Journal of Epidemiology.* 1999 May;149(10):943–49.

80 **You'll be a vision** Stringham, JM, et al. "The influence of dietary lutein and zeaxanthin on visual performance." *Journal of Food Science.* 2010 January–February;75(1):R24–29.

81 **Broccoli nutrition by the numbers** USDA National Nutrient Database

for Standard Reference, USDA Agriculture Research Service, Nutrient Data Laboratory. http://www.nal.usda.gov/fnic/foodcomp/search.

82 **it contains nutrients that animal studies**   Vaughn, N, et al. "Intracerebroventricular administration of soy protein hydrolysates reduces body weight without affecting food intake in rats." *Plant Foods for Human Nutrition.* 2008 March;63(1):41–46.

83 **researchers from the Federal University of Viçosa**   Alfenas, RC, et al. "Effects of protein quality on appetite and energy metabolism in normal weight subjects." *Brazilian Archives of Endocrinology and Metabolism.* 2010 February;54(1):45–51.

83 **Another study published in** *British Journal of Nutrition*   Lin, Y, et al. "Plant and animal protein intake and its association with overweight and obesity among the Belgian population." *British Journal of Nutrition.* 2011 April;105(7):1106–16.

84 **In one ten-week trial**   Te Morenga, L, et al. "Effect of a relatively high-protein, high-fiber diet on body composition and metabolic risk factors in overweight women." *European Journal of Clinical Nutrition.* 2010 November;64(11):1323–31.

85 **A note about soy and breast cancer**   Hilakivi-Clarke, Leena. Email to Beth Janes. July 21, 2011.

85 **the beans' load**   Sacks, FM, et al. "Soy protein, isoflavones, and cardiovascular health: An American Heart Association Science Advisory for Professionals from the Nutrition Committee." *Circulation.* 2006 February;113(7):1034–44.

85 **Researchers from Yao Municipal Hospital**   Hoshida, S, et al. "Different effects of isoflavones on vascular function in premenopausal and postmenopausal smokers and nonsmokers: NYMPH study." *Heart and Vessels.* 2011 January; published online.

85 **The beans are a boon**   Castelo-Branco, C, et al. "Isoflavones: Effects on bone health." *Climacteric.* 2011 April;14(2):204–11.

86 **PMS won't be such a pain**   Bryant, M, et al. "Effect of consumption of soy isoflavones on behavioural, somatic and affective symptoms in women with premenstrual syndrome." *British Journal of Nutrition.* 2005 May;93(5):731–39.

86 **Edamame nutrition by the numbers**   USDA National Nutrient Database for Standard Reference, USDA Agriculture Research Service, Nutrient Data Laboratory. http://www.nal.usda.gov/fnic/foodcomp/search.

87 **Lab research from the Harvard Medical School**   da-Silva, WS, et al. "The small polyphenolic molecule kaempferol increases cellular energy expenditure and thyroid hormone activation." *Diabetes.* 2007 March;56(3): 767–76.

87 **Researchers at Japan's National Institute of Health and Nutrition**   Murakami, K, et al. "Hardness (difficulty of chewing) of the habitual diet in

relation to body mass index and waist circumference in free-living Japanese women aged 18–22 y." *The American Journal of Clinical Nutrition.*
2007 July;86(1):206–13.

88 **Eating flavonoid-containing fruits** Hughes, LAE, et al. "Higher dietary
flavone, flavonol, and catechin intakes are associated with less of an increase in BMI over time in women: A longitudinal analysis from the Netherlands Cohort Study." *The American Journal of Clinical Nutrition.* 2008
November;88(5):1341–52.

89 **a study in** *The Journal of Nutrition* Beydoun, MA, et al. "Serum antioxidant status is associated with metabolic syndrome among U.S. adults in
recent national surveys." *The Journal of Nutrition.* 2011 May;141(5):903–13.

89 **People with a history** Hughes, MC, et al. "Food intake and risk of squa-
mous cell carcinoma of the skin in a community: The Nambour Skin
Cancer Cohort Study." *International Journal of Cancer.* 2006 October;119(8):1953–60.

89 **Kale's multitude of antioxidant** Martin, Keith. Email to Beth Janes. August 2, 2011.

90 **You'll maintain a youthful brain** Kang, JH, et al. "Fruit and vegetable
consumption and cognitive decline in aging women." *Annals of Neurology.*
2005 May;57(5):713–20.

91 **Kale nutrition by the numbers** USDA National Nutrient Database for
Standard Reference, USDA Agriculture Research Service, Nutrient Data
Laboratory. http://www.nal.usda.gov/fnic/foodcomp/search.

92 **savory taste that experts say** Cheskin, Lawrence. Email to Beth Janes.
April 15, 2011.

92 **When researchers at Johns Hopkins** Cheskin, LJ, et al. "Lack of energy
compensation over 4 days when white button mushrooms are substituted
for beef." *Appetite.* 2008 July;51(1):50–57.

93 **The more water-rich foods** Murakami, K, et al. "Intake from water
from foods but not beverages, is related to lower body mass index and
waist circumference in humans." *Nutrition.* 2008 October;24(10):925–32.

93 **You'll boost your immunity** Reyes, Maridel. "Shed years & pounds in 7
days." *SELF.* August 2010, p. 146.

93 **Mushrooms could put a cap** Zhang, M, et al. "Dietary intakes of mushrooms and green tea combine to reduce the risk of breast cancer in Chinese
women." *International Journal of Cancer.* 2009 March;124(6):1404–8.

93 **Lab studies conducted at Arizona State University** Martin, K. "Both
common and specialty mushrooms inhibit adhesion molecule expression
and in vitro binding of monocytes to human aortic endothelial cells in a
pro-inflammatory environment." *Nutrition Journal.* 2010 July;9:29.

94 **Use this chart** "The Mushrooms Story: Varieties Overview." Mushroom
Council. http://mushroominfo.com/varieties.

95 **Exposing mushrooms** Roberts, J, et al. "Vitamin D_2 formation from

post-harvest UV-B treatment of mushrooms (*Agaricus bisporus*) and retention during storage." *Journal of Agricultural and Food Chemistry.* 2008 June;56(12):4541–44.

95 **researchers from University Medical Center Freiburg** Urbain, P, et al. "Bioavailability of vitamin D_2 from UV-B-irradiated button mushrooms in healthy adults deficient in serum 25-hydroxyvitamin D: A randomized controlled trial." *European Journal of Clinical Nutrition.* 2011 August;65(8):965–71.

95 **up to 77 percent of Americans** Ginde, AA, et al. "Demographic differences and trends of vitamin D insufficiency in the U.S. population, 1988–2004." *Archives of Internal Medicine.* 2009 March;169(6):626–32.

97 **Mushroom nutrition by the numbers** USDA National Nutrient Database for Standard Reference, USDA Agriculture Research Service, Nutrient Data Laboratory. http://www.nal.usda.gov/fnic/foodcomp/search.

99 **when researchers at Tufts University** Howarth, NC, et al. "Dietary fiber and weight regulation." *Nutrition Reviews.* 2001 May;59(5):129–39.

99 **After eating both a breakfast and a lunch** Bodinham, CL, et al. "Acute ingestion of resistant starch reduces food intake in healthy adults." *British Journal of Nutrition.* 2010 March;103:917–22.

99 **Center for Science** Center for Science in the Public Interest. "10 worst and best foods." *Nutrition Action Healthletter.* http://www.cspinet.org/nah/10foods_bad.html.

99 **Sweet spuds are heart studs** Osganian, SK, et al. "Dietary carotenoids and risk of coronary artery disease in women." *The American Journal of Clinical Nutrition.* 2003 June;77(6):1390–99.

99 **Researchers from Harvard** Zhang, S, et al. "Dietary carotenoids and vitamins A, C, and E and risk of breast cancer." *Journal of the National Cancer Institute.* 1999 March;91(6):547–56.

100 **In skin, sweet potatoes' beta-carotene** Janes, Beth. "The great-skin diet." *SELF.* October 2008, p. 221.

101 **Sweet potato nutrition by the numbers** USDA National Nutrient Database for Standard Reference, USDA Agriculture Research Service, Nutrient Data Laboratory. http://www.nal.usda.gov/fnic/foodcomp/search.

Chapter 4: Super Legumes and Grains

105 **People who ate a balanced meal** Higgins, JA, et al. "Resistant starch consumption promotes lipid oxidation." *Nutrition & Metabolism.* 2004 October;1(1):8.

105 **about what you get** Murphy, MM, et al. "Resistant starch intakes in the United States." *Journal of the American Dietetic Association.* 2008 January;108(1):67–78.

105 **After eight weeks** Crujeiras, AB, et al. "A hypocaloric diet enriched in

legumes specifically mitigates lipid peroxidation in obese subjects." *Free Radical Research.* 2007 April;41(4):498–506.

106 **Overweight subjects**   Venn, BJ, et al. "The effect of increasing consumption of pulses and wholegrains in obese people: A randomized controlled trial." *Journal of the American College of Nutrition.* 2010 August;29(4): 365–72.

106 **Fiber and other compounds**   Adebamowo, CA, et al. "Dietary flavonols and flavonol-rich foods intake and the risk of breast cancer." *International Journal of Cancer.* 2005 April;114(4):628–33.

106 **eating roughly 1 cup**   Villegas, R, et al. "Legume and soy food intake and the incidence of type 2 diabetes in the Shanghai Women's Health Study." *The American Journal of Clinical Nutrition.* 2008 January;87(1):162–67.

106 **Choose lentils for a healthy digestive system**   Fuentes-Zaragoza, E, et al. "Resistant starch as prebiotic: A review." *Starch.* 2011 July;63(7):406–15.

108 **Lentil nutrition by the numbers**   USDA National Nutrient Database for Standard Reference, USDA Agriculture Research Service, Nutrient Data Laboratory. http://www.nal.usda.gov/fnic/foodcomp/search.

109 **research suggests its beta-glucan**   Beck, EJ, et al. "Increases in peptide Y-Y levels following oat beta-glucan ingestion are dose-dependent in overweight adults." *Nutrition Research.* 2009 October;29(10):705–9.

109 **Dieters who ate 3 cups**   Maki, KC, et al. "Whole-grain ready-to-eat oat cereal, as part of a dietary program for weight loss, reduces low-density lipoprotein cholesterol in adults with overweight and obesity more than a dietary program including low-fiber control foods." *Journal of the American Dietetic Association.* 2010 February;110(2):205–14.

109 **Researchers from Maastricht University**   van de Vijver, LPL, et al. "Whole-grain consumption, dietary fibre intake and body mass index in the Netherlands cohort study." *European Journal of Clinical Nutrition.* 2009 January;63(1):31–38.

110 **Their heart-healthy benefits**   Jonnalagadda, SS, et al. "Putting the whole grain puzzle together: Health benefits associated with whole grains summary of American Society for Nutrition 2010 Satellite Symposium." *The Journal of Nutrition.* 2011 May;141(5):1011S–22S.

110 **given permission by the FDA**   "Federal Register 62 FR 3583, January 23, 1997   Food Labeling: Health Claims; Oats and Coronary Heart Disease; Final Rule." Food and Drug Administration Website. http://www.fda .gov/food/labelingnutrition/labelclaims/healthclaimsmeetingsignificant scientificagreementssa/ucm074719.htm. Updated April, 30, 2009.

110 **Research from Tufts University**   Chen, C, et al. "Avenanthramides and phenolic acids from oats are bioavailable and act synergistically with vitamin C to enhance hamster and human LDL resistance to oxidation." *The Journal of Nutrition.* 2004 June;134(6):1459–66.

110 **Oats help your immune system**   Sherry, CL, et al. "Sickness behavior in-

duced by endotoxin can be mitigated by the dietary soluble fiber, pectin, through up-regulation of IL-4 and Th2 polarization." *Brain, Behavior, and Immunity.* 2010 May;24(4):631–40.

110 **Your risk for diabetes**   de Munter, JSL, et al. "Whole grain, bran, and germ intake and risk of type 2 diabetes: A prospective cohort study and systematic review." *PLoS Medicine.* 2007 August;4(8):e261.

112 **Oatmeal nutrition by the numbers**   USDA National Nutrient Database for Standard Reference, USDA Agriculture Research Service, Nutrient Data Laboratory. http://www.nal.usda.gov/fnic/foodcomp/search.

113 **Women who ate low-GI carbs**   Stevenson, EJ, et al. "Fat oxidation during exercise and satiety during recovery are increased following a low-glycemic index breakfast in sedentary women." *The Journal of Nutrition.* 2009 May;139(5):890–97.

114 **swapping refined grains**   Harland, JI, et al. "Whole-grain intake as a marker of healthy body weight and adiposity." *Public Health Nutrition.* 2008 June;11(6):554–63.

114 **people who eat two**   Kris-Etherton, Penny. Email to Beth Janes. August 1, 2011.

117 **Dieters who ate five servings**   Katcher, HI, et al. "The effects of a whole grain–enriched hypocaloric diet on cardiovascular disease risk factors in men and women with metabolic syndrome." *The American Journal of Clinical Nutrition.* 2008 January;87(1):79–90.

117 **Study subjects who were told**   Osterholt, KM, et al. "Incorporation of air into a snack food reduces energy intake." *Appetite.* 2007 May;48(3): 351–58.

117 **It's one of the best things**   Harris, KA, et al. "Effects of whole grains on coronary heart disease risk." *Current Atherosclerosis Reports.* 2010 November;12(6):368–76.

117 **Women who ate**   Larsson, SC, et al. "Whole grain consumption and risk of colorectal cancer: A population-based cohort of 60,000 women." *British Journal of Cancer.* 2005 May;92(9):1803–7.

118 **Popcorn helps zap zits**   Smith, RN, et al. "A low-glycemic-load diet improves symptoms in acne vulgaris patients: A randomized controlled trial." *The American Journal of Clinical Nutrition.* 2007 July:86(1):107–15.

120 **a cup without butter**   Center for Science in the Public Interest. "Movie theaters fill buckets . . . and bellies." *Nutrition Action Healthletter,* December 2009:1–5.

120 **Popcorn nutrition by the numbers**   USDA National Nutrient Database for Standard Reference, USDA Agriculture Research Service, Nutrient Data Laboratory. http://www.nal.usda.gov/fnic/foodcomp/search.

121 **In a study of middle-aged**   McKeown, NM, et al. "Whole- and refined-grain intakes are differentially associated with abdominal visceral and subcutaneous adiposity in healthy adults: The Framingham Heart

Study." *The American Journal of Clinical Nutrition.* 2010 November;92(5):1165–71.

123 **Subjects following a reduced-calorie**   Layman, DK, et al. "A moderate-protein diet produces sustained weight loss and long-term changes in body composition and blood lipids in obese adults." *The Journal of Nutrition.* 2009 March;139(3):514–21.

123 **Researchers in Sydney**   McMillan-Price, J, et al. "Comparison of 4 diets of varying glycemic load on weight loss and cardiovascular risk reduction in overweight and obese young adults: A randomized controlled trial." *Archives of Internal Medicine.* 2006 July;166(14):1466–75.

124 **when obese, prediabetic people**   Solomon, TPJ, et al. "A low–glycemic index diet combined with exercise reduces insulin resistance, postprandial hyperinsulinemia, and glucose-dependent insulinotropic polypeptide responses in obese, prediabetic humans." *The American Journal of Clinical Nutrition.* 2010 December;92(6):1359–68.

124 **Quinoa nutrition by the numbers**   USDA National Nutrient Database for Standard Reference, USDA Agriculture Research Service, Nutrient Data Laboratory. http://www.nal.usda.gov/fnic/foodcomp/search.

126 **In a study of nearly forty-five hundred**   Merchant, AT, et al. "Carbohydrate intake and overweight and obesity among healthy adults." *Journal of the American Dietetic Association.* 2009 July;109(7):1165–72.

126 **Increasing one's intake of whole grains**   Koh-Banerjee, P, et al. "Changes in whole-grain, bran, and cereal fiber consumption in relation to weight gain among men." *The American Journal of Clinical Nutrition.* 2004 November;80(5):1237–45.

126 **Researchers at Wake Forest University**   Mellen, PB, et al. "Whole grain intake and cardiovascular disease: A meta-analysis." *Nutrition, Metabolism & Cardiovascular Diseases.* 2008 May;18(4):283–90.

127 **A study in the** *Archives of Internal Medicine*   Brinkworth, GD, et al. "Long-term effects of a very low-carbohydrate diet and a low-fat diet on mood and cognitive function." *Archives of Internal Medicine.* 2009 November;169(20):1873–80.

129 **Whole-grain pasta nutrition by the numbers**   USDA National Nutrient Database for Standard Reference, USDA Agriculture Research Service, Nutrient Data Laboratory. http://www.nal.usda.gov/fnic/foodcomp/search.

Chapter 5: Super Nuts, Seeds, and Oil

130 **Research shows that replacing**   Mattes, RD. "The energetics of nut consumption." *Asia Pacific Journal of Clinical Nutrition.* 2008;17(S1):337–39.

131 **a portion will stay trapped**   Mattes, Richard D. Email to Beth Janes. June 8, 2011.

131 **Dieters who ate almonds** Wien, MA, et al. "Almonds vs. complex carbohydrates in a weight reduction program." *International Journal of Obesity.* 2003 November;27(11):1365–72.

132 **Women who added 344 calories' worth** Hollis, J, et al. "Effect of chronic consumption of almonds on body weight in healthy humans." *British Journal of Nutrition.* 2007 September;98(3):651–56.

133 **but when people ate almonds** Jenkins, DJ, et al. "Effect of almonds on insulin secretion and insulin resistance in nondiabetic hyperlipidemic subjects: A randomized controlled crossover trial." *Metabolism.* 2008 July;57(7):882–87.

133 **help your ticker** Jenkins, DJ, et al. "Assessment of the longer-term effects of a dietary portfolio of cholesterol-lowering foods in hypercholesterolemia." *The American Journal of Clinical Nutrition.* 2006 March;83(3):582–91.

133 **Research suggests almonds** Wien, MA, et al. "Almond consumption and cardiovascular risk factors in adults with prediabetes." *Journal of the American College of Nutrition.* 2010 June;29(3):189–97.

133 **Almond butter may function** Mandalari, G, et al. "Potential prebiotic properties of almond (*Amygdalus communis L.*) seeds." *Applied and Environmental Microbiology.* 2008 July;74(14):4264–70.

133 **You'll help your body** Avery, NG, et al. "Effects of vitamin E supplementation on recovery from repeated bouts of resistance exercise." *Journal of Strength and Conditioning Research.* 2003 November;17(4):801–9.

135 **They also stimulate** Little, TJ, et al. "Modulation by high-fat diets of gastrointestinal function and hormones associated with the regulation of energy intake: Implications for the pathophysiology of obesity." *The American Journal of Clinical Nutrition.* 2007 September;86(3):531–41.

135 **Unsaturated fat oxidizes** Mattes, Richard D. Email to Beth Janes. June 8, 2011.

135 **one theory** Soares, Mario J. Email to Beth Janes. August 8, 2011.

135 **Omega-3s** Buckley, Jon. Email to Beth Janes. June 29, 2011.

136 **Healthy fats extinguish** Weil, Andrew. "The healthiest way to eat." *SELF.* November 2005, p. 98.

136 **a diet heavy in palmitic acid** Benoit, SC, et al. "Palmitic acid mediates hypothalamic insulin resistance by altering PKC-theta subcellular localization in rodents." *Journal of Clinical Investigation.* 2009 September;119(9):2577–89.

137 **A study from Harvard University** Field, AE, et al. "Dietary fat and weight gain among women in the Nurses' Health Study." *Obesity.* 2007 April;15(4):967–76.

137 **trans fats are the most significant** Kavanagh, K, et al. "Trans fat diet induces abdominal obesity and changes in insulin sensitivity in monkeys." *Obesity.* 2007 July;15(7):1675–84.

139 **Almond butter nutrition by the numbers** USDA National Nutrient Database for Standard Reference, USDA Agriculture Research Service, Nutrient Data Laboratory. http://www.nal.usda.gov/fnic/foodcomp/search.

141 **trading up to monounsaturated fats** Piers, LS, et al. "Substitution of saturated with monounsaturated fat in a 4-week diet affects body weight and composition of overweight and obese men." *British Journal of Nutrition.* 2003 September;90(3):717–27.

141 **Studies show that eating like a Greek** Bes-Rastrollo. Email to Beth Janes. July 20, 2011.

141 **Subjects who ate a diet** Piers, LS, et al. "Substitution of saturated with monounsaturated fat in a 4-week diet affects body weight and composition of overweight and obese men." *British Journal of Nutrition.* 2003 September;90(3):717–27.

141 **Dieters who followed** Aude, WY, et al. "The National Cholesterol Education Program Diet vs. a diet lower in carbohydrates and higher in protein and monounsaturated fat: A randomized trial." *Archives of Internal Medicine.* 2004 October 25;164(19):2141–46.

142 **One more *major* reason** Lopez-Miranda, J, et al. "Olive oil and health: Summary of the II International Conference on Olive Oil and Health consensus report, Jaen and Cordoba (Spain), 2008." *Nutrition, Metabolism & Cardiovascular Diseases.* 2010 May;20(4):284–94.

143 **For California oils** Darragh, Patricia. California Olive Oil Council. Interview with author.

143 **Restaurant diners who** Wansink, B, et al. "Interactions between forms of fat consumption and restaurant bread consumption." *International Journal of Obesity.* 2003 July;27(7):866–68.

144 **Olive oil nutrition by the numbers** USDA National Nutrient Database for Standard Reference, USDA Agriculture Research Service, Nutrient Data Laboratory. http://www.nal.usda.gov/fnic/foodcomp/search.

146 **In a study of almost nine thousand people** Bes-Rastrollo, M, et al. "Nut consumption and weight gain in a Mediterranean cohort: The SUN Study." *Obesity.* 2007 January;15(1):107–16.

146 **Eating a quick-digesting** Johnston, Carol. Email to Beth Janes. May 2, 2011.

146 **People following a diet** McManus, K, et al. "A randomized controlled trial of a moderate-fat, low-energy diet compared with a low fat, low-energy diet for weight loss in overweight adults." *International Journal of Obesity.* 2001 October;25(10):1503–11.

146 **They're a super snack** Li, TY, et al. "Regular consumption of nuts is associated with a lower risk of cardiovascular disease in women with type 2 diabetes." *The Journal of Nutrition.* (2009) July;139(7):1333–8.

147 **nuts' niacin** Morris, MC, et al. "Dietary niacin and the risk of incident

Alzheimer's disease and of cognitive decline." *Journal of Neurology, Neurosurgery, and Psychiatry.* 2004 August;75(8):1093–99.

147 **vitamin E may lower** Devore, EE, et al. "Dietary antioxidants and long-term risk of dementia." *Archives of Neurology.* 2010 July;67(7): 819–25.

147 **Peanuts make a great** "Tryptophan." MedlinePlus Website. U.S. National Library of Medicine, National Institutes of Health. http://www.nlm .nih.gov/medlineplus/ency/article/002332.htm. Updated October 13, 2011.

148 **Peanut nutrition by the numbers** USDA National Nutrient Database for Standard Reference, USDA Agriculture Research Service, Nutrient Data Laboratory. http://www.nal.usda.gov/fnic/foodcomp/search.

150 **You need the mineral** He, Ka. Email to Beth Janes. June 15, 2011.

150 **most women in the United States** Ford, ES, et al. "Dietary magnesium intake in a national sample of U.S. adults." *The Journal of Nutrition.* 2003 September;133(9):2879–82.

150 **Women who ate a diet** Lejeune, M, et al. "Ghrelin and glucagon-like peptide 1 concentrations, 24-h satiety, and energy and substrate metabolism during a high-protein diet and measured in a respiration chamber." *The American Journal of Clinical Nutrition.* (2006) January;83(1):89–94.

150 **As a woman's intake of magnesium** Ford, ES, et al. "Intake of dietary magnesium and the prevalence of the metabolic syndrome among U.S. adults." *Obesity.* 2007 May;15(5):1139–46.

151 **rich in phytosterols** "Phytosterols." Micronutrient Information Center Website. Oregon State University, Linus Pauling Institute. http://lpi.oregonstate.edu/infocenter/phytochemicals/sterols/#disease_prevention. Updated September 2008.

152 **The seeds may ease headaches** McLaughlin, L. "Eat to beat." *SELF.* April 2010, p. 121.

152 **They could reduce your risk** Kim, DJ, et al. "Magnesium intake in relation to systemic inflammation, insulin resistance, and the incidence of diabetes." *Diabetes Care.* 2010 December;33(12):2604–10.

153 **Pumpkin seed nutrition by the numbers** USDA National Nutrient Database for Standard Reference, USDA Agriculture Research Service, Nutrient Data Laboratory. http://www.nal.usda.gov/fnic/foodcomp/search.

Chapter 6: Super Fish and Meat

154 **Research suggests that omega-3s** Buckley, JD, et al. "Long-chain omega-3 polyunsaturated fatty acids may be beneficial for reducing obesity: A review." *Nutrients.* 2010 December;2(12):1212–30.

155 **Sardines' calcium** Zemel, Michael. Interview with author.

155 **Among a group of overweight** Kabir, M, et al. "Treatment for 2 mo with

omega-3 polyunsaturated fatty acids reduces adiposity and some athero-genic factors but does not improve insulin sensitivity in women with type 2 diabetes: A randomized controlled study." *The American Journal of Clinical Nutrition.* 2007 December;86(6):1670–79.

155 **As a woman's intake of calcium** Jacqumain, M, et al. "Calcium intake, body composition, and lipoprotein-lipid concentrations in adults." *The American Journal of Clinical Nutrition.* (2003) June;77(6):1448–52.

155 **Dieters who ate** Due, A, et al. "Effect of normal-fat diets, either medium or high in protein, on body weight in overweight subjects: a randomised 1-year trial." *International Journal of Obesity.* 2004 October;28(10):1283–90.

156 **American Heart Association recommends** "Fish and Omega-3 Fatty Acids." American Heart Association Website. http://www.heart.org/ HEARTORG/General/Fish-and-Omega-3-Fatty-Acids_UCM_303248 _Article.jsp. Updated September 7, 2010.

156 **Omega-3s may also** Reyes, Maridel. "Shed years & pounds in 7 days." *SELF.* August 2010, p. 146.

156 **Women who consumed one** Christen, WG, et al. "Dietary omega-3 fatty acid and fish intake and incident age-related macular degeneration in women." *Archives of Ophthalmology.* 2011 July;129(7):921–29.

156 **omega-3s tamp down** Goldberg, RJ, et al. "A meta-analysis of the analgesic effects of omega-3 polyunsaturated fatty acid supplementation for inflammatory joint pain." *Pain.* 2007 May;129(1–2):210–23.

156 **one of the least contaminated** Cohen, Arianne. "Green special: Shopping smarter." *SELF.* April 2008, p. 52.

156 **And those caught in the Pacific** Cascorbi, Alice. "Seafood Watch seafood report: Sardines, volume 1." Monterey Bay Aquarium. February 10, 2004.

157 **Your skin may get softer** Chen, Joanne. "The food lover's guide to great skin." *SELF.* September 2010, p. 106.

160 **Sardine nutrition by the numbers** USDA National Nutrient Database for Standard Reference, USDA Agriculture Research Service, Nutrient Data Laboratory. http://www.nal.usda.gov/fnic/foodcomp/search.

161 **an amount research shows** Paddon-Jones, D, et al. "Protein, weight management, and satiety." *The American Journal of Clinical Nutrition.* (2008) May;87(suppl):1558S–61S.

161 **In order to break down** Johnston, CS, et al. "Postprandial thermogenesis is increased 100% on a high-protein, low-fat diet versus a high-carbohydrate, low-fat diet in healthy, young women." *Journal of the American College of Nutrition.* 2002 February;21(1):55–61.

161 **About 40 percent of those pounds** Yu, Winnie. "Losing weight?" *SELF.* May 2010, p. 108.

162 **It may enhance the effect** Micco, Nicci. "Eating made easy." *SELF.* October 2005, p. 170.

162 **Only about the first 30 grams** Symons, TB, et al. "A moderate serving of

high-quality protein maximally stimulates skeletal muscle protein synthesis in young and elderly subjects." *Journal of the American Dietetic Association.* 2009 September;109(9):1582–86.

164 **Studies routinely find** Noakes, M. "The role of protein in weight management." *Asia Pacific Journal of Clinical Nutrition.* 2008;17(S1):169–171.

164 **Between 9 and 16 percent** McLaughlin, Leah. "Eat to beat." *SELF.* April 2010, p. 125.

165 **Women on a diet that included** Noakes, M, et al. "Effect of an energy-restricted, high-protein, low-fat diet relative to a conventional high-carbohydrate, low-fat diet on weight loss, body composition, nutritional status, and markers of cardiovascular health in obese women." *The American Journal of Clinical Nutrition.* 2005 June;81(6):1298–306.

165 **Overweight people who regularly** Batterham, M, et al. "High-protein meals may benefit fat oxidation and energy expenditure in individuals with higher body fat." *Nutrition & Dietetics.* 2008 December;65(4):246–52.

165 **Researchers from the University of Illinois** Layman, DK, et al. "Dietary protein and exercise have additive effects on body composition during weight loss in adult women." *The Journal of Nutrition.* 2005 August;135(8):1903–10.

165 **You could strengthen** "How to Boost Your Immune System." Harvard Health Publications Website. Harvard Medical School. http://www.health.harvard.edu/flu-resource-center/how-to-boost-your-immune-system.htm.

165 **Steak may encourage clear** Chen, Joanne. "The food lover's guide to great skin." *SELF.* September 2010, p. 104.

167 **according to the USDA** USDA. "The Food Guide Pyramid." http://www.nal.usda.gov/fnic/Fpyr/pmap.htm.

169 **Steak nutrition by the numbers** USDA National Nutrient Database for Standard Reference, USDA Agriculture Research Service, Nutrient Data Laboratory. http://www.nal.usda.gov/fnic/foodcomp/search.

170 **Having higher levels** Zemel, Michael. Interview with Beth Janes.

170 **In a study analyzing the diets** Cade, JE, et al. "The UK Women's Cohort Study: Comparison of vegetarians, fish-eaters and meat-eaters." *Public Health Nutrition.* 2004 October;7(7):871–78.

171 **Overweight subjects who consumed** Hill, AM, et al. "Combining fish-oil supplements with regular aerobic exercise improves body composition and cardiovascular disease risk factors." *The American Journal of Clinical Nutrition.* (2007) May;85(5):1267–74.

171 **Researchers at the University of Minnesota** Moore, Rick. "Vitamin D and weight loss." *UM News Features.* University of Minnesota. http://www1.umn.edu/news/features/2009/UR_CONTENT_165066.html.

171 **Only 36 percent** Perry, Marge. "Get hooked on salmon." *SELF.* April 2011, p. 152.

171 **your best bet**   Austin, Sara. "Full nets, empty oceans." *SELF.* June 2011, pp. 159–62.

175 **Wild salmon nutrition by the numbers**   USDA National Nutrient Database for Standard Reference, USDA Agriculture Research Service, Nutrient Data Laboratory. http://www.nal.usda.gov/fnic/foodcomp/search.

Chapter 7: Super Eggs and Dairy

176 **eat eggs in the a.m.**   Vander Wal, JS, et al. "Egg breakfast enhances weight loss." *International Journal of Obesity.* 2008 October;32(10):1545–51.

177 **After eight weeks**   Ibid.

178 **Overweight women who ate**   Vander Wal, JS, et al. "Short-term effect of eggs on satiety in overweight and obese subjects." *Journal of the American College of Nutrition.* 2005 December;24(6):510–15.

178 **They won't harm your heart**   Kritchevsky, SB. "A review of scientific research and recommendations regarding eggs." *Journal of the American College of Nutrition.* 2004 December;23(6 suppl):596S–600S.

178 **Eggs are a beauty**   Chen, Joanne. "The food lover's guide to great skin." *SELF.* September 2010, p. 107.

180 **Egg nutrition by the numbers**   USDA National Nutrient Database for Standard Reference, USDA Agricultural Research Service, Nutrient Data Laboratory. http://www.nal.usda.gov/fnic/foodcomp/search.

181 **Most women don't get**   Zemel, Michael. Interview with Beth Janes.

182 **Compared with those who ate less**   Zemel, MB, et al. "Effects of calcium and dairy on body composition and weight loss in African-American adults." *Obesity Research.* 2005 July;13(7):1218–25.

182 **Women who ate an ounce**   Rosell, M, et al. "Association between dairy food consumption and weight change over 9-y in 19,352 perimenopausal women." *The American Journal of Clinical Nutrition.* (2006;) 84:1481–8 8.

182 **Without it**   Zemel, Michael. Interview with Beth Janes.

182 **Calcium helps maintain**   Janes, Beth. "The beauty diet." *SELF.* October 2006, p. 201.

184 **Parmesan nutrition by the numbers**   USDA National Nutrient Database for Standard Reference, USDA Agricultural Research Service, Nutrient Data Laboratory. http://www.nal.usda.gov/fnic/foodcomp/search.

185 **When your calcium intake**   Zemel, Michael. Interview with Beth Janes.

186 **People on a low-calorie diet**   Ibid.

186 **Subjects who ate**   Ping-Delfos, WC, et al. "Diet induced thermogenesis, fat oxidation and food intake following sequential meals: Influence of calcium and vitamin D." *Clinical Nutrition.* 2011 June;30(3):376–83.

186 **Women who increased**   Gunther, CW, et al. "Fat oxidation and its relation to serum parathyroid hormone in young women enrolled in a 1-y

dairy calcium intervention." *The American Journal of Clinical Nutrition.* (2005;) 82:1228–34.

187 **A review of studies**   Ralston, RA, et al. "A systematic review and meta-analysis of elevated blood pressure and consumption of dairy foods." *Journal of Human Hypertension.* 2011 February 10 [e-pub ahead of print].

187 **PMS sufferers who took**   Khajehei, M, et al. "Effect of treatment with dydrogesterone or calcium plus vitamin D on the severity of premenstrual syndrome." *International Journal of Gynecology & Obstetrics.* 2009 May;105(2):158–61.

189 **Yogurt nutrition by the numbers**   USDA National Nutrient Database for Standard Reference, USDA Agricultural Research Service, Nutrient Data Laboratory. http://www.nal.usda.gov/fnic/foodcomp/search.

Chapter 8: Super Tasty Extras

190 **The caffeine in a cup**   Janes, Beth. "Brava java." *SELF.* August 2009, pp. 128–31.

190 **Caffeine in coffee seems**   Wasmer Andrews, Linda. "Fire up your metabolism." *SELF.* December 2005, p. 83.

190 **block signals of muscle fatigue**   Jenkins, NT, et al. "Ergogenic effects of low doses of caffeine on cycling performance." *International Journal of Sport Nutrition & Exercise Metabolism.* 2008 June;18(3):328–42.

191 **the chlorogenic acid found in**   Van Dam, R, et al. "Coffee, caffeine, and risk of type 2 diabetes: A prospective cohort study in younger and middle-aged U.S. women." *Diabetes Care.* 2006 February;29(2):398–403.

191 **Study subjects who consumed**   Belza, A, et al. "The effect of caffeine, green tea and tyrosine on thermogenesis and energy intake." *European Journal of Clinical Nutrition.* 2009;63:57–64.

191 **A study in *The American Journal of Clinical Nutrition***   Lopez-Garcia, E, et al. "Changes in caffeine intake and long-term weight change in men and women." *The American Journal of Clinical Nutrition.* (2006;) 83:674–80.

191 **The day after stimulating their**   Jenkins, NT, et al. "Ergogenic effects of low doses of caffeine on cycling performance." *International Journal of Sport Nutrition & Exercise Metabolism.* 2008 June;18(3):328–42.

191 **It benefits your bean**   Janes, Beth. "Brava java." *SELF.* August 2009, p. 129.

192 **The brew boosts heart health**   Ibid.

192 **Phytoestrogens, antioxidant flavonoids**   Ibid.

192 **pancreatic cancers**   Dong, J, et al. "Coffee drinking and pancreatic cancer risk: A meta-analysis of cohort studies." *World Journal of Gastroenterology.* 2011 March 7;17(9):1204–10.

192 **It could help you dodge**   Van Dam, R, et al. "Coffee, caffeine, and risk of

type 2 diabetes: A prospective cohort study in younger and middle-aged U.S. women." *Diabetes Care.* 2006 February;29(2):398–403.

192 **These additives may reverse**   Arciero, Paul. Email to Beth Janes. January 24, 2009.

193 **Your body can build a tolerance**   Wasmer Andrews, Linda. "Fire up your metabolism." *SELF.* December 2005, p. 83.

195 **330: Milligrams caffeine**   Janes, Beth. "Brava java." *SELF.* August 2009, p. 131.

195 **2: Calories**   USDA National Nutrient Database for Standard Reference, USDA Agricultural Research Service, Nutrient Data Laboratory. http://www.nal.usda.gov/fnic/foodcomp/search.

196 **stearic acid, a portion of which**   Kris-Etherton, Penny. Email to Beth Janes. August 1, 2011.

196 **Stearic acid also doesn't**   Kelly, FD, et al. "A stearic acid–rich diet improves thrombogenic and atherogenic risk factor profiles in healthy males." *European Journal of Clinical Nutrition.* 2001;55:88–96.

196 **may improve insulin sensitivity**   Grassi, D, et al. "Short-term administration of dark chocolate is followed by a significant increase in insulin sensitivity and a decrease in blood pressure in healthy persons." *The American Journal of Clinical Nutrition.* 2005;81:611–14.

196 **eating dark chocolate daily**   Martin, FP, et al. "Metabolic effects of dark chocolate consumption on energy, gut microbiota, and stress-related metabolism in free-living subjects." *Journal of Proteome Research.* 2009;8: 5568–79.

197 **After snacking on about**   Sorensen, LB, et al. "Comparison of the effect of dark and milk chocolate on appetite and energy intake." *International Journal of Obesity.* 2007;31(suppl 1):S89.

197 **When women were deprived**   Polivy, J, et al. "The effect of deprivation on food cravings and eating behavior in restrained and unrestrained eaters." *International Journal of Eating Disorders.* 2005 December;38(4): 301–9.

197 **People who treated themselves**   O'Neil, CE, et al. "Candy consumption was not associated with body weight measures, risk factors for cardiovascular disease, or metabolic syndrome in U.S. adults: NHANES 1999–2004." *Nutrition Research.* 2011;31:122–30.

197 **Antioxidant-loaded dark chocolate**   Ding, EL, et al. "Chocolate and prevention of cardiovascular disease: A systematic review." *Nutrition & Metabolism.* 2006 January 3;3:2.

198 **Dark chocolate cuts off cancer cells**   Patz, Aviva. "Slash your cancer risk in minutes a day." *SELF.* October 2008, p.164.

198 **The flavonols in dark chocolate**   Field, DT, et al. "Consumption of cocoa flavonols results in an acute improvement in visual and cognitive functions." *Physiology & Behavior.* 2011 June 1;103(3–4):255–60.

198 **The antioxidant flavonols** Heinrich, U, et al. "Long-term ingestion of high flavonol cocoa provides photoprotection against UV-induced erythema and improves skin condition in women." *The Journal of Nutrition.* 2006 June;136(6):1565–69.

198 **The flavonols help increase** Janes, Beth. "The great-skin diet." *SELF.* October 2008, p. 223.

200 **Dark chocolate nutrition by the numbers** USDA National Nutrient Database for Standard Reference, USDA Agricultural Research Service, Nutrient Data Laboratory. http://www.nal.usda.gov/fnic/foodcomp/search.

Chapter 9: Thirty-one Days to Slim! The No-Diet Superfood Weight Loss Plan

206 **breakfast eaters are up to 50** Pereira, Mark A. "Eating breakfast may reduce risk of obesity, diabetes, heart disease." Study presented at the American Heart Association's 43rd Annual Conference on Cardiovascular Disease Epidemiology and Prevention, Miami, Florida, March 6, 2003.

206 **increasing your fiber intake** Baer, DJ, et al. "Dietary fiber decreases the metabolizable energy content and nutrient digestibility of mixed diets fed to humans." *The Journal of Nutrition.* 1997 April;127(4):579–86.

207 **most Americans eat only** American Dietetic Association. "Position of the American Dietetic Association: Health implications of dietary fiber." *Journal of the American Dietetic Association.* 2008;108:1716–31.

208 **When people ate vegetables** Bell, EA, et al. "Energy density of foods affects energy intake across multiple levels of fat content in lean and obese women." *The American Journal of Clinical Nutrition.* 2001 June;73(6): 1010–18.

209 **the more often you hit restaurants** Timmerman, GM. "Restaurant eating in nonpurge binge-eating women." *Western Journal of Nursing Research.* 2006 November;28(7):811–24.

210 **women who increase their produce** He, K, et al. "Changes in intake of fruits and vegetables in relation to risk of obesity and weight gain among middle-aged women." *International Journal of Obesity.* 2004;28:1569–74.

211 **Behavior-based bonuses** Paul-Ebhohimhen, V, et al. "Systematic review of the use of financial incentives in treatments for obesity and overweight." *Obesity Reviews.* 2008 July;9(4):355–67.

211 **the ratio of slimming unsaturated** USDA, Agriculture Research Service. "Energy intakes: Percentages of energy from protein, carbohydrate, fat, and alcohol, by family income (in dollars) and age." What We Eat in America. NHANES 2007–2008. http://www.ars.usda.gov/ba/bhnrc/fsrg.

214 **people who used them** Fowler, SP, et al. "Fueling the obesity epidemic? Artificially sweetened beverage use and long-term weight gain." *Obesity.* 2008 August;16(8):1894–900.

214 **People who had an**   Fitzgerald, Matthew. "Flip your hunger switch." *SELF.* October 2007, p. 133.

217 **People who had a meal**   Blatt, AD, et al. "Hidden vegetables: An effective strategy to reduce energy intake and increase vegetable intake in adults." *The American Journal of Clinical Nutrition.* 2011 April;93(4): 756–63.

Chapter 10: The Drop 10 Menu: Five Weeks of Satisfying, Fat-Melting, Superfood-Packed Breakfasts, Lunches, Snacks, and Dinners

230 **Women who took twenty-nine minutes**   "URI study confirms popular dietary lore: Eating slowly really does inhibit appetite." University of Rhode Island Press Release. November 15, 2006. http://www.uri.edu/ news/releases/?id=3771.

230 **Some relaxing every day**   Reyes, Maridel. "What's your weight fate?" *SELF.* August 2009, p. 86.

230 **Dieters who weighed themselves**   Vanwormer, JJ, et al. "The impact of regular self-weighing on weight management: A systematic literature review." *International Journal of Behavioral Nutrition and Physical Activity.* 2008 November;4(5):54.

231 **Americans guzzle**   Duffey, KJ, et al. "Shifts in patterns and consumption of beverages between 1965 and 2002." *Obesity.* 2007 November;15(11): 2739–47.

231 **Getting fewer than seven**   Spiegel, K, et al. "Brief communication: Sleep curtailment in healthy young men is associated with decreased leptin levels, elevated ghrelin levels, and increased hunger and appetite." *Annals of Internal Medicine.* 2004 December;141:846–51.

231 **Adding a favorite topping**   "Eat-right flash." *SELF.* March 2008, p. 112.

232 **Regularly munching after eight**   "The *SELF* Jump Start Diet." *SELF.* January 2006, p. 55.

249 **Research suggests that working out**   MacLean, Paul. Email to Beth Janes. July 27, 2011.

249 **Regular exercise sessions**   Thomas, JG, et al. "The National Weight Control Registry: A study of 'successful losers.'" *Health & Fitness Journal.* 2011;15(2):8–12.

249 **when researchers at Pennsylvania State University**   Rolls, BJ, et al. "The effect of large portion sizes on energy intake is sustained for 11 days." *Obesity.* 2007 June;15(6):1535–43.

250 **Emotional eaters**   Ozier, AD, et al. "Overweight and obesity are associated with emotion- and stress-related eating as measured by the Eating and Appraisal Due to Emotions and Stress Questionnaire." *The Journal of the American Dietetic Association.* 2008 January;108(1):49–56.

250 **Our brain is more rational**   Milkman, KL, et al. "I'll have the ice cream soon and the vegetables later: A study of online grocery purchases and order lead time." Working Paper 07–078, Harvard Business School. April 2007.

251 **Women who had dropped**   Wing, RR, et al. "A self-regulation program for maintenance of weight loss." *The New England Journal of Medicine.* 2006 October 12;355(15):1563–71.

251 **women ate about 120 more calories**   Pomerleau, M, et al. "Effects of exercise intensity on food intake and appetite in women." *The American Journal of Clinical Nutrition.* 2004 November;80(5):1230–36.

Chapter 11: The Drop 10 Recipes: Simple, Fat-Fighting, Superfood-Loaded Meals and Snacks for the Whole Family

253 **Research shows that cooking**   "What's your weight fate?" *SELF.* August 2009, p. 84. Also see "2010 Jump Start Plan." *SELF.* January 2010, p. 104.

254 **A lack of time is one**   "2008 *SELF* challenge: Slim down for good!" *SELF.* May 2008, p. 116.

Chapter 12: Treat Tracking: How Your Favorite Foods Fit into the Drop 10 Diet

307 **A study in *Physiology & Behavior***   Rolls, BJ, et al. "Variety in a meal enhances food intake in man." *Physiology & Behavior.* 1981 February;26(2): 215–21.

317 **Researchers at Princeton University**   Lewis, MJ, et al. "Galanin and alcohol dependence: Neurobehavioral research." *Neuropeptides.* 2005 June; 39(3):317–21.

331 **research suggests that downing**   Fowler, SP. 65th Annual Scientific Sessions, American Diabetes Association, San Diego, California, June 10–14, 2005. Abstract 1058-P. University of Texas Health Science Center School of Medicine, San Antonio. http://www.uthscsa.edu/hscnews/singleformat2.asp?newID=1539.

Chapter 13: Superworkouts to Zap Fat Even Faster

339 **increase the size**   Gingerich Mackenzie, Natalie. "Fire up your burn." *SELF.* October 2010, p. 88.

340 **An overview of weight loss studies**   Amorim Adegboye, AR, et al. "Diet or exercise, or both, for weight reduction in women after childbirth." *Cochrane Database of Systematic Reviews.* 2007 July 18;(3):CD005627.

340 **Almost 90 percent of adults**   Catenacci, VA, et al. "Physical activity pat-

terns in the National Weight Control Registry." *Obesity*. 2008 January;16(1):153–61.

340 **Women who did three strength-training** Bocalini, DS, et al. "Strength training preserves the bone mineral density of postmenopausal women without hormone replacement therapy." *Journal of Aging and Health*. 2009 June;21(3):519–27.

340 **Women who mixed sprints** Trapp, EG, et al. "The effects of high-intensity intermittent exercise training on fat loss and fasting insulin levels of young women." *International Journal of Obesity*. 2008 April;32(4):684–91.

341 **Tabata intervals** Karras, Tula. "Easy exercise!" *SELF*. April 2011, p. 107.

341 **Moves that call on** Mickle, Kelly. "3 Steps to your best summer body!" *SELF*. June 2011, p. 138.

351 **you may need to down** Garrard, Cathy. "Water world." *SELF*. May 2011, p. 188.

358 **Pressing "play"** Karras, Tula. "Get a rockin' body." *SELF*. July 2011, p. 98.

358 **When the tempo of music** Waterhouse, J, et al. "Effects of music tempo upon submaximal cycling performance." *Scandinavian Journal of Medicine & Science in Sports*. 2010 August;20(4):662–69.

358 **People who worked out** Feltz, DL, et al. "Buddy up: The Köhler effect applied to health games." *Journal of Sport & Exercise Psychology*. 2011 August;33(4):506–26.

359 **thinking about when** Chandon, P, et al. "When does the past repeat itself? The interplay of behavior prediction and personal norms." *Journal of Consumer Research*. 2011 October;38(3):420–30.

359 **confidence-building cues** Hatzigeorgiadis, A, et al. "Self-talk and sports performance: A meta-analysis." *Perspectives on Psychological Science*. 2011 July;6(4):348–56.

Chapter 14: Superfood Swaps When Dining Out: How to Tap the Fat-Melting Powers of Superfoods Anywhere

364 **America's most popular restaurants** "R&I 2009 top 400 restaurant chains." *Restaurants & Institutions*. July 15, 2009.

365 **restaurant servings can be** Rouss, Shannan. "Size matters." *SELF* Dishes Summer 2007, p. 51.

405 **People who dined** Chandon, P, et al. "The biasing health halos of fast-food restaurant health claims: Lower calorie estimates and higher side-dish consumption intentions." *Journal of Consumer Research*. 2007 October;34(3):301–14.

406 **When blindfolded** Barkeling, B, et al. "Vision and eating behavior in obese subjects." *Obesity*. 2003 January;11(1):130–34.

Index